Modern Developments in the Principles and Practice of Chiropractic

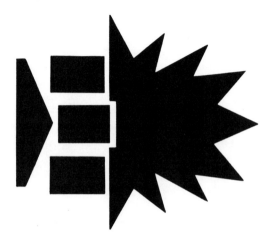

Based on a conference sponsored by
the International Chiropractors Association,
Anaheim, California, February 1979

Modern Developments in the Principles and Practice of Chiropractic

edited by

Scott Haldeman, D.C., Ph.D., M.D.
Department of Neurology
University of California
Irvine, California

APPLETON-CENTURY-CROFTS/New York

80 81 82 83 84 / 10 9 8 7 6 5 4 3 2 1

Prentice-Hall International, Inc., London
Prentice-Hall of Australia, Pty. Ltd., Sydney
Prentice-Hall of India Private Limited, New Delhi
Prentice-Hall of Japan, Inc., Tokyo
Prentice-Hall of Southeast Asia (Pte.) Ltd., Singapore
Whitehall Books Ltd., Wellington, New Zealand

Library of Congress Cataloging in Publication Data

Main entry under title:

Modern developments in the principles and practice
   of chiropractic.

   Includes index.
   1. Chiropractic—Congresses. I. Haldeman, Scott.
II. International Chiropractic Association.
RZ213.M62   615.5'34   80-12312
ISBM 0-8385-6350-3

PRINTED IN THE UNITED STATES OF AMERICA

Contents

Contributors

Leon R. Coelho, D.C., Ph.D.
Chief Administrative Assistant
International College of Chiropractic–Preston
Institute of Technology
Bundoora, Victoria, Australia

John H. Coote, Ph.D.
Reader in Physiology
The Medical School
University of Birmingham
Birmingham, England

H.F. Farfan, M.D., C.M., F.R.C.S. (C)
Orthopedic Surgeon
Clinical Investigation Unit
St. Mary's Hospital
Montreal, Canada

Richard A. Gerren, Ph.D.
Postdoctoral Fellow
Department of Psychobiology
University of California
Irvine, California

Russell W. Gibbons, B.A.
Writer and editor
Pittsburgh, Pennsylvania

Ronald Gitelman, D.C., F.C.C.S. (C)
Professor of Chiropractic Sciences
Department of Clinical Chiropractic
Canadian Memorial Chiropractic College
Toronto, Canada

Adrian S. Grice, D.C., F.C.C.S. (C)
Director
Division of Chiropractic Sciences
Canadian Memorial Chiropractic College
Toronto, Canada

Scott Haldeman, D.C., Ph.D., M.D.
Department of Neurology
University of California
Irvine, California

Andries M. Kleynhans, D.C.
Head, Chiropractic Program
International College of Chiropractic–Preston
Institute of Technology
Bundoora, Victoria, Australia

Marvin W. Luttges, Ph.D.
Assistant Professor
Department of Aerospace Engineering Sciences
University of Colorado
Boulder, Colorado

Reed B. Phillips, D.C., D.A.C.B.R.
Director of Research
Foundation for Chiropractic Education
and Research
Des Moines, Iowa

Aiko Sato, M.D.
Head, 2d Department of Physiology
Tokyo Metropolitan Institute of Gerontology
Tokyo, Japan

Chung Ha Suh, Ph.D.
Professor
Department of Mechanical Engineering
University of Colorado
Boulder, Colorado

Sydney Sunderland, M.D., D.Sc.,
F.R.A.C.P., F.A.A.
Professor Emeritus
Department of Experimental Neurology
University of Melbourne
Melbourne, Australia

John J. Triano, D.C.
Research Associate
Los Angeles College of Chiropractic
Glendale, California
Chiropractor in private practice
Boulder, Colorado

Walter I. Wardwell, Ph.D.
Professor
Department of Sociology
University of Connecticut
Storrs, Connecticut

Henry G. West, Jr., D.C., F.I.C.C.
Faculty
Department of Orthopedics
Los Angeles College of Chiropractic
Glendale, California

Preface

The placing of hands on the spine and paraspinal tissues and the adjustment or manipulation of these tissues is one of the oldest and most widely used healing arts. Terminology, explanations, and techniques have varied considerably, depending on the period in time and the clinical training of the practitioner. Recent years have seen the development of the general term *spinal manipulative therapy* (SMT), which describes all procedures whereby the hands are placed on the spine or paraspinal tissues with the object of improving a patient's health. Such procedures include the specific spinal adjustment, the nonspecific long-lever spinal manipulation, mobilization of the joints of the spine, soft tissue massage, trigger-point manipulation, and manual traction. The term describes all manipulative techniques irrespective of the training of the practitioner or the specific reason for carrying out the procedure. The public and most clinicians have equated the practice of SMT with chiropractic since chiropractors currently make up the largest, most skilled, and best organized body of health care professionals offering this service. In addition, chiropractic is the only profession that has made spinal manipulative therapy the basis of its training, service, and research.

Over the past ten years there has been a rapid increase in sociological, experimental, and clinical research that is relevant to chiropractic. This, in turn, has resulted in the development of a rational approach to the theory and practice of chiropractic. This volume is a product of the work of leading authorities in the fields of history, sociology, neurophysiology, spinal biomechanics, and clinical chiropractic. The authors have been asked to review the research in their respective fields and present an accurate picture of the current status of the principles and practice of chiropractic. The book has been compiled with the aim of producing a text for undergraduate students of chiropractic to use as an overview of specific courses; for the practicing clinician who wishes to be brought up to date with the latest developments in this field; and as an introduction to the current principles and practice of chiropractic for members of the other healing professions.

The production of this text and the conference on which it was based could not have taken place without the financial and moral support of Dr. Joseph Mazzarelli and the Board of Control of the International Chiropractors Association (ICA). Their support is deeply appreciated. Special appreciation must also be given to Dr. Jerry McAndrews, Executive Vice-President of the ICA, for his undaunting assistance in solving many of the problems which inevitably arise when embarking on a venture of this magnitude. The work and dedication of Dr. Harold Hughes and his convention committee, especially Ruth Schimmelpfenig, who were responsible for the organization of the conference is gratefully acknowledged. I give special thanks to my wife, Joan, for her tremendous patience, valuable advice, and the many hours she has spent discussing and reviewing material in preparation for this text. Finally, neither the conference nor this text would have been possible were it not for the support of those practicing chiropractors who have demonstrated their interest in and support of the scientific evaluation of their theories and methods of practice.

Scott Haldeman

SECTION ONE
Social Aspects

CHAPTER ONE

The Evolution of Chiropractic: Medical and Social Protest in America
Notes on the Survival Years and After

RUSSELL W. GIBBONS

Like so many institutions particular to the American experience, it has taken an observer from a detached European vantage point to measure the significance of one of them in both medical and social history. Brian Inglis, a distinguished British historian, commentator, and author of a two-volume work, *The History of Medicine,* has declared: "The rise of chiropractic . . . has been one of the most remarkable social phenomena in American history . . . yet it has gone virtually unexplored." (Inglis 1965)

It is not the purpose of this chapter to analyze the absence of serious scholarship by historians of marginal medicine, but rather to trace that phenomenon, and to suggest that in spite of its humble origins and formulative years, chiropractic has had a decided impact on the evolution of health care attitudes in the United States, and to some degree in other parts of the Western world.

I will offer this caveat, however, to those medical historians who so far have almost totally succeeded in ignoring the significance of the chiropractic story, in quoting that very succinct and perceptive commentator of our times, author Murray Kempton:

A man's spirit can be marked most clearly in its passage from the reform to the revolutionary impulse at the moment when he decides that his enemy will no longer write his history. (Kempton 1975)

Reflect, for a few moments, on that injunction with what we know of chiropractic. We are in a watershed period of transition in the United States, where established doctrines and traditional concepts are under assault or have fallen from entrenched positions of respectability. Attitudes toward health care are changing as are those toward politics, religion, and virtually every aspect of our culture. The Western view of the world is changing, and our view of life, health, and disease is also changing.

In this context, the survival of chiropractic becomes almost a happening. For over three-quarters of a century, it has fought for literal survival, overcoming a systematic persecution and prosecution, in what Inglis said was a "virulence unequaled in the annals even of the medical profession." Commentators have described the medical lobby as the most potent, the most established instrument of influence in the modern political process, an appropriate extension of the fact that the health care industry has now become the largest private employer in the United States.

That a group of "rag-tag marginal healers," as one disgruntled regular-school writer described them, should be able to overcome the concerted assault on their continued existence and to arrive, very much alive, at the front door of medicine, is worthy enough of attention. The front door metaphor recalls the often-quoted declaration by the late Morris Fishbein, long-time editor of the *Journal of the American Medical Association,* who considered chiropractic as almost a personal affront: "If osteopathy is essentially a method of entering medicine by the back door . . . chiropractic by contrast is an attempt to arrive through the cellar." (Fishbein 1925)

The story of chiropractic survival is one of dramatic passions, even of revolutionary impulses within the meaning of the Kempton declaration. For it has been a reform movement in health care attitudes and delivery in North America. And chiropractors, like so many other forces for change within our social experience, have allowed their history to be neglected, forgotten, or stolen. They should not, however, allow the Fishbeins and other adversaries to write their history.

For if medical historians pay cognizance to chiropractic at all, they usually relegate it to a footnote reference as something like the surviving limb of the sectarian tree. And to do further metaphorical violence, they consign homeopathy and eclecticism as dead branches of medicine and osteopathy as a successful—though separate but equal—fusion to the medical "trunk." Yet chiropractic is something more than just successful medical dissent. It also represents a very real social protest in the first half of this century. What remains to be traced, however, are the "survival years" from 1895 through 1913 to the death of D. D. Palmer, the ascendency and dominance of the emerging profession by B. J. Palmer through the 1924 Lyceum-neurocalometer debacle, and the roots of the ideological split which has existed with modern chiropractic to the present.

Passions and Actions: "Straights Versus Mixers"

One of the better contributions in the recent sociology of chiropractic has been a clarification of the nomenclature, something which has plagued observers from outside the profession since chiropractic became a subject for social observation and commentary. The designation of spinal manipulative therapy (SMT) made at the National Institutes of Health seminar in 1975 cleared the air for many.

The literature of chiropractic abounds in superlatives and subjectives, and after three-quarters of a century, the terms "straight" and "mixer" serve only to rekindle old passions and actions. A newer generation of practitioners and students has little identification with the terms, and considering the lack of public understanding may consider them as but unfortunate aberrations of the professionalization of chiropractic.

Accordingly, alternate designations are suggested in this chapter, which may please no one in the profession but which will at least be a recognition that professional maturation demands something better than the impassioned labeling of the past. Straight, hands-only chiropractic is, after all, pure chiropractic. In this chapter, "straights" will become "purists."

The even more offensive "mixer" deserves a better description, and because by definition of its adversaries as well as its advocates it is a broad scope of practice. It can be designated as simply "broad scope" chiropractors. Incidentally, I will touch upon the difficulties of absolutes in discussing purist versus broad scope, for as we know there is a neofundamentalist faction within chiropractic today which seriously believes that clinical and physical diagnosis and even counseling about hygiene and sanitation are departures from the purist concept.

The survival of chiropractic contains virtually all of the ingredients of social protest and reform movements within American history. Like the abolitionists, they were the victims of a systematic persecution and were literally driven from one town to another. Like the feminists and suffragettes, they were ridiculed and ostracized in the community. Like the union organizers, they were arrested on trumped-up charges and jailed. And like the civil rights workers, they were intimidated and subverted by *agents provocateurs*. In the finest tradition of reform movements, they were imprisoned for their beliefs, as this account from California recalls:

In just one year [1921], 450 of approximately 600 chiropractors were hauled into court and convicted of practicing without a license. They were given jail sentences or the alternative of a fine. They chose to go to jail. (Inglis 1965)

This vendetta, of course, turned around in favor of the persecuted minority, and a chiropractic initiative act was passed the next year by a majority of 145,000 votes. If this history is disquieting to those who believe that the merits of any healing art should be decided in the dispassionate surroundings of science and inquiry, and not in the fickle and uninformed court of public opinion, then let us recall that the ascendency of "scientific medicine" came in the early part of this century not through the rational persuasions of the laboratory but through the political process. It was the landmark watershed indictment of medical education by the Rockefellers, through Abraham Flexner, which resulted in the emergence of the regular school of medicine as a political presence (Flexner 1967).

Consider some of the *dramatis personae* of chiropractic, and then again reflect upon the absence of any real history of its survival, with only 15 years short of its centennial.

Daniel David Palmer, The Discoverer (Fig. 1). D. D. is still an enigma to those who practice his healing art, which has outraged the keepers of orthodoxy in medicine and science for most of this century. Without formal training, unlettered, and at times given to both eccentricity and genius, he was as contentious with his followers as with allopathic medicine. He was imprisoned for practicing without a license and became the spiritual forerunner of thousands of chiropractors who would go to jail between the world wars. His premise—that illness is essentially functional and becomes organic only as an end process—is finding wider acceptance today. Scorned as a charlatan in his time, he may yet occupy a chapter of significance in the history of Western medicine.

Bartlett Joshua Palmer, The Developer (Fig. 2). B. J. may have been the last great entrepreneur of folk medicine in the United States. Taking over his father's fledgling infirmary and school when only 25, he built within a decade the country's largest nonmedical institution, as-

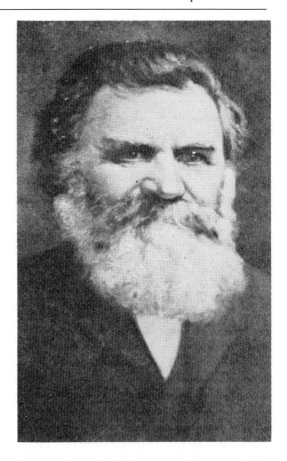

FIG. 1. **Daniel David Palmer (1844–1913): An unlettered, contentious, and at times eccentric healer who gave birth to the last surviving protest school in medicine.**

sembled the world's largest osteological museum, started the nation's second commercial broadcasting station, provided a forum for some of the greatest dissenters of the first quarter century, and established himself as the Prophet of Chiropractic, with the Iowa river town of Davenport as its mecca. He was Elbert Hubbard, Titus Oakes, Baron Munchausen, and P. T. Barnum all rolled into one—yet to his research clinic at mid-century would come "hopeless" and terminal cases—some on referral from the Mayo and Cleveland clinics—to leave apparently cured.

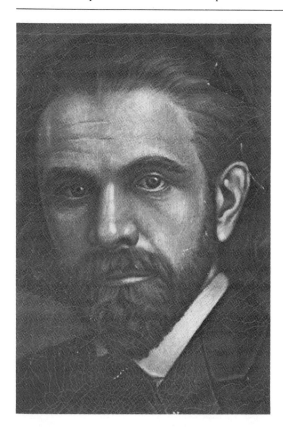

FIG. 2. **Bartlett Joshua Palmer (1881-1961): Controversial and colorful, he outraged his detractors in both medicine and chiropractic as much with this style as with his propositions, yet provided an environment for legitimate spinal research and its development.**

Andrew Taylor Still. A Kansas country doctor, he was almost two decades ahead of D. D. Palmer in announcing discovery of a new theory of health and disease, yet within his lifetime he saw the school of the bearded merchant from Davenport—a onetime patient and house guest—overshadow osteopathy. He outlived Palmer long enough to see his distinct healing art succumb to the wiles of mainline medicine. Like D. D., the "Old Doctor" had metaphysical and spiritualistic origins for his

discovery and both would meet at a "bonesetter's summit" which has since been forgotten or disavowed by both professions.

Willard Carver. As an Iowa lawyer, he brought chiropractic to the Indian Territory and founded his own school, eventually claiming title as the Constructor in opposition to B. J. For almost four decades he would engage in bitter philosophical debate with both Palmers as to the merits of the various chiropractic thrusts. A man of cultured experiences and letters, he presided over four institutions in as many different cities at the same time, bestowing doctorates in philosophy as well as chiropractic. His pupils, like those of the Palmers and other early chiropractic schools, came from the most humble of circumstances.

There were many others whose stars shot across the chiropractic and manipulative sky. Many of them lit up the horizon of medical dissent for extended periods, others only exploding and disappearing from sight. The egocentric character of chiropractic leadership, both in its early training institutions and in its volatile technique debates, may have evolved from the charismatic nature of the Palmers, and it was no doubt fueled by the sense of isolation from the mainstream of the health and scientific communities, with whom their fledgling profession was in a constant combative stage of open war.

A fuller appreciation of the evolution of chiropractic should be related to its first two watershed periods: The first was the three decades from its founding in 1895 to the neurocalometer debacle of 1924, which represented both the survival years and the early growth years. The second watershed period embraced the half century from the 1924 Lyceum, in which B. J. made his self-fulfilling historic address, "The Hour Has Struck," to 1974, when chiropractic approached the threshold of initial acceptance in the health delivery system on three significant fronts. The social forces which were underway in the United States in those 80 years cannot be divorced from the founding, survival, toleration and quasi-acceptance of chiropractic as a form of social protest and medical dissent.

There are periods of hidden American history that have a bearing on the chiropractic story, and they have remarkable parallels to today's new movement toward holistic self-healing, popular nutrition, and the consciousness of consumers as buyers in the health market, seeking alternative forms to traditional medicine (Baumen 1978).

The Popular Health Movement: Rebellion to Heroic Medicine

The healing business was in a state of difficult evolution to professionalization and the establishment of a scientific base in the second half of the nineteenth century, a period which would be climaxed with the emergence of the Still and Palmer schools. "Heroic" medicine, so-called because physicians of the regular school would employ therapy that was drastic, was the rule of the day. The regimen from their bags included bloodletting and purges, many times used until the patient fainted. Recitation of the primitive state of medicine in that period is limited only to the observation that it produced an understandable outrage that crystalized into a medical protest movement.

The feminist writers Ehrenreich and English (1978) have called it the Popular Health Movement, and have linked it to the early women's movement of the 1830s and the Workingmen's party of the same period. Swapping medical horror stories, women's circles moved on to swapping not recipes but their own home remedies and then sought more systematic ways to build their knowledge and skills. Today's "know your body" courses had their distant roots in the "Ladies Physiological Societies" of the pre–Civil War period, in which the one universal ideology was a distrust of the regular medical school.

Fanny Wright, who predated the more fa-mous Mother Jones by several decades, was an intellectual leader and rouser of workers' rights and women's suffrage. She established a People's Hall of Science in New York's Bowery where public instruction in physiology was one of the most popular offerings. And at the same time a poor New Hampshire farmer was piecing together a healing system that would become the main basis of the first real alternative to the regular school.

Samuel Thomson had watched his wife suffer and his mother die at the hands of the regulars' heroic therapy. He reacted by reconstructing the folk medicine he had learned as a farm boy from a female lay healer and midwife. His system was a success with the people he visited because most of them had experienced similar disaster with the regular physicians.

Thomson's medical philosophy involved much more than a set of techniques. His goal was to remove healing from the market and utterly democratize it: every person should be his or her own healer. To this end he set out to spread his healing system as widely as possible among the American people. He set up hundreds of "Friendly Botanical Societies," in which people met to share information and study the Thomsonian system. Five Thomsonian journals were published, and at its height the Thomsonian movement claimed 4 million adherents out of a total United States population of 17 million (Ehrenreich and English 1978).

Other healing systems followed the Thomsonians, including the first true drugless alternative—the Hygienic movement of Sylvester Graham, who called for the eating of raw fruits and vegetables and whole grain breads and cereals. Although ignominiously recalled today only through the cracker named after him, his forces combined with the Thomsonians to triumph over orthodoxy. "It was a disastrous chapter for the regulars, one that contemporary medical historians often prefer to forget," said Ehrenreich and English, who added:

Every state that had a restrictive physician-licensing law softened it or repealed it in the 1830s.

Some, like Alabama and Delaware, simply changed their laws to exempt Thomsonian and other popular kinds of irregular healers from prosecution. This was an enormous victory for "people's medicine." At least one of the movement's principles—anti-monopolism—had been driven home. (Ehrenreich and English 1976)

The eclipse of the Thomsonians and the Hygienic movements occurred about the same time but for different reasons. The various botanic societies and institutes began to compete with the regular schools through training practitioners, and were ultimately no match for orthodoxy. As one historian recalls, "They easily succumbed to the very forces they set out to challenge." The Hygienic protest faded away, but only after forcing the regulars to incorporate most of its precepts—in the best tradition of the reform movement in America. Lamented one of its surviving journals:

> People learned to bathe, to eat more fruits and vegetables, to ventilate their homes, to get daily exercise, to avail themselves of the benefits of sunshine, to cast off their fears of night air, damp air, cold air and draughts, to eat less flesh and to adopt better modes of food preparation. It has now been forgotten who promulgated these reforms; the record has been lost of the tremendous opposition to these reforms that the medical profession raised; it is believed that the medical profession was responsible for the decline of disease and death, the decline of the infant death rate, the inauguration of sanitation, and the increased life-span. The credit for these benefits must go to Natural Hygiene. (Ehrenreich and English 1976)

From the Thomsonian and botanical periods came the first organized school to compete with the now emerging allopathic majority. Eclectic medicine, which at one time represented about one-tenth of all practitioners, became popular in the Midwest as well as the eastern seaboard states. Its adherents, like all reformers, often spent as much time in conflict with each other as with the allopaths who held them in universal contempt. One such classic confrontation in

1856 may be cited to gain an insight into the passions which could rise over such controversies as the efficacy of certain concentrated remedies.

In this instance, the faculty, staff, and student body of the Eclectic Medical Institute of Cincinnati, Ohio—then considered one of the top six American medical institutions and the training school for a quarter of the physicians in Ohio—were engulfed in a dispute between two faculty adversaries, Cleaveland and Newton, that soon reached the boiling point:

> The election in April, 1856, of two separate boards of trustees, each claiming legal right to the institute, was the signal for open warfare. Newton and a band of allies quickly occupied the college building, but were promptly beseiged by Cleaveland's forces wielding knives, pistols, chisels, bludgeons, and blunderbusses. At one point the "usually staid" Prof. Buchanan was heard exhorting the troops outside with cries of "On, on! my brave lads." But to no avail. For over twenty-four hours the siege dragged on, until the appearance of a six-pound cannon at the institute's entrance convinced the Cleavelandites it might be more expedient to retire to the neutral ground of a courtroom. A prolonged and lively court battle ended in victory for the Newtonians, whereupon the defeated professors, in typical 19th-century fashion, opened their own school, the Eclectic College of Medicine. (Numbers 1972)

The eclectics proceeded to establish more schools and hospitals, many times in competition with those of their larger reform school rivals, the homeopaths. Better organized, and with a strong European tradition which centered around their founder, Samuel Hahnemann, homeopathy flourished in the United States for much of the nineteenth century. Rich patrons enabled homeopaths to endow many hospitals, and they had several schools. They reflected the unique combination of attaining respectability in the profession while holding unorthodox views—as Benjamin Rush and Oliver Wendell Holmes had dramatized. Yet with the Flexner report in 1910, all but their better institutions succumbed to rising standards, and the frontal allopathic assault on their very ideology resulted in the last homeopathic school eroding from the scene within two decades. Its hospitals were forced to become orthodox, and only the hospital in Philadelphia bearing the founder's name recalls their once influential role in medicine (Kaufman 1971).

The reform movement in medicine seemed to be following the syndrome of the biggest fish—the health dissidents were swallowed up, their palatable heretical doctrine digested or discarded, and the allopathic whale continued to swim undisturbed in the health sea. While this was continuing, as the last quarter of the nineteenth century began, the seedbed for the manipulative protest schools was being laid in the prairie states of Iowa, Kansas, and Missouri.

Still and Palmer: The Manipulative Protest Schools

Andrew Taylor Still was a country doctor with only a few months training at one of the Kansas City schools that was long closed when Flexner denounced virtually all of medical education. An epidemic of spinal meningitis took the lives of three of his children, and like Thomson and Hahnemann he turned from regular therapy and sought an alternative system. In June, 1874, in the small northeast Missouri town of Kirksville, he "flung to the breeze the banner of osteopathy." It took 18 years for Still, who by then was 66, to open his American School of Osteopathy.

Closer to the Mississippi River, another healer was making his reputation. Daniel David Palmer, born in the Canadian backwoods in 1845, had been an itinerant tradesman, taught school, and was involved in making and losing several small mercantile fortunes in Illinois and Iowa before he became a magnetic healer in Burlington, Iowa in 1886. Within the next decade, he would attract patients from throughout the Midwest and he began his own study of the

anatomy and physiology of the human body, ignoring the popular view that he was a local quack (Homola 1963).

Palmer was 50 that hot September day in 1895 when Harvey Lillard came into his office in the Putnam Building on the south end of Brady Street in Davenport's tenderloin district (Fig. 3). That day the creative act was said to have been laid for chiropractic, soon named by the Reverend Samuel H. Weed, a Palmer patient.

The early growth years began in 1896 when D. D. began instruction on the fourth floor of the Putnam building as Dr. Palmer's School and Cure, and later as the Palmer Institute and Chiropractic Infirmary. Through 1902 only 15 graduates sat under "Old Dad Chiro." Among those obtaining a degree that year was B. J., who had just turned 21.

D. D. began to collect the notes and papers that he would publish in 1910 in Portland, Oregon as *The Chiropractor's Adjuster. The Dictionary of American Biography* (1934) would quote one friendly historian who found it

> Mosaic in its dicta and Platonic in its thoroughness . . . flaying allopathy in particular, he denounced the use of drugs and discussed the cure of almost every disease from abasia to zymosis . . . [it] teemed with maxims, controversy, satire, poetry and irrelevancies, but withal, revealed a genius that must have impressed his offended colleagues.

Offended colleagues there would be for all of the three decades in the public life of D. D. Palmer as healer, evenly divided between both centuries. Like the doctrines which he published about his new school, his movements were erratic. After divesting his interest in the school, infirmary, and osteological collection to his son, the Founder left Davenport as an itinerant—proselytizing, practicing, and teaching. He carried it to the Indian Territory, to California, to Oregon and finally Canada, returning to Davenport in 1913 as a tragic discoverer denied. He died in Los Angeles three months after being struck by an automobile in the school lyceum parade. The car was driven

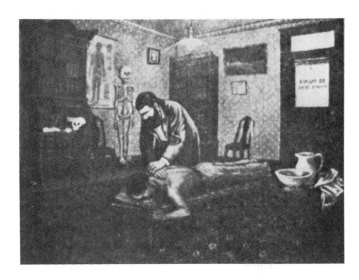

FIG. 3. **The first chiropractic adjustment on September 18, 1895 in Palmer's office in Davenport's Ryan Building. The restoration of the hearing of Harvey Lillard was central to the evolution of the new school. Courtesy of Thomas and Chester Paciorek.**

by B. J., and largely unsubstantiated charges of patricide would linger for years (DAB 1934; Gibbons 1976).

It is difficult to discuss chiropractic history without relating the life, the eccentricities, and the exceptional charisma of Bartlett Joshua Palmer. Though he was a font of endless words, authored at least thirty volumes of varying lengths, edited two of chiropractic's earliest publications for over half a century, and contributed thousands of hours in a crisp, incisive spoken word over the medium of the radio and television industries that he helped to pioneer, B. J. in many ways remains an enigma as his father was a riddle in the greater story.

B. J. Palmer:
Barnum with Science

B. J.'s accomplishments, his controversies, and his leadership tyranny are well known to those who have explored chiropractic. He was a self-described genius of chiropractic, and upon reflection, there is some currency in that assertion to stand the test of history. His brilliant organizational mind left little room for dissenters and

he ruthlessly cast out those who opposed him on critical issues he saw affecting the profession. From the inception of the Palmer properties on Brady Street Hill, there was an injunction to write only to Dr. B. J. Palmer, or "address all correspondence to firm and not individuals." He maintained control to a suffocating degree, yet at the same time retained the passionate loyalty of most of those who were on his staff and faculty (Gibbons 1978).

B. J. jealously watched over the ideological flame which he maintained he alone was to keep, and his financial judgment and decision making were absolute. He was the maximum leader of chiropractic's first school—the Fountainhead—and for a good part of two decades he was the undisputed leader of the profession. Yet from 1924 to his death in 1961 he was a titular leader only, keeping the flame for a fundamentalist minority and doing battle with most of the profession, which he saw as inevitably following the osteopathic moth into the seductive medical flame.

Those who had experienced B. J. at a Palmer School lyceum or had encountered him in the early days reported a religious-like experience. Almost from the first days of his presidency of the PSC, B. J. wore his hair long, flowing over his shoulders. He was invariably attired in a white linen suit, and his long, black, silk bow tie hung halfway to the waist. "He was a striking figure," wrote fellow iconoclast Elbert Hubbard, and it was that figure which would dominate the chiropractic landscape for three-quarters of its existence. B. J. was "into" counterculture when most others sought conformity. He emulated Hubbard and was also P. T. Barnum in telling the chiropractic school story.

His school printing presses produced literally millions of tracts every year, and for those faithful who wanted a life-size bust of the maximum leader or eight portraits "in various thought-poses"—these too were available (Hubbard 1916).

Yet B. J. the entrepreneur provided the environment which advanced both the physical and biological sciences in the Davenport mecca of chiropractic (Fig. 4). The osteological laboratory and museum which were started by the Founder were expanded to the point that an investigating team from the Council on Medical Education and Hospitals of the AMA declared in 1928 that it "was without doubt, the best col-lection of human spines in existence." The X-ray laboratories which B. J. established only 13 years after Roentgen made his discovery were among the first and the finest in healing institutions. In 1934, in cooperation with physiologists and a medical team in Dresden, Germany he secured the first wet specimen showing a transparency of the spinal canal in the upper cervical region. And the next year he established a research clinic in the school's class-room building, where he received the most dif-ficult of medically diagnosed diseases. The equipment and facilities of the clinic made it one of the finest in the Midwest with a full med-ical and nursing staff, a complete diagnostic laboratory, and a physical medicine section. B. J. also secured ownership of Clear View Sanitarium and operated it as a chiropractic facility for mental patients, with clinical oppor-tunities for senior Palmer students, for some 20 years. His 1935 instrument for reading brain waves and their conduction through the spinal cord was a prototype of today's EEG used in clinical diagnosis (American Medical Associa-tion 1928).

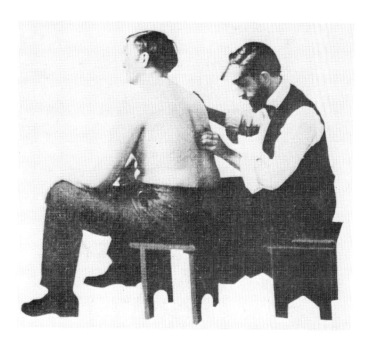

FIG. 4. **B.J. examining a patient, circa 1912. His philosophy allowed for little dissent as to the chiropractic thrust, evolving from atlas–axis, to meric, and finally to HIO ("hole-in-one").**

Science was always in conflict with hucksterism during B. J.'s tenure as the neo-Developer. "I will sell chiropractic, serve chiropractic, and save chiropractic if it will take me twenty lifetimes to do it," he would write. The Palmer School "gave birth of Specific, Pure and Unadulterated Chiropractic," and B. J. set forth to sell, serve, and save in the best of Barnum tradition.

In August, 1924, under the tent which was erected on the east end of the campus, B. J. announced the neurocalometer, a pioneer heat-sensing device that was a double-pronged instrument to determine the existence of a subluxation. B. J.'s lyceum address was given an advance billing as "The Hour Has Struck," and chiropractors who came by the thousands were led to believe that the very future of the profession would be decided at this historic occasion. A critical view agreed that it was historic, but only in that it marked the decline of B. J.'s unquestioned leadership:

> Who shall forget that torrid night under the tent when B. J. spoke . . . in that philippic he maligned chiropractic . . . said many ugly things to the field. It was the hour that nearly rimracked and slaughtered and destroyed chiropractic. (Bealle 1947)

A massive wave of defections of purist followers came after the 1924 lyceum, although a hard core of believers would hold to B. J.'s assertion that "no chiropractor can practice chiropractic without an NCM (neurocalometer) . . . no chiropractor can render an efficient, competent or honest service without the NCM." (B. J. Palmer 1933) The difficulty in quoting B. J. would be the same in quoting anyone who published 39 volumes and separate papers well in excess of 10,000 pages on chiropractic: contradictions and absurdities abound.

The senior Palmer, in writing of the claimed first chiropractic adjustment on Harvey Lillard on September 18, 1895, was emphatic in saying that "I replaced the displaced fourth dorsal vertebra by one move, which restored his hearing fully." (D. D. Palmer 1910) Yet B. J. would maintain years later that "[we] consistently and repeatedly have said that it was not fourth dorsal vertebra but was Axis that was adjusted in Harvey Lillard . . . why do I say it was Axis? Because I was there and saw what he [D. D.] did, where he did it—and it was the Axis." (B. J. Palmer 1957) The assertion was in keeping with B. J.'s derision of anything but "Palmer specific" adjusting technique, promulgated in the late 1930s.

Did a 13-year-old Bart stand in the wings of D. D.'s office and make an observation about a manipulative thrust which was still not fully understood by his father at the time? William A. Seely, the homeopath who graduated under the Founder in 1898 wrote to D. D. in 1906, referring to B. J. as "that little unruly kid that was in knickerbockers when you taught me the principles of the science of chiropractic." (B. J. Palmer 1957)

The "unruly kid," however, would ultimately give chiropractic purpose, direction, and a distinct identity around which to gather and survive. The life and times of B. J. Palmer is much of chiropractic, and the two cannot be divorced. His superpure ideology was embraced within this proposition: "that everything within the chiropractic philosophy, science and art works from above-down, inside-out. Anything and everything outside that scope is medicine, whether you like it or not." (B. J. Palmer 1958)

Those trained in the basic sciences today will find gross errors relative to anatomy and physiology in the writings of D. D. Palmer, although they remain remarkable considering he was self-taught in these sciences. They may appear to be minor, however, when contrasted with some of those within the many published works of his son, very little of which would survive any scientific scrutiny today.

The evangelical character of early chiropractic may have been expressed by this contribution in the January 1915 issue of *The Chiropractor,* the monthly journal of the Palmer School. Howard Nutting, who was an uncle of Willard Carver and a close associate of B. J. Palmer, urged practitioners to "keep bravely on until the flag of chiropractic is unfurled in every town and hamlet; on until every asylum for the insane, for the inebriate and for the feeble minded shall be without occupants, or until the penitentiaries and reformatories are deserted and their crumbling walls and rusted bolts stand only as silent testimonials to the success of chiropractic." (Nutting 1915)

Bonesetting Cousins: The Osteopathic Controversy

Yet if there was dissent between the founding father and his son, who lost little time in proclaiming himself as the Developer, it was only a prelude to a constant state on internal controversy which would surround the endless debates over scope of practice, the most effective chiropractic thrust, and the education of practitioners. Part of that debate was the often-repeated assertion in much of the early literature that D. D. Palmer had "stolen" his concepts from the Father of Osteopathy, A. T. Still, and the criticism which was made of D. D. by his early medical associates and others whose orthodox training had led them to a qualified acceptance of the chiropractic principle.

Palmer himself believed otherwise, declaring in his 1910 tome, *The Chiropractor's Adjustor,* that he was "more than pleased to know that our cousins, the osteopaths, are adopting chiropractic methods and advancing along scientific and philosophical lines." The osteopathic connection has yet to be documented, but it is plausible not only in the proximity of Davenport to the seat of osteopathy, but the eclectic pattern of D. D. in seeking out anything from contemporary schools who held out cures. An early house historian of the Palmers, Dye, wrote that turn-of-the-century druggists in Davenport recall the Founder writing prescriptions, although it would have been in violation of the medical practice act that was passed in Iowa when D. D. was practicing magnetic healing (Dye 1939).

Kirksville would have been only a day's jour-

ney down the river and overland to north-central Missouri and, despite the assertions by both Palmers and their followers, it is more than probable that the senior Palmer made the trip on several occasions. Andrew T. Still had "unfurled the banner of osteopathy" in Kirksville in 1874 and was known widely as a teacher of a new manipulative concept of health. It is conceivable that Palmer would have made the "Still connection," and Charles Still, a son of the founder of osteopathy, contended that Palmer had even been a guest in Still's home. Several Missouri chiropractors who visited the original Still homestead on the campus of what is now the Kirksville College of Osteopathic Medicine had reported seeing D. D.'s name in the guest book in the early 1890s. The younger Still also wrote that an osteopath by the name of Obie Stother had passed on the manipulative techniques of the Old Doctor to the senior Palmer (Booth 1924).

B. J. Palmer wrote in 1931 that "my father never was in Kirksville, never attended that or any other osteopathic school. It is true that he met and talked with Andrew T. Still at Clinton, Iowa at the spiritualist camp meeting on several occasions." Regardless of whether D. D. was in Kirksville, the osteopaths bitterly denounced chiropractic as a "pure steal," one 1913 condemnation even declaring that the Developer had incorporated the Still reference to Kirksville as the "Fountain Head" and his school shibboleth of "find it, fix it, leave it alone" into the Davenport litany. Adjustment of the spinal column was an original Still precept, claimed the fundamentalist osteopaths, but they were soon in a minority as leaders of the reform school courted allopathic recognition as "separate but equal" providers. In Kansas, Missouri, and many of prairie states in the early part of the century, both D.O.'s and D.C.'s were known as "rubbing doctors," and the proliferation of chiropractors moved the American Osteopathic Association to court those who sought broader practice.

A 1921 resolution submitted at the convention of the American Osteopathic Association was adopted which declared "that all osteopathic colleges be opened to those . . . with a high school diploma and eighteen months or more of chiropractic training, these individuals to be given nine or more months of advanced standing." The osteopaths were trading two hours of chiropractic training for one of theirs at a time when the Palmer School was conducting a separate "physicians and osteopaths course" in which licensed M.D.'s and D.O.'s could pick up a D.C. after four months of study and clinic (Booth 1924).

Both founders, incidentally, had strong metaphysical learnings, and one account by B. J. Palmer has the senior Palmer and Still meeting at a "bonesetter's summit," in Clinton, Iowa after the turn of the century. Still outlived Palmer by only a few years, but long enough to see his reform school of medicine already succumbing to the wiles of orthodoxy.

Despite his acceptable medical credentials, Still would in time become an embarrassment to any of those who would become a part of the profession to which he gave birth. This mini-controversy has relevance only in that orthodoxy applied a blanket condemnation to both manipulative schools for much of the first quarter of this century. This condemnation was also applied equally to both Still with his limited medical training and Palmer with his nonmedical background. Martin Gardner, an author whose books on psuedoscientific activities are still widely read, lumps both in his bag of "medical follies." To him, Still was but a "medical illiterate." The original osteopathic proposition earned the same violent scorn from the regular school, and its adoption of allopathic medicine and surgery was seen as but an affirmation of this judgment (Gardner 1957).

The Old School Converts: Medical Allies and Critics

More to the point were the observations of some of the senior Palmer's early medical associates and other orthodox practitioners who found his lack of formal training in the sciences as an occasion to record their reservations about total acceptance of the Founder's healing ideology. Much of D. D.'s book is given to this debate, especially with A. P. Davis—a homeopathic physician who was one of Still's first graduates and who later taught at his Kirksville school prior to taking up chiropractic under D. D.—who in 1903 made a sworn statement that the two schools were distinct and separate in theory and application (D. D. Palmer 1910).

Another early Palmer medical associate, Alvah A. Gregory, conducted a school with the Founder in Oklahoma City while it was still the Indian Territory. He later broke with Palmer in a dispute over the nature of the spinal subluxation, arguing that instead of displaced vertebrae, there was a "relaxation of spinal ligaments." It was in his 1910 book on *Spinal Adjustment* that Gregory, a regular school M.D., expressed his reservations concerning Palmer's unorthodoxy:

It might be well to state that the practice of spinal adjustment was introduced in this country by a man almost wholly unacquainted with Pathology, Symptomatology, or Etiology, and one who knew practically nothing of Anatomy and but little of Physiology. Consequently so many of the teachings in connection with the philosophy and science of spinal adjustment have been freely mixed with error and superstition and this fact has greatly hindered its investigation and reception by the medical world. Some of the medical profession and others of the better educated class of people have felt that because spinal adjustments were first introduced by a man who was wholly uneducated in therapeutic lines, he could not have made any discovery of much consequences or importance as a therapeutic auxiliary; but this does not, by any means, follow. (Gregory 1910)

Another physician, Arthur L. Forster, president of the National School which had begun after a curriculum dispute with B. J. in 1906, expressed similar qualifications:

Palmer, however, fell into one serious error. He did as so many before him have done. He became overzealous. He claimed that all disease is due to subluxations of the vertebrae and that all diseases could be eradicated by adjustment of the vertebrae. Naturally, such views could not be subscribed to by anyone with a liberal training in the sciences underlying the art of healing, and especially, one with a knowledge of pathology. This preliminary training Palmer lacked; and it goes without saying that had he possessed such knowledge, he would not have made the claims which he did.

He derided all other forms of therapy, and persisted in his original views to the end. Nevertheless, while the advancement made in chiropractic technique has been very great, and broader views now obtain among the profession as a whole, still to Palmer must be given the credit for furnishing the impetus which carried chiropractic to a recognition of its wonderful possibilities. (Forster 1915)

If the elder Palmer had limitations in his training, it apparently was little deterrent in the presentations which he made in orthodox circles, limited though they may have been. In May 1906, in Kansas City, Missouri, D. D. claimed to have stolen the show at a meeting of regulars. In a letter to John A. Howard, a former student who was soon to embark on a career as a chiropractic school head, the Founder wrote:

I cannot let your letter go until I tell you of the M.D.'s meeting yesterday. They have a county society which meets once a month. I attended although I do not do so at home [Davenport]. A paper was read; each member discussed its merits. I asked to have a say. They reluctantly voted me five mintues. When the five minutes were up several said, "Go on." So they voted me another five minutes. By that time all the rules were forgotten and I occupied most of the afternoon . . . Dr. Martin said that he had a headache. I offered to cure it by one touch. He accepted. I seated him in front of the audience. He showed his surprise and admitted that the headache was gone. Several questions were asked for me to answer. Chiropractic captured the meeting. (D. D. Palmer, quoted in Natl Chiropr J, 1936)

Howard founded the second significant rival school in Davenport that same year.

The Early Medical Presence: Chicago's National School

In 1905, the American School of Chiropractic in Cedar Rapids was founded by one of D. D.'s earliest graduates, Solon Langsworthy, along with a former medical student, Oakley Smith, and a chiropractor-midwife who claimed the first license in Illinois, Minoria Paxton. They authored a two-volume text, *Modernized Chiropractic,* which may have preceded B. J.'s premature *Science of Chiropractic* in early 1906. Howard began his school because B. J. evidenced little interest in obtaining unfortunates from the county morgue to provide anatomy students with a dissection class. The National School moved to Chicago in 1908, which at the time was to Flexner "the plague spot to medical education in the country." When Illinois passed one of the first so-called Drugless Practitioners Acts, the state became a fertile ground for medical dissenters of every persuasion. Soon the administration of the National School passed into the hands of a group of physicians, who became officers of the institution and occupied the majority of the titles listed as professorships.

By the time Howard left the National College in 1916, the faculty boasted six doctors of medicine who also listed the D.C. degree. The dean of the faculty was an 1897 graduate of Rush Medical College, William C. Schulze. A native of Germany, he graduated from a small liberal arts college in Missouri before entering Rush, which was the medical department of the Universtiy of Chicago. After practicing in Wisconsin and after a five-year tour as medical director of the Chicago Zander Institute, Schulze joined the National faculty in 1910, taking the chairs of Obstetrics and Gynecology. His publication included *A Text Book of the Diseases of Women* (Gibbons 1977).

Arthur L. Forster, who taught diagnosis, authored one of the first texts, *Principles and Practices of Spinal Adjustment.* His degree was from the medical department of the University of Illinois. The other M.D.'s listed on the National Faculty in 1915 included graduates of Northwestern University Medical School, Bennett, Loyola, Chicago Hospital, and the Chicago College of Medicine and Surgery. The Schulze-Forster administration at the National College was to produce one of the more unique instances of a chiropractic intrusion into the traditional orthodox territorial imperative. Although the lost or strayed repositories of records have yet to reveal the connection, apparently sometime during 1914 through 1925 there was an arrangement for senior students at the National Institution, then located in a massive stone structure on Ashland Avenue, to visit the wards of Cook County Hospital. The connection could have been any one of the six M.D.'s who were listed as professors in the school catalogue for those years, but considering that the majority of the eleven regular and irregular Illinois schools surveyed by Flexner in 1910 had similar formal or informal arrangements at Cook County—and that he recommended the closing of all but three—the relationship might not have been that surprising (Gibbons 1977; Flexner 1967).

The National–Cook County experience was one of the few instances in chiropractic where its students had access to orthodox hospitals and an inpatient experience, one of the consistent criticisms leveled against its training. For an insight into the natural history of pathology, a clinician must have that opportunity, regular critics maintained, while at the same time removing any possibilities for such an experience by the school that they had consigned to quackery. Denied the right to have its students make rounds in public hospitals (whether unaware of the tax-supported arguments or uninterested in the legal fight to secure such rights, this course was never pursued by any of the major chiropractic lobbies, the Universal, National, International, and American associations), they resigned themselves to maintaining public clinics for an outpatient experience (Gibbons 1977).

Only a few comparatively brief inpatient relationships existed with chiropractic hospitals, whose limitations must have reflected the prejudices and discrimination applied to all irregular institutions by health agencies directed by regular school administrators. During the same

period as the National–Cook County association, Carver College in Oklahoma City listed an affiliation with the "D. D. Palmer Memorial Hospital" in that city, and through the 1950s had an obstetrical connection in a private hospital conducted by John Hubbard, a physician-chiropractor. A similar arrangement in Los Angeles existed for some years.

Chiropractic hospitals and sanitariums existed, if not flourished, for most of the period from 1920 to 1960. There were notable experiments with inpatient facilities for mental illness, the Chiropractic Psychiatric Hospital at Forest Park preceding the Clear View Sanitarium, both in Davenport. Worthy of more attention, however, were those chiropractic institutions built for general hospital facilities, usually in rural areas and with an associated visiting staff of regular physicians and surgeons. The Wisconsin General Chiropractic Hospital and the Bakkum Chiropractic Hospital in Iowa functioned with maternity wards and surgeries as well as adjustment rooms, and if official sanctions were visited upon their allopathic staff in those depression and World War II years, its chiropractic administrations did not report them.

Two pioneers in chiropractic hospitalization did feel the wrath of orthodoxy and the weight of hostile state authorities. George Hariman built the first chiropractic hospital in North Dakota, the result of his Cook County rounds in 1914, but experienced removal of its tax exemption and prejudices by the nurses' registry in securing an adequate nursing staff. Leo Spears, a 1921 Palmer graduate who built the profession's largest hospital, opened a 200-bed unit at the height of World War II and in 1949 opened a second 600-bed unit dedicated to D. D. Palmer (the first was named after Willard Carver). Before his death in 1956, Spears had broken ground and erected the shell of a third unit, a massive three-block structure that was advertised to have 2100 beds. A stormy petrel who was in Colorado courts as much as his hospital wards, Spears had a penchant for testimonial advertising that embarrassed as many chiropractors as it outraged his medical detractors. Yet when his hospital flourished, it was a unique experience in the profession's history. William S. Rehm, an intern during 1956, recalled that

> there were so many patients that they occupied beds in the halls of both the Palmer and Carver buildings . . . the pediatrics ward always had a waiting list. It was the time when Dr. Leo [Spears] was doing his "cancer work" and most of the 30 interns and 24 residents were occupied with changing dressings as much as with treatment. (Interview with the author, 1978)

As with so many institutions in chiropractic, Spears' hospital experienced a demise after its founder died. Injunctions, denial of a permit by the state health board, quarantine, and public charges of "murder" when an inpatient died did not close Spears, but the denial of hospitalization payments by insurance carriers for all purposes did. The Carver unit is closed and the planned "Chiropractic Pioneers" unit has long since been sold and is now a nursing facility. The surviving D. D. Palmer unit today has an occupancy only a shadow of its capacity when Leo Spears died.

The classic case of harassment and neglect by both the public sector and orthodox health agencies toward a chiropractic facility may be in Louisville, Kentucky, where a nonprofit, charitable institution utilizing chiropractic has struggled for more than 23 years to remain open. The Kentuckiana Childrens Center, founded and still administered by a woman chiropractor, Lorraine Golden, has served thousands of long-term, physically and emotionally handicapped children without cost in temporary World War II–period quarters built for a veterans' hospital. Yet because of its chiropractic service, it has been excluded from mainline funding and federal assistance, existing on a monthly budget met through voluntary contributions and community support.

The disappearance of chiropractic hospitals is in contrast to its schools, which have experienced a growth phase since 1974, with the chartering of five new colleges, and the acquisition of as many new campuses by some of the older institutions since that watershed year when the

U.S. Department of Health, Education and Welfare recognized the chiropractic accrediting agency. An overview of chiropractic's initial training schools and their evolution to higher educational institutions is necessary to comprehend its survival.

Training the Adjustor: The Bootstrapping of Chiropractic

To understand the saga of chiropractic schooling requires total objectivity from any historical vantage point toward at least the recognition that in its primitive period through the first two decades of this century it was more training in imparting the art of the adjustor, rather than any exposure to an education in the biological sciences within a classical framework. Any understanding of those efforts should be compartmentalized with the Palmer School experience from 1912 through 1924 and the serious non-Palmer institutions which must be sifted from the proliferation of schools which began in that period (Fig. 5).

The description "serious" is used because it was apparent that there were persons of competence, coming to chiropractic with formal and liberal educations, who sought to advance the fledgling healing art with an academic experience that was superior to the training school concept that was dominant in Davenport. Not a few of them were with medical backgrounds, and there is evidence that despite the eccentricities of B. J. Palmer, a gradual evolution of didactic curriculum and classroom opportunities took place under Alfred Baker Hender, M.D., during his 31 years as dean of the Palmer School of Chiropractic (1912–43).

Hender's counterpart in the bastions of mixing was William Charles Schulze, a German-born graduate of Rush Medical College who was president of the National School—and later the National College for 23 years (1915–38). Both were practicing physicians as well as chiropractic school administrators, both occupied the chairs of obstetrics and gynecology in their respective institutions, both maintained

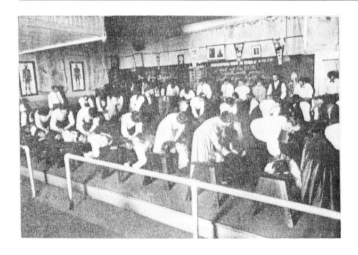

FIG. 5. **Palpation and nerve tracing class, circa 1919. The Palmer School student population rose from a dozen in 1906 to 800 by 1916, and the school soon became the country's largest nonmedical institution.**

hospital associations and regular medical affiliations, and both were known as frequent spokesmen for chiropractic before state legislative committees of that period when licensure was being sought.

Much has been written about the fly-by-night character of the early chiropractic schools, the worst of which were crass "diploma mills"; many were merely efforts to achieve a production line of practitioners under the guise of a scholastic environment. Their existence served to delay the legislative sanctions that the profession needed in the survival years, but they also functioned as a conduit for hundreds—perhaps thousands—of ill-trained technicians of the art of spinal adjustment, who seeped into the licensed states as well as flooded the so-called "open" jurisdictions where a vehement medical lobby refused to buckle.

Recalling the existence of some of these institutions only serves to remind us of the particularly American aspect of chiropractic's social history, for its early growth period was very much identified with the interior revolution that took place within the professions following World War I. "The art and mystery of the scientific machine," wrote critic H. L. Mencken at the time, "has been closed to all but the sons of the wealthy."

The social consequences of the Flexner report, which tended to further restrict openings into orthodox healing schools, were combined

with the many backwashes of the war. The European experience of thousands of Americans tended to provide for more tolerance for alternative forms of medicine, and indeed the United States provided the first government subsidy to chiropractic by paying for the schooling of those veterans who went to Davenport and the revived chiropractic institutions in Oklahoma City, Chicago, Los Angeles, New York, and other cities.

Some did not wish to spend the eighteen months resident study required in the better schools and sought an even quicker entry route. Here is the carrot offered by one such place, with the impressive title of "American University," in an advertisement that appeared in popular publications (e.g., *The Electrical Experimenter*) during 1919 and 1920:

BE A CHIROPRACTOR. LEARN AT HOME. By the American University system of instruction, you can become a Doctor of Chiropractic by studying in spare time at home or in class at the university. You do not require special talent or advanced education.

Technically, this institution was not a diploma mill, for it conducted courses in Chicago's Manierre Building and had a "home study" correspondence course. How many graduated D.C.'s went "into the field" from this experience is conjecture, but they eventually were accepted to sit for state boards in some states and were licensed under grandfather provisions in others. Even the fundamentalist Universal Chiropractors Association accepted them into membership.

The eclectic philosophy of chiropractic education led it toward the inevitable course of disparate approach to both instruction and the selection of the student body. While payment of a matriculation fee was the chief requirement in many schools, some were selective. A Seattle, Washington institution demanded probationary residence on campus and election by the student body as a prerequisite to full acceptance. According to the school's circulars, a student at Palmer would be expected to subscribe to "P., S. & U." chiropractic—B. J.'s acronym for "Pure, Straight and Unadulterated"—and their counterparts at the Oklahoma City school of rival Willard Carver would, as freshmen requirements, read "Carver's Scientific Catechism."

B. J., ever the publicist, knew little restraint in broadcasting the attributes of his Fountainhead, which he declared to be "universally recognized as the hub of all things chiropractic." His contemporaries demonstrated similar approaches, implying that one need not visit the Davenport mecca to become knowledgeable about the emerging healing art. Attorney-chiropractor Carver, noting B. J.'s self-proclamation as the Developer, termed himself "the Constructor of the Science of Chiropractic," and his college prospectus declared it: "The institution of excellence. Presided over by the longest-time student of chiropractic alive." (Carver n.d.)

T. F. Ratledge, another early chiropractic school founder—at whose Los Angeles institution D. D. Palmer had lectured—was equally emphatic: "The Ratledge School is superior, gives superior instruction, and equips for the successful practice of a superior profession." (Ratledge 1922)

Few institutions offering the D.C. degree in the first half of this century could afford not to succumb to such salesmanship. With the exception of the late 1940s, when the United States government again provided direct subsidy to all institutions of advanced instruction, the student populations of chiropractic's proprietary schools were in regional competition with each other. The curve lines of chiropractic population in the 1920 and 1930 decades, which can only be based upon states wtih full licensure—and estimating an additional 20 to 25 percent in the "open" states (New York, Texas, and four others, with jurisdictions such as Ohio and Illinois having both licensed and unlicensed)—generally reflect the student bodies of the larger schools, some of which descended to dangerous levels in the war years. The Fountainhead itself, following the neurocalometer debacle of 1924, experienced a rollercoaster descent from the 3100 students of 1922 to fewer than 300 in the depression year of 1929. B. J.'s son, David D. Palmer, returned to Davenport that summer following his graduation from the University of Pennsylvania, where

> I found the PSC virtually bankrupt and under the control of the First National Bank of Davenport . . . the school was operating in virtual receivership [and] the bank had complete charge of our school operations. (David D. Palmer 1976)

The second floor auditorium of the D. D. Palmer Memorial Building was converted into a skating rink during the worst of those lean years, and other mercantile endeavors devised by the third generation Palmer returned the school to stable financial condition. The Palmer fiscal footnote is cited because it is correctly identified as the most stable and permanent of the pioneer chiropractic institutions, yet it came close to receivership at a time when its owner was recognized as a millionaire owner of broadcasting and real estate in Iowa.

The economics of survival of chiropractic education deserves a fuller exploration than any superficial treatment here can accord. Yet it stands as one of the more remarkable achievements of the chiropractic story. With few exceptions, the continuing schools that emerged between the two world wars were proprietary institutions and stock corporations, rarely with any but chiropractors serving as trustees. Decisions of any academic or clinical nature were largely made by the owner or co-owners, and only in a few instances were any efforts made toward nonprofit incorporations with a relationship to the profession.

Those notable exceptions, where some sort of endowment was secured as a nonprofit venture, were by Frank Dean, whose Columbia Institute founded in 1919 continues as the New York Chiropractic College, a part of the State University of New York, and Hugh B. Logan, whose college founded in suburban Lombardy near St. Louis in 1936 became the surviving institution of the Carver College. The efforts of John J. Nugent, the tireless Director of Education of the National Chiropractic Association, resulted in the surrender of equities in 19 chiropractic schools by some 46 owners by 1939 (Stanford Research Institution 1960).

Yet all of these institutions continued to graduate the practitioners that maintained chiropractic as the second largest and the primary alternative health care provider group in these years. Without any federal or state assistance they survived, sustained the student decline between the middle 1950s and the late 1960s, merged, went through the final throes of the change from private to professional ownership, and succeeded in meeting the influx of the new breed of chiropractic student that began at the threshold of approval by the Department of Health, Education and Welfare.

It is noteworthy that every existing North American chiropractic college has either acquired wholly new campuses or undertaken major additions to existing physical plants within the past decade, again without any assistance from public agencies. The standardization of its curriculums, expansion of libraries and laboratories, and the acquisition of top teaching faculties represent a long step from the limited educational experience in chiropractic in the decade following the death of the Founder.

Perimeters of Practice:
The "Chiropractic G.P."

It may be appropriate here to continue from the educational experience to a little-known sector in the evolution of the chiropractic scope of practice controversy. As evidence of the perimeters of broad practices which many in the profession had achieved in the third decade of its existence, the rather remarkable example of a California institution chartered as the College of Chiropractic Physicians and Surgeons (CCPS) may be offered. Founded in 1931, it operated for 15 years on West Ninth Street in Los Angeles, when it merged with the present Los Angeles College of Chiropractic.

The CCPS was nonprofit and professionally owned, but what made it unique despite its name was its stress upon general practice and specialties which have all but disappeared from the chiropractic scene today. The college announcements for 1933, under "Physicians and Surgeons Post Graduate Course," offered "an advanced course in medicine and surgery extending over a period of two years open to graduate chiropractors, who desire to increase their knowledge of therapeutics and who can present to the College Credential Committee proper credentials of having completed a one-year course of college grade in physics, chemistry, and biology. At the completion of this course, the chiropractor is in a position to intelligently give advice when called upon to do so. Surgery and surgical specialties are taught in such a manner that the student learns to distinguish between cases which do and do not require surgical care. The general management of surgical cases with the possibilities and disadvantages of surgical methods are made clear."

While the college qualified that those chiropractors granted its "Physicians and Surgeons Certificate" would "not be expected to become qualified as surgical specialists," the course totaled 2060 hours in general medicine and surgery, including 50 hours of anesthesiology and 154 hours in a course called "Clinical Chiropractic Surgery." The clinical experience was not limited to the two outpatient facilities associated with CCPS, but through an inpatient teaching arrangement with an affiliated hospital: "Through the facilities of the Bellevue Hospital, a 60-bed general hospital owned and operated by the Chiropractic Profession, the student receives direct instruction by the attending staff in the care of surgical and obstetrical cases, together with a wide variety of acute and chronic diseases. This is in addition to the practical work which the student secures in the College Clinic." Bellevue, one of half a dozen chiropractic hospitals in Los Angeles that long ago succumbed in the undertow of private hospitalization, was known as a maternity facility. The extensive Obstetrical Department at the college included a service in the college clinic, a department in Bellevue and a service for home maternity cases. The announcement stressed the emphasis on this specialty:

> There is also established the obstetrical clinic in the college where the pre-natal examination of the patient is conducted by the student under the supervision, at all times, of one of the instructors of this department. The treatment prescribed is given by the student and the general welfare of the patient is closely watched so that a normal completion of the term of pregnancy may be expected.

Chiropractic obstetrics, which survives today within the legal scope of practice only in Oregon, once enjoyed a specialty status in California and half a dozen other states, notably Oklahoma.

Broad Scope Flirtations with "Fringe Medicine"

Surprisingly, even purist schools and leaders accepted pregnancy as a natural process within the biological functions, and did not look upon pregnancy as a disease, with technological-surgical delivery its treatment. This approach can be attributed to the Palmers themselves with a pioneer reference by the Founder in *The Chiropractor's Adjustor,* in which he declares that "a chiropractor should be able to care for any condition which may arise in the families under his care, the same as a physician ... [during pregnancy] many have their vertebrae displaced in this critical period, causing acute and chronic diseases. If the accoucheur is a chiropractor, he can adjust, thereby preventing disease." (D. D. Palmer 1910)

The Palmer School's instruction in obstetrics under A. B. Hender was "sufficient to qualify the student to pass any of the state examining board's examinations on midwifery ... we teach the art of the practical part of the work in so far as we can obtain obstetrical cases outside." Completion of clinical work in obstetrics was a prerequisite to graduation at Carver College as well as the leading institutions such as National, Los Angeles, and Western States colleges through the early 1960s.

"Birth without violence" advocate Frederick Leboyer (1975) may have asked the question which many early chiropractic obstetricians considered with a knowledge of the subluxations of the spinal column. "Why, when the vulnerable spine has always been curved," asked Leboyer, "do we insist on holding the newborn infant upside down and jerking the back straight?"

The demise of chiropractic obstetrics, like the disappearance of chiropractic hospitals and sanitariums, was closely interrelated to the ascendency of medical economics and the spiralling costs of health care in America. Private hospitals closed their doors or went public or professional when the cost of having a baby rose from $16 per hospital day in 1950 to $175 in 1976, with other inpatient costs rising comparably.

Denied hospital access, those D.C.'s who continued to practice the specialty were restricted to home deliveries (in Oregon, as late as 1976, ten percent of the nonhospital births in the state were delivered by chiropractors). The medical solution to the "midwife problem," however, was another instance of regular school imperialism asserting its domain in every sector of the art of healing.

This was an extension of the rise of orthodoxy after its first success in overcoming the Popular Health Movement, of its internal skirmishes with the eclectic and homeopathic schools, its warfare with A. T. Still's reform school, all in the second half of the nineteenth century, to the Flexner investigations of 1910. For by the turn of the century, 50 percent of the babies born in the United States were still delivered by midwives, who did not accept childbirth as a pathological event requiring the intervention of a physician.

American medicine, giving no quarter in its battle with the irregular schools, would settle for nothing less than the final solution to the midwife question: they would be eliminated and outlawed. One medical journal urged:

> Surely, we have enough influence and friends to procure the needed legislation. Make yourselves heard in the land, and the ignorant, meddlesome midwife will soon be a thing of the past. (Ehrenreich and English 1976)

Thus in the same growth decades of chiropractic—between 1900 and 1930, midwives were almost eliminated from the country, outlawed in many states, and harassed by local health authorities in other places. The campaign against them utilized much of the same rhetoric in the antichiropractic wars. "She is the most virulent bacteria of them all," declared one diatribe against midwifery, recalling the proceedings of the New York State Medical Society in 1949, when one distinguished participant said " . . . we are not talking about the licensing of chiropractors . . . we are talking about the destruction of chiropractors, the elimination of murderers." (Proceedings 1949) Eventually, obstetrics became big business in the health care community, with an estimated $4 billion annual expenditure in 15 to 20 million days of hospital care.

The flirtation with general medical practice may have had its origins in the intense purist–broad scope debates of the 1920s, when Drugless Practitioner Acts were enacted in Illinois, Pennsylvania, and a few other states, in the liberal scope of the pioneer law in Oregon in 1915, and following the California initiative referendum of 1922. It must be recognized, however, that the faction which adhered to manipulative doctrine the least had an interlocking relationship with fringe medicine for most of the first half century.

For definition of this overview, fringe medical practice would have included the remnants of the two surviving nineteenth century reform schools, homeopathy and eclectic medicine—the last of whose schools closed, respectively, in 1923 and 1938—and those osteopathic practitioners who did not disdain such associations as "cultist slumming." It would also have included those regular practitioners who had avoided or circumvented the official wrath of the mainline by practicing in private hospitals not seeking accreditation, and whose lack of state society affiliations did not affect their licenses.

The literature of broad scope publications from 1930 to 1960 provides insight into these relationships, the bridge for which was naturopathy. Naturopathic medicine has all but departed from the healing arts scene, with active licensure remaining in only a few states and with only two small training institutions surviving. The larger broad scope chiropractic schools also offered naturopathic degrees under separate charters until the late 1950s. While they existed, however, the naturopaths provided the catalyst for several attempts to merge the various reform sects under one unlikely holistic umbrella (Wardwell 1978).

The limbo of lost organizations of fringe medicine remains as a monument to these efforts. Among them may be recalled the International Society of Liberal Physicians and the National Medical Society, the latter a conglomerate of M.D. dissenters of all schools as well as naturopaths, osteopaths, chiropractors, and physiotherapists. In the early 1950s, the Society was seeking a charter from Congress to establish a medical school that would offer degrees in all of the healing arts. The world of fringe medicine in these years included those followers of Albert Abrams, whose diagnostic "boxes" caused him to be drummed out of the regular profession where he had gained an international reputation as a neurologist; the advocates of "zone therapy," and the acupuncture that prior to 1974 had only a foothold in American-Chinese medicine; herbalists and nutritionists outside of the mainline, and the cult followings which grew around the various cancer cures such as Harry Hoxsey and Andrew Ivy's Krebiozen. Ivy, it may be recalled, was like Abrams, a man of some distinguished reputation in the mainline before his "cancer cure." (Gardner 1957)

The outrage which such activities evoked at the Fountainhead only reinforced the hardline purists, who were convinced that anything but hands-only chiropractic would combine to destroy the legacy of the Palmers. The end-result of the flirtations of that part of extreme broad scope practitioners—the "supermixers" if we were to revert to that description—has been a dead end in the therapeutic road. Naturopathic medicine, unable to provide a central distinctive focus like manipulative therapy, has all but followed the fate of homeopathic and eclectic medicine. And while osteopathy claims that it has survived as separate and distinct, governmental agencies usually lump medical and osteopathic physicians together. Graduates of osteopathic colleges are trained not as competent manipulators, says Wardwell (1956), but as competent allopathic physicians.

Prosecutions and Persecutions to Threshold Acceptance

If chiropractic's survival is to be credited to its own ideology as much as the social factors which developed to its advantage, then it must be attributed not to the broad scope advocates so much as to the purists. To B. J. Palmer and the fundamentalist school must be accorded the motivation which did stamp it with a distinctive label within the therapeutic marketplace, something recognized by public identification as well as by begrudging allopathic condemnation. For while broad scope advocates may have elevated its practice closer to the threshold of respectability and subsequent acceptability by the scientific mainline, the purist concept provided the separate identity during a period when its continued existence was doubted by many. Morris Fishbein liked to predict "an early relapse and a not far-distant end" when lecturing on what he called the "medical cults." Yet the year he died, the chiropractors that he held in such abject contempt were to rub professional elbows with orthopedists, neurophysiologists, and manipulative specialists at an international conference sponsored by the National Institutes of Health.

That day, however, was not to come until the doors of countless jailhouses, county lockups, and prison farms were to close on the practitioners of the last surviving reform school of healing. Beginning with the trial, conviction, and imprisonment of D. D. Palmer for "practicing medicine without a license" in Scott County, Iowa in 1906, thousands would face the courts on the same charge, and hundreds would go to jail. *The Chiropractor and Clinical Journal* through most of the 1920s and into the 1930s carried a monthly page of the "Crusaders"—those D.C.'s who had been convicted and were serving time, asking readers to write them at their prison addresses.

The prosecutions continued through the early 1960s, with investigators from the medical boards in New York and Massachusetts, the last bastions of orthodoxy, seeking arrests whenever the legislative initiative of the medical lobby called for them. A mass arrest of 100 chiropractors in New York City in 1922 followed the abortive California prosecutions and helped to launch the laymen's movement, called the American Bureau of Chiropractic (ABC). Led by William Werner, this group marshalled enough support to fill Madison Square Garden in 1935, cheering such chiropractic boosters as Happy Chandler, the populist lieutenant governor of Tennessee (and later baseball commissioner) and Edward Lodge Curran, a priest-attorney who was a prominent follower of the late Father Coughlin. Yet as late as 1949, a well-known Manhattan husband-and-wife team—whose patients included the late Ambassador Joseph Kennedy—was sent to jail after their refusal to tell the court that they would "desist in the practice of medicine without a license." From the Women's House of Detention, Katherine (Kitty) Scallon would write a friend of her concern for her husband, Mack Scallon, who was serving his time on Hart's Island:

> Being here is sometimes like a bad dream, when you think of it being for nothing but doing good. . . . I felt down-hearted when the news came that Mabel [Palmer] died, but I would always perk up when I thought of chiropractic and the many people it had helped . . . and then I'd throw my shoulders back and be ready and willing to make any sacrifice to help free our beloved science. (Scallon 1949)

The administration building at one of the new

chiropractic institutions, Sherman College, is named after the Scallons.

Yet the dissenters persisted and endured. The passion for justice, the courage that comes to all minorities when they are the object of assault by established orthodoxy, be it politics or medicine, came to those followers of Palmer. Their legacy was part of that tragic destiny of America, which is hidden in its virtue: that which the physician signer of the Declaration of Independence, Benjamin Rush, had warned of when he said "to restrict the art of healing to one class and deny equal privilege to others constitutes the bastile of medical science."

Chiropractic has survived. As it approaches its centennial, those who inherit the legacy can look back at one of the more remarkable instances of successful social and medical protest in North American history.

REFERENCES

American Medical Association: Report of Investigations Council on Medical Education and Hospitals. JAMA 99:20, 1928

Bauman E: Holistic Health Handbook. Berkeley, CA, And/Or Press, 1978

Bealle M: Medical Mussolini. Washington, Columbia, 1947

Booth ER: History of Osteopathy. Kirksville, MO, 1924

Carver W: Chiropractic Red Book. Oklahoma City, Carver College, n.d.

Dictionary of American Biography [DAB], vol. 14. New York, Charles Scribner, 1934

Dye AA: The Evolution of Chiropractic. Philadelphia, 1939

Ehrenreich B, English D: For Her Own Good. New York, Anchor/Doubleday, 1978

Ehrenreich B, English D: Witches, Midwives and Nurses. Old Westbury, NY, Feminist Press, 1976

Fishbein M: The Medical Follies. New York, Boni & Liveright, 1925

Flexner A: Medical Education in the United States. New York, Times-Arno Press, 1967 [orig 1910]

Forster AL: Principles and Practice of Spinal Adjustment. Chicago, National School of Chiropractic, 1915

Gardner M: Fads and Fallacies in the Name of Science. New York, Dover Publications, 1957

Gibbons RW: The historical conflicts of cultism and science. Popular Culture 11:3, 1978

Gibbons RW: Physician-chiropractors: Medical presence in the evolution of chiropractic. Presentation, 50th Annual Meeting, American Association for the History of Medicine, May 1977

Gregory AL: Spinal Adjustment. Oklahoma City, Palmer-Gregory College, 1910

Harriman EA: Correspondence with the author, 1975

Homola S: Bonesetting, Chiropractic, and Cultism. Panama City, FL, Critique Books, 1963

Hubbard E: The Science of Keeping Well, East Aurora, NY, Roycrofters Press, 1914

Inglis B: The Case for Unorthodox Medicine, New York, G.P. Putnam, 1963

Kaufman M: Homeopathy in America: The Rise and Fall of a Medical Heresy. Baltimore, Johns Hopkins Press, 1971

Kempton M: The Briar Patch, New York, Dutton, 1975

Kett J: The Formation of the American Medical Profession, 1780-1860. New Haven, Yale University Press, 1968

Leboyer F: Birth Without Violence. New York, Alfred A. Knopf, 1975

Mencken HL: Prejudices. New York, Alfred A. Knopf, 1927

Numbers R: The making of an eclectic physician. Bulletin of the History of Medicine 47:2, 1972

Nutting H: A glorious future. The Chiropractor 11:1, 1915

Palmer BJ: Chiropractic Clinic. Davenport, IA, Palmer School of Chiropractic Press, 1949

Palmer BJ: Comments by B.J. The Fountainhead News, December 1933

Palmer BJ: History in the Making. Davenport, IA, Palmer School of Chiropractic, 1957

Palmer BJ: Shall Chiropractic Survive? Davenport, IA, Palmer School of Chiropractic, 1958

Palmer DD: The Chiropractor's Adjuster. Portland, OR, Portland Publishing Co., 1910

Palmer DD: Letter. National Chiropractic Journal 6:3, 1936

Palmer David D: The Palmers. Davenport, IA, Baldwin Brothers, 1976

Proceedings of the House of Delegates, Medical Society of the State of New York, New York State Journal of Medicine, September 1, 1949

Ratledge TF: Profession with a future. California Backbone 1:11, 1922

Scallon K to M Garfunkle, April 1949, Sherman College Library Collection, Spartanburg, SC

Stanford Research Institute, Chiropractic in California, Los Angeles, 1960

Wardwell W: Social factors in the survival of chiropractic. Sociological Symposium, no. 22, Spring 1978

CHAPTER TWO
The Present and Future Role of the Chiropractor

WALTER I. WARDWELL

The past and the future are separated by the present. The present itself has no duration but is simply "now." What is past is history, and what will happen in the future can only be known after the fact.

Although our best guide for the future is the past, even Santayana's famous maxim, "Those who forget the past are doomed to repeat it," provides no clear indication as to how the past is to be used. What kind of guidance can it give? If by history we mean only the bare chronology of events, it may profit us little to study it. We need a systematic frame of reference that facilitates analysis of the processes we are interested in, in order to comprehend the forces influencing events.

For example, a persistent American value is the goal of making the world a better place in which to live through overcoming the many adversities that beset man—pests, pestilence, floods, poverty, crime, and so on. Our conviction that we can conquer these evils impels us to seek more knowledge, better science, and improved technology. But new theories and techniques must compete for survival with those already in existence. Innovation and change are opposed by tradition, habituation, and vested interests in established dogmas, power, and prestige. Out of the clash of values and interests will come some future resolution, but it is impossible to predict exactly what. Extraneous forces seemingly unrelated to the problem at hand often exert the decisive influence.

In the health field an example of an extraneous force is the East–West conflict, which has an impact not only on our religious and cultural values but also on the availability of economic resources for delivering health care. Another example is the large-scale migration of people from rural areas to cities, from cities to suburbs, and from developing societies to industrial societies. Still another is the increasing education and sophistication of people everywhere in matters of health, nutrition, disease prevention, and environmental problems, especially those pertaining to clean water, air, food, and energy. Finally, we should not overlook the increasing American acceptance of the role of government in protecting the environment, controlling the use of energy, planning the economy, and regulating the many other aspects of our lives as workers, employers, and consumers. This is not a complete list of extraneous factors affecting our health care system but it will do for a start.

Selected Trends in American Health Care

Central to providing health care for the American people is the consensus that health care is a right, not merely a privilege. No longer is poverty accepted as justification for denying treatment to those who need it. Indeed, planners now focus attention precisely on the role that poverty plays in producing diseases through depriving the poor of adequate nutrition, housing, and sanitation, and adequate knowledge of the techniques of health maintenance and disease prevention. They are trying to devise programs to identify previously undiscovered causes of disease. An impressive example of such trends is federal legislation to provide renal dialysis free of charge to all who need it.

The concern with unmet health needs and medically underserved populations, both rural and central city, has become a major thrust of health planning. Legislation mandating Health Systems Agencies (HSAs) establishes grass roots structures to implement the new social value that good health and health care is a right of all Americans. Some call this trend a "drift toward socialism." But hostility toward that phrase should not blind us to the broader significance of increased federal expenditures for health care. In this respect the early opposition to Medicare by the American Medical Association (AMA) was insightful, for Medicare was indeed the foot in the door—the entering wedge—leading to other national programs to implement the new consensus that health and health care are everyone's rights. Whether the phrase used is "national health service" or "national health insurance," or something else, massive federal appropriations bring federal regulation in their wake. For even if our health care system remains a "mixed system" including private insurance companies, and even if quality is controlled by peer review systems such as PSROs (Professional Standards Review Organizations), the federal government, as the principal payer for services, inevitably will increasingly dominate the system.

If the United States had adopted socialized medicine in the 1940s (as did Great Britain) before Medicare and Medicaid and the extensive proliferation of private health insurance plans had occurred, the change to socialized medicine could have been made more easily at that time than it could be now. From an economic point of view it might make little difference if the federal government should take over health care completely, or merely regulate it. For even if the government were to socialize health care completely, it would have to rely on existing experts and leaders to administer it and on existing practitioners to staff it. The percentage of our gross national product going to health care (which is now 8.8 percent) might not increase very much, although a larger proportion of it undoubtedly would come from federal taxes and a smaller proportion from personal resources. The presumed inefficiency of the large federal bureaucracy that would be required to administer it might not require many more dollars than does the present confusing variety of administrative forms and regulations needed to obtain reimbursements from Medicare, Medicaid, Workmen's Compensation, and private insurance companies. Even if the United States should adopt some form of socialized medicine or merely modify the present system to mandate insurance coverage for workers while itself paying the premiums for the poor, the aged, and the unemployed, thus merely reallocating the burden of paying the costs of health care. In neither case would the type of health care being delivered be fundamentally changed as long as organized medicine dominates it.

However, there is little likelihood that the United States will soon adopt socialized medicine. The entrenched interests of private medicine and of the private insurance and pharmaceutical industries practically guarantee that it will not happen. And the greater the proportion of health care services that are reimbursed by a system requiring specific authorization of payment for each treatment of each patient of each practitioner, the more entrenched the fee-for-service system becomes.

About the only fundamental change in the present system of delivering health care that seems at all likely to occur is expansion of the prepaid comprehensive health care delivery model represented by Health Maintenance Organizations (HMOs), a model pioneered by the Kaiser Plans and several others very popular on the West Coast. Because they are not run by the federal government but on the initiative of private groups, they are compatible with our free enterprise ideology. And since they involve the insurance principle of prepaid care and the assumption of entrepreneurial risk, they are compatible with insurance company practices. But to the extent that they involve comprehensive care, continuity of care, efficient record keeping, easily available interaction with diagnostic and therapeutic specialists and assistants, early identification of health problems and pathologies, health education, disease prevention, and reduced hospitalization rates, HMOs represent a sharp break with traditional fee-for-service practice. This is particularly true of the "staff model" HMOs, where nearly all providers are on salary. Health Maintenance Organizations decrease the amount of paperwork associated with health insurance since one fee from the client covers almost everything. The most significant point about HMOs is that the financial incentive to contain costs which they offer to providers increases pressure for them to become more effective in health education and disease prevention and thereby to eliminate unnecessary diagnostic and therapeutic procedures, especially surgery and other in-hospital treatment.

Potentially, HMOs could radically change the landscape of health care delivery in the United States, especially if they should become inclusive of all health care services—dental, optical, audiometric, and chiropractic—and if ways could be found to include the elderly and the indigent as well. If and when most Americans become covered by HMOs, it is conceivable that the federal government would assume full responsibility and take over the entire system. Such a scenario for the evolution of HMOs to socialized medicine does not appear likely at the present time, since they service only about 3 percent of the American population and the proportion of the population that is covered is expanding very slowly, despite a federal policy of encouraging new HMOs. However, the scenario provides food for thought concerning possible future developments.

How Do Chiropractors Fit Into the Evolving Health Care System?

How might chiropractors fit into the American health care delivery system in the future? The starting point must necessarily be where they are now, and where they have come from. Gibbons (Chapter 1, this volume) has performed an invaluable service for chiropractors, historians, social scientists, and public health planners with his pioneering analysis documenting the history of chiropractic. Within the past generation,

chiropractors have attained public acceptance and the legal standing of certified and licensed practitioners in all of the United States and in most of the other countries where they practice. The distribution of chiropractors in the United States and in the Canadian provinces is shown in Table 1. Their uneven distribution is apparent. Ratios vary from 2:100,000 in Virginia and in the Canadian maritime provinces to 33:100,000 in New Hampshire, with the highest ratios in the West North Central, Pacific, and Mountain states and in the Canadian province of Alberta. In all of Europe it has been estimated that there are about 800 chiropractors with about 120 in Switzerland, 150 in Denmark, and 30 in Norway (Sparlin 1978). There are also significant numbers in Great Britain, Germany, South Africa, Australia, and New Zealand.

In 1974 the United States Office of Education authorized the Council on Chiropractic Education (CCE) of the American Chiropractic Association (ACA) to establish an accrediting commission for chiropractic colleges. Initially CCE identified only four colleges that met its standards, but as of this writing there are seven fully accredited colleges; three others are "recognized candidates for accreditation." Among the seven remaining colleges in the United States are four very new ones. Three colleges located outside the United States hold "affiliate member" status with the CCE. The 20 colleges, their total enrollments as of October 1978, and the total number of degrees awarded in 1978 are listed in Table 2.

Programs of study in chiropractic colleges parallel those in medical colleges except that chiropractic theory and practice replace surgery and materia medica. Most of the student's fourth year is devoted to practice in the college clinic. Several colleges contract to have some nonclinical subjects taught by the faculty of accredited colleges (e.g., New York Chiropractic College) or are negotiating to become affiliated components of them (e.g., Canadian Memorial Chiropractic College). The International College of Chiropractic in Australia is affiliated with the Preston Institute of Technology. The two-year preprofessional academic

TABLE 1. Numbers of Chiropractors and Population Ratios: United States and Canada, January 1, 1978

Area	Licensed Chiropractors	Resident Chiropractors	Resident Chiropractors per 100,000 Population
United States	30,530	22,100	11
New England			
Maine	192	73	7
New Hampshire	494	286	33
Vermont	245	46	9
Massachusetts	390	280	5
Rhode Island	42	33	4
Connecticut	150	106	4
Total	1513	825	7
Middle Atlantic			
New York	1467	1400	8
New Jersey	962	817	12
Pennsylvania	1268	1077	9
Total	3697	3294	9
East North Central			
Ohio	646	610	6
Indiana	444	378	7
Illinois	1143	961	9
Michigan	1013	865	9
Wisconsin	645	538	12
Total	3891	3352	8
West North Central			
Minnesota	687	579	15
Iowa	1279	686	24
Missouri	1717	1305	27
North Dakota	116	30	5
South Dakota	168	109	16
Nebraska	133	78	5
Kansas	739	468	20
Total	4839	3255	19
South Atlantic			
Delaware	57	23	4
Maryland	282	164	4
District of Columbia	12	6	1
Virginia	137	98	2
West Virginia	128	72	4
North Carolina	514	320	6
South Carolina	222	222	9
Georgia	581	387	9
Florida	1833	1084	13
Total	3766	2376	8
East South Central			
Kentucky	1509	384	11
Tennessee	274	155	4
Alabama	534	289	8
Mississippi	300	100	4
Total	2617	928	7

TABLE 1. (*cont.*)

Area	Licensed Chiropractors	Resident Chiropractors	Resident Chiropractors per 100,000 Population
West South Central			
Arkansas	262	181	8
Louisiana	307	280	7
Oklahoma	742	395	14
Texas	1259	1087	8
Total	2570	1943	9
Mountain			
Montana	171	98	13
Idaho	121	97	11
Wyoming	72	51	12
Colorado	392	298	11
New Mexico	306	182	15
Arizona	591	385	17
Utah	174	174	14
Nevada	231	68	11
Total	2058	1353	13
Pacific			
Washington	719	595	16
Oregon	401	328	14
California	4292	3782	17
Alaska	39	33	8
Hawaii	96	36	4
Total	5547	4774	16
Puerto Rico	239	19	0.5
Canada			
Prince Edward Island*	2	2	2
Nova Scotia	19	19	2
New Brunswick	20	16	2
Quebec	485	477	8
Ontario*	880	880	10
Manitoba*	62	62	9
Saskatchewan	60	57	6
Alberta	308	262	14
British Columbia	230	230	9
Total	2066	2005	9

*"Total licensed" figures for these provinces are for 1979 and were provided by President Donald Sutherland of Canadian Memorial Chiropractic College. They were also used in the "resident" column to calculate the total for Canada and the population ratios for the three provinces.
From Federation of Chiropractic Licensing Boards, Glendale, CA,: 1978-79 Official Directory of Chiropractic and Basic Science Examining Boards, with Licensure and Practice Statistics, plus other sources. Population data from Metropolitan Life Insurance Company: Statistical Bulletin 59:11, 1978.

TABLE 2. **Chiropractic Colleges, Accreditation Status, Enrollments and Graduates, 1978**

College (year founded)	Total Enrollment (October 1978)	Graduates (1978)
Accredited colleges		
Logan College of Chiropractic Chesterfield, Missouri (1935)	557	140
Los Angeles College of Chiropractic Glendale, California (1911)	689	134
National College of Chiropractic Lombard, Illinois (1906)	880	204
New York Chiropractic College Glen Head, New York (1919)	645	226
Northwestern College of Chiropractic St. Paul, Minnesota (1941)	387	85
Palmer College of Chiropractic Davenport, Iowa (1895)	1848	548
Texas Chiropractic College Pasadena, Texas (1908)	309	60
Total	5315	1397
Recognized candidates for accreditation		
Cleveland Chiropractic College Kansas City, Missouri (1922)	231	63
Life Chiropractic College Marietta, Georgia (1974)	861	140
Western States Chiropractic College Portland, Oregon (1903)	498	87
Total	1590	290
Other United States colleges		
Adio Institute of Straight Chiropractic Levittown, Pennsylvania (1978)	70	0
Cleveland Chiropractic College Los Angeles, California (1908)	311	87
Northern California College of Chiropractic Palo Alto, California (1978)	90	0
Pacific States Chiropractic College San Lorenzo, California (1978)	18	0
Sherman College of Straight Chiropractic Spartanburg, South Carolina (1973)	404	85
Southwestern Chiropractic College Sweetwater, Texas (1979)	0	0
University of Pasadena College of Chiropractic Pasadena, California (1973)	193	81
Total	1086	253
Total United States	7991	1940

TABLE 2. (*cont.*)

College (year founded)	Total Enrollment (October 1978)	Graduates (1978)
Affiliate member colleges (outside U.S.)		
Anglo-European College of Chiropractic Bournemouth, England (1965)	120	26
Canadian Memorial Chiropractic College Toronto, Ontario, Canada (1945)	580	128
International College of Chiropractic Melbourne, Australia (1975)	245*	0
Total	945	154
GRAND TOTAL	893	2094

*Data for April 1979
From Council on Chiropractic Education.

requirement prevails in all chiropractic colleges while approximately half of the students enter with a baccalaureate.

In 1974 four major events signaled acceptance of chiropractic as an established health profession in the United States. Besides the establishment of an accrediting procedure for the colleges, the last remaining state to license chiropractors (Louisiana) did so. In the same year Congress authorized Medicare payments to chiropractors for services rendered to persons 65 years of age and over, and Congress directed that $2 million be used for a study of "the scientific basis of chiropractic." An immediate result was that in February 1975 the National Institute for Neurological and Communicative Diseases and Stroke (NINCDS) of the United States Public Health Service sponsored a historic conference in Bethesda, Maryland which focused on the more appropriate topic of "the scientific basis of spinal manipulative therapy," at which world leaders in neurophysiology and spinal biomechanics plus medical, osteopathic, and chiropractic practitioners of spinal manipulative therapy presented scientific papers (Goldstein 1975). The consensus of the 58 participants was that spinal manipulative therapy clearly benefits many patients, especially those with neuromusculoskeletal conditions, but that the reasons why it does so are not yet well understood and require further research.

Today the typical chiropractor is a white male who practices either solo or with one or two other chiropractors employing one or more chiropractic assistants. In 1977 he charged an average fee of $11 for a routine office visit and $56 for the initial visit of a new patient, including laboratory work, x-rays, and chiropractic adjustment. In 1976 his median gross annual income approached $50,000, with, of course, considerable variation around that figure. When physiotherapy is used, the most frequently procedures are, in descending order, ultrasound, diathermy, low-voltage electrotherapy, traction, radiant heat, and massage (Velie 1979).

A survey conducted by the ACA in 1973 based on a 25 percent random sampling of its members drew a 58 percent response rate and 1074 usable returns (Shenk 1974). The results showed that 85 percent own an x-ray machine, two-thirds always take a case history on a new patient, and two-thirds use no instruments for spinal examination; 90 percent refer patients to M.D.'s while 65 percent receive referrals from M.D.'s. Approximately 80 percent provide counseling and vitamin or mineral supplements. The average number of patients seen per week was 103, with an average of 17 minutes devoted to each patient. Any one patient received an average of 14 treatments in a year. Only 1 percent of all treatments were given in patients' homes.

A 1972 profile of chiropractic students at the five then ACA-accredited colleges revealed that

93 percent were male, the average age was 26.4 years, 50 percent were married with an average of one child per family, 64 percent had been a chiropractic patient for an average of 9.5 years before becoming a student, 26 percent had earned a baccalaureate prior to entering chiropractic college, and 57 percent worked at least part-time while attending school. One in seven had a chiropractor father, and one in four had a relative who was a chiropractor (Shenk 1973).

The United States Health Interview Survey in 1974 produced estimates that about 3.6 percent of the United States population (i.e., 7.5 million persons) had consulted a chiropractor during the preceding 12-month period (Table 3). Variations between regions of the country ranged from 2.5 percent in the South to 5 percent in the West, and from 2.4 percent in urban centers to 6.6 percent on farms. Other frequent users of chiropractic revealed in Table 3 are whites in comparison with blacks, middle-aged in comparison with young and aged, and middle-income persons compared to those with low or high incomes. In a random sampling of 1000 persons in Wisconsin, a state with a moderate chiropractor-to-population ratio, Duffy (1979) found that 12.5 percent had utilized the services of a chiropractor within the previous 2 years and that 35.8 percent had at some time in their lives been examined or treated by a chiropractor. When asked about their most recent experience with a medical doctor and with a chiropractor, 73 percent of those who had consulted a chiropractor, compared to 90 percent of those who had consulted a medical doctor, felt that their treatment was either somewhat or very effective; 93 percent were satisfied with their chiropractor in general compared to 97 percent for their medical doctor. Several other studies have documented overall patient satisfaction with treatment by chiropractors and their acceptance by the general public as health providers (Baum 1971; Harding 1977; Parker and Tupling 1976).

Third-party payment for chiropractors' services is now practically universal under workmen's compensation legislation. In addition, many states require payments for chiropractors' services by Blue Shield or other private insur-

ance carriers. In view of several studies showing that total payment for chiropractors' treatments are less than for medical treatments for comparable conditions (Kane 1974; Cichoke and West 1978) it is not surprising that insurance companies for many years have underwritten chiropractors' services even without a legal mandate to do so. In fiscal year 1978, the federal government paid $30,530,924 to chiropractors for reimbursement of services under Medicare.

Since 1974 several significant developments have occurred that justify the conclusion that chiropractic is now a well-established part of the American health care delivery system. Applications and enrollments to chiropractic colleges have increased in quantity and quality. The colleges have strengthened their faculties and improved their physical facilities and equipment. Interprofessional contacts in research and academic settings, scientific conferences, and health planning organizations occur more frequently, as does the sharing of support facilities such as laboratories. The AMA's Committee on Quackery and its Bureau of Investigation, each of which had devoted the majority of its time and resources to the effort to contain (if not destroy) chiropractic, have been abolished.

In 1976 the AMA, the American Osteopathic Association, ten other medical organizations, and four officials of the AMA were named in a mammoth antitrust lawsuit entered by Dr. Chester Wilk and four other chiropractors who asked for damages and injunctive relief charging:

> The defendants have attempted to monopolize, and conspired to monopolize, health care services in the United States and conspired to unreasonably restrain duly licensed chiropractic doctors including the plaintiffs herein from competing with medical doctors and osteopathic doctors in the delivery of health care services to the general public in the United States, and moreover, have been and are engaged in a combination and conspiracy to first isolate and then eliminate the chiropractic profession in the United States (Wilk et al. 1976).

In addition to monetary damages and injunctive relief the suit asks the court that:

TABLE 3. **Persons Receiving Chiropractic Services in the United States, 1974**

	Number of Persons Receiving Service (thousands)			Persons Receiving Services as Percent of Total Population		
	Male	Female	Total	Male	Female	Total
All persons*	3,811	3,715	7,527	3.8	3.5	3.6
Age						
Under 6 years	69	61	130	0.7	0.6	0.7
6–16 years	336	197	533	1.5	0.9	1.2
17–24 years	478	488	966	3.4	3.2	3.3
25–44 years	1,229	1,206	2,345	5.0	4.6	4.8
45–64 years	1,326	1,325	2,650	6.5	5.9	6.2
65 years and over	374	438	812	4.4	3.6	3.9
Color						
White	3,680	3,572	7,252	4.2	3.8	4.0
All other	132	143	275	1.1	1.0	1.0
Family income						
Less than $2,000	52	156	208	2.0	3.3	2.8
$2,000–$3,999	192	314	506	3.0	3.2	3.1
$4,000–$6,999	504	559	1,064	3.7	3.6	3.7
$7,000–$9,999	494	592	1,086	3.7	4.3	4.0
$10,000–$14,999	1,111	1,005	2,115	4.2	4.0	4.1
$15,000 or more	1,303	927	2,229	4.1	3.0	3.5
Usual activity status†						
Going to school	486	352	837	1.8	1.3	1.6
Working	2,669	1,389	4,058	5.3	4.8	5.1
Keeping house	—	1,856	1,856	—	4.7	4.7
Retired	482	15	497	5.6	2.0	5.3
Other	105	43	148	3.3	2.1	2.8
Geographic region						
Northeast	837	808	1,645	3.6	3.1	3.3
North Central	1,156	1,198	2,353	4.3	4.2	4.2
South	818	839	1,657	2.6	2.5	2.5
West	1,001	870	1,871	5.5	4.5	5.0
Place of residence						
SMSA‡	2,189	2,078	4,266	3.2	2.8	3.0
Central city	794	737	1,531	2.7	2.2	2.4
Outside central city	1,394	1,341	2,735	3.6	3.2	3.4
Outside SMSA	1,623	1,638	3,260	5.1	5.0	5.1
Nonfarm	1,340	1,419	2,760	4.8	4.9	4.9
Farm	282	218	500	7.2	6.0	6.6

*Includes unknown income.
†Excludes children under 6 years of age.
‡Standard metropolitan statistical area.
From: Utilization of selected medical practitioners: United States, 1974. Vital and Health Statistics of the National Center for Health Statistics, No. 24, 1978.

Defendants be ordered to rectify the adverse effects on public health care flowing proximately from their illegal acts including establishment and maintenance for ten years, at defendants' sole expense and at a cost to defendants of no less than $1,000,000 per year, of an interprofessional research institute controlled equally by medical doctors and Doctors of Chiropractic for promoting inter-professional research and educational programs, and for developing a common lexicon.

Among the early results of the suit has been a reversal of AMA policy toward professional interrelationships between M.D.'s and chiropractors. In March 1977 the AMA's Judicial Council announced:

A physician may refer a patient for diagnostic or therapeutic services to another physician, a limited practitioner, or any other provider of health care services permitted by law to furnish such services, whenever he believes that this may benefit the patient. As in the case of referrals to physician-specialists, referrals to limited practitioners should be based on their individual competence and ability to perform the services needed by the patient (American Medical News 1977).

Thus the AMA's public opposition to chiropractic was muted almost overnight. And the AMA's strategy toward chiropractic appears to have changed from one of opposition on all fronts (legislative, media campaigns, professional ostracism, etc.) to one of containment.

Despite these advances chiropractic remains a divided profession. Although studies reveal nearly unanimous agreement among the rank and file that the ACA and the International Chiropractors Association (ICA) should merge (NYSCA Newsletter 1972) the leaders of the two associations have not found it possible to achieve organizational unity. In view of the wide agreement among practicing chiropractors as to what chiropractic is, it is perhaps surprising that the ancient shibboleths of the extremists still govern much of the dialogue within the profession—i.e., "pure and unadulterated straight chiropractic" on one side, and allegations of "mixing chiropractic with naturopathy or medicine" on the other. Two of the newest colleges have even incorporated the

word "straight" into their titles and have refused to seek accredited status with the ACA-dominated CCE. While those "mixer" colleges that earlier (three as late as 1948) taught naturopathy alongside chiropractic and offered both D.C. and N.D. degrees no longer do so, chiropractic mixers tend to use such medical terms as "diagnosis," "portal of entry," "physician," etc. Although ACA members outnumber ICA members by about three to one, the ICA has recently exhibited renewed vitality by moving its offices to Washington, by actively supporting the antitrust suit against organized medicine, and by winning the federal contract for its Foundation for the Advancement of Chiropractic Tenets and Science (FACTS) to conduct a nationwide study of the cost of chiropractic education, the supply and demand for chiropractic services and manpower, and the cost of those services (Mazzarelli 1978). While the ACA earlier won the competition to have its accrediting agency (CCE) designated by the United States Office of Education to set standards for all chiropractic colleges, the ICA's Palmer College continues to attract and to graduate by far the largest number of students. Although organizational unity would produce many benefits for chiropractors, it may require a new generation of chiropractic leaders.

Relations Between Medicine and Chiropractic

Although it is too early to predict whether organized medicine will ever give up its active opposition to chiropractors, begin to cooperate with them, and admit them to true professional communion, as it has done with osteopathy, such complete acceptance seems not likely to occur. Were it to happen, it could result in the "co-optation" or swallowing up of chiropractic into medicine that B. J. Palmer feared and struggled against so valiantly. But it is not likely that chiropractors will be offered that temptation even if they should desire it. The medical opposition has always been so intense and so well organized that chiropractors have had little choice but to fight back.

Certainly it is unlikely that many physicians will themselves want to become skilled in chiropractic adjusting. Despite the existence of a small group of medical practitioners in the North American Academy of Manipulative Medicine, it is not likely that many medical generalists or specialists will ever want to become competent manipulators. The medical curriculum is already so crowded that there is simply not enough time to develop manipulative skills in the average physician. The alternative of training orthopedists, neurologists, or physiatrists as competent manipulators would not only be a diversion for them but the small numbers of those specialists would not comprise enough practitioners to treat more than a small fraction of the patients who need manipulative therapy.

There are several other possible future types of relationships between chiropractic and organized medicine. One, which can be easily dismissed, would be for chiropractors to practice under medical supervision as physical therapists do. Following medical diagnosis the physical therapist often exercises considerable independent judgment as to the appropriate therapy. One judgment that more and more physical therapists are making these days is that they should include manipulative therapy in their repertoire. James Cyriax, M.D., offers such instruction in short courses calling it "orthopaedic medicine," and so does the physical therapist Stanley Paris, who prefers the designation "orthopaedic physical therapy." But chiropractors, who are already licensed doctors, some of whom call themselves "chiropractic physicians," are not about to subordinate themselves to medical prescription, which would reduce them to the status of ancillaries to medical doctors. Chiropractors have been autonomous practitioners and have functioned at a so much higher level than physical therapists in the diagnosis and treatment of illness for too long for them to be willing to regress to the lower status of physical therapists.

An alternative arrangement that would probably be preferred by most physicians would be for any manipulative treatment to be done by physical therapists under medical supervision.

But that alternative would not work for several reasons. First, physicians would have to develop expertise in areas that they do not well understand, such as when to prescribe manipulative therapy, when it is contraindicated, when it should be modified during the course of treatment, etc. Only if physicians had as much knowledge as chiropractors would they be qualified to make such judgments. As for the physical therapists, if they were to make such decisions under the loose kind of medical supervision that they now function under, they would need more expertise than they typically acquire in their present baccalaureate programs. They would need so much more diagnostic, clinical, and manipulative skill that they would in effect be chiropractors. Although physical therapists have been encouraged by both James Cyriax and Stanley Paris to move in this direction, it has not yet become a major trend in physical therapy education or practice.

A Parallel Profession?

Chiropractors could maintain their present stance vis-à-vis medicine but become even more the equals of physicians and therefore a profession parallel to medicine. This alternative involves continuing to emphasize the differences between medicine and chiropractic, the uniqueness of chiropractic treatment, the contrasting philosophical approaches of health maintenance versus therapy, and the alternative terminology that chiropractors have traditionally preferred (for example, "analysis" instead of "diagnosis" and "adjustment" instead of "treatment"). It also requires chiropractic colleges independent of medical control and chiropractic licensing boards dominated by chiropractors. It views chiropractors as "primary care providers" with a concern for patients' problems nearly as broad in scope as that of physicians. Although the distinction from mixers that chiropractic straights have long insisted upon limits the range of therapies that chiropractors offer to adjustment of the spine (plus occasionally that of other osseous segments) using hands only, straights have nevertheless generally been reluctant to limit very much the range of conditions which they believe chiropractors should treat. Mixers, on the other hand, while they have sometimes maintained that naturopathic remedies and physiotherapy devices fall within the purview of chiropractic, have sometimes been more likely than straights to consider the range of conditions that chiropractors should properly treat as quite limited.

In any case, the distinction between straights and mixers has become less important than it used to be, perhaps as a result of the waning of B. J. Palmer's personal influence. Chiropractors can now acknowledge what was probably always the case—that the distribution of chiropractors on the "straight-mixer" dimension has never really been bimodal (that is, with most chiropractors at one extreme or the other) but closer to what statisticians call a normal distribution, with the majority falling in the middle, between the two extremes. Nevertheless the split between the ICA and the ACA has been very real and it has been in the interest of the leaders of the two associations to maximize the differences between them and to maintain the fiction that chiropractors divide neatly into two distinct practitioner groups.

Despite their rivalry, the following forces are bringing the ICA and the ACA closer together:

1. The need to cooperate in the political arena, first most noticeable in the joint preparation of Chiropractic's White Paper (1969) following the 1967 Surgeon General's study of the question of including chiropractic under Medicare;
2. General acceptance of the Chiropractic Council on Education as the agency which sets uniform standards for the accreditation of chiropractic colleges;
3. Increasingly uniform requirements set by state laws and licensing boards;
4. Development of peer review standards for the payment of chiropractors' services by third-party payers;
5. A speculative point: the public's anticipation of what a chiropractor treats and how he

goes about doing so which may tend to standardize what chiropractors do.

If chiropractic continues on its present course toward becoming a health profession parallel to medicine, certain negative consequences should not be overlooked. To the extent that the differences from medicine are emphasized and special kinds of education, examining, and licensing are retained, the contrast between chiropractic and the other health professionals integrated with orthodox medicine will remain great. The negative trade-off is that differences between professions usually result in ranking of those professions on a scale of desirability or prestige. Since organized medicine is so strong and prestigious, other health professions benefit from being related to it, including those subordinated to it and the so-called "limited" medical professions such as dentistry, podiatry, optometry, and psychology. The latter have escaped domination by medicine by claiming only a limited part of the therapeutic enterprise as their own, without attacking medicine's basic theories concerning the nature of disease or the physician's dominant role in treating systemic or life-threatening illnesses. By limiting their expertise to a particular part of the human body (i.e., teeth, feet, eyes, or personality) and to a relatively narrow range of techniques, the limited medical professions have avoided threatening organized medicine, and hence have been able to survive through being accepted and tolerated in their limited roles.

Chiropractors cannot have their cake and eat it too. To the extent that they reject the basic conceptions of medical science as fundamentally wrong, and propound chiropractic as a completely different philosophy and science capable of treating nearly the entire range of human ailments, they inevitably find great difficulty in convincing the mass of informed citizens that medicine's evaluation of chiropractic is wrong. Such citizens, unless persuaded by personal experience, are unlikely to view chiropractic as scientific or chiropractors as qualified doctors. Lack of acceptance by the public and rejection by orthodox medical authorities explains why the word "marginal" has been used to describe the chiropractic profession ever since 1952 (Wardwell 1952). However, from being "marginal," chiropractic could evolve, as has osteopathy, to being "parallel" to medicine if it becomes the equal of medicine in education, scientific research, public acceptance, and success in therapy. The questions would then be: What would happen at that point? Would chiropractic tend to merge with orthodox medicine, as osteopathy is beginning to do? Or could it remain equal but separate?

Should Chiropractors Become Limited Medical Practitioners?

Still another possible role for chiropractic would be for it to become a limited medical profession. The best examples have already been cited—dentistry, podiatry, optometry, and psychology—to which could be added speech therapy and audiology. These professions limit both the range of the therapeutic techniques they employ and the parts of the body they treat. And they do not challenge medicine's basic theories of disease and therapy, although they often contend with medicine over the relative importance of the body parts they treat or over the details of preferred treatment. In recent years they have attained a reasonably stable relationship with organized medicine—a modus vivendi (Wardwell 1979). Among the reasons why the limited medical professions have escaped medical domination are such historical factors as lack of interest by regular physicians in the problem area, shortage of physicians, or lack of money to be made treating trivial conditions (e.g., corns) or chronic symptoms (e.g., psychoneuroses).

Although they are not primary care providers, limited medical practitioners are "portals of entry" to the health care system, since they typically are the point of first contact for patients who have not undergone a medical diagnosis. Hence they must be able to recognize conditions beyond their competence to treat and be willing to refer them to someone who can, usu-

ally a medical doctor. Nowadays the limited professions receive sufficient training in diagnosis so that they seldom fail to identify problems which should be referred to an alternative provider. Although they often feel pressure to expand their scope of practice (e.g., for optometrists to use dilating drops in the eyes; or for podiatrists to treat subcutaneous pathologies), limited medical practitioners generally experience little difficulty in keeping within their specified limits.

The question is whether limited medical practitioners offer chiropractors an appropriate model for a relationship with organized medicine that both groups can find acceptable. Opposition is certain to arise from those chiropractors who are unwilling to limit their scope of practice to less than the full range of human illnesses. For those who are willing to limit their scope of practice, the question is: What limits would they agree to? And what limits would organized medicine insist upon? Opposition would probably also arise from chiropractors who prescribe biologicals, practice obstetrics, set fractures, or perform minor surgery—those chiropractors whose conceptions of the breadth of chiropractic practice sometimes disturb other chiropractors as well as medical specialists in orthopedics or obstetrics.

Despite opposition from both sides, redefinition of the chiropractor's role along the lines of limited medicine would offer chiropractic some advantages. If agreement could be reached between chiropractors and physicians as to chiropractic's legitimate scope, and if physicians were convinced that chiropractors are competent to identify problems requiring referral to physicians, the following benefits might accrue:

1. Medical opposition to chiropractors should cease.
2. The public's image of chiropractors should improve.
3. Payments to chiropractors for services rendered within their scope of practice should be more readily made.
4. The number of referrals to chiropractors by other types of practitioners should increase.
5. Chiropractors should have gained an even

more secure place in the American health care system.

Among the pressures currently pushing chiropractors in the direction of the limited medicine model are:

1. Chiropractors in fact devote most of their time to the alleviation of neuromusculoskeletal symptoms.
2. These conditions are the kinds that the public believes that chiropractors can treat best.
3. It is for such conditions that physicians and other providers are most likely to refer patients to chiropractors.
4. Third-party payers are most willing to reimburse chiropractors for treating such conditions.
5. There is a more obvious and direct relationship between chiropractic adjustments and such conditions.
6. If a chiropractor is especially cautious or concerned about his image, it is no doubt safer for him to restrict his practice to neuromusculoskeletal conditions than to attempt to treat systemic conditions or those involving internal organs.

What are some of the forces resisting this redefinition of the chiropractor's role? The general objections by organized medicine to any recognition of chiropractic or chiropractors are too well known to deserve repetition. Many chiropractors would also resist such a change, for a variety of reasons. Some may feel that chiropractic is nearly unlimited in its potentialities. Others may not be willing to accord recognition to the role that medical doctors play in therapy. Still others may feel that being a parallel profession to medicine is the preferred goal; or that rivalry and hostility between the two competing professions is more desirable than any kind of accommodation between them.

In the final analysis, as the Swiss chiropractor Sandoz (1977) said so well in a recent article:

Chiropractic does not and should not belong to chiropractors, to M.D.'s or to anyone else except to the sick. . . . Chiropractic should be in the hands of those who can get the most out of it for the benefit of the sick. It is finally a question of who is and who will render the most efficient service with it.

A brief comparison with what has happened to osteopathy and naturopathy will help clarify the alternatives for chiropractic.

Comparison With Osteopathy and Naturopathy

The evolution of osteopathy to medical respectability is continuing. The decision by the California College of Osteopathic Physicians and Surgeons in 1961 (by a margin of one vote) to become the University of California College of Medicine, Irvine was a severe blow to osteopathy. The previous graduates of the college were invited, in return for a small fee and a brief didactic exposure, to accept an M.D. degree. They could then become licensed M.D.'s provided they did not also call themselves osteopaths. Simultaneously the California state medical and osteopathic societies merged. In 1962 a California law prohibited the licensing of any new osteopaths. (However, the law was successfully challenged in the courts and finally voided by the California Supreme Court in 1974—Bruce et al. 1975). Also in 1961 the House of Delegates of the American Medical Association decreed that henceforth each state medical society could decide for itself whether to accept osteopaths as professional equals. However, their remaining antipathy toward osteopathy was revealed in their phrasing of the directive, "The test should be the question: Does the individual doctor of osteopathy practice osteopathy or does he in fact practice a method of healing founded on a scientific basis?" (Judicial Council 1961)

Perhaps not surprisingly the effect of these developments was to reinvigorate in the American Osteopathic Association (AOA) sentiments of hostility toward organized medicine. The AOA reacted by chartering a new osteopathic state association in California, and it successfully opposed the attempted merger of the two professions in Washington state. In 1967 the AOA House of Delegates accused the AMA of seeking "to dominate or control all aspects of American health care—a role that the AMA neither merits nor has the moral or legal right to enforce. . . . The osteopathic profession stands together in vigorously opposing this arrogant policy of academic piracy" (White Paper: 1968). Since then nine new osteopathic colleges have been opened including a new one in California. It is clearly current AMA policy to incorporate osteopathy within the medical fold. Government publications now combine M.D.'s and D.O.'s in most tabulations, separating them only for special purposes. Graduates of osteopathic colleges can now compete for medical residencies and ultimate board certification as medical specialists. The intent of these policy changes on the part of the AMA seems to be to draw a sharp line between M.D.'s and osteopaths on one side and chiropractors on the other. However, since many of the remaining osteopaths retain a strong sense of professional identity, are proud of their manipulative skills and resentful of medicine's strategems, it seems safe to conclude that so far the AMA has not been much more successful in absorbing osteopaths than in its efforts to prevent the growth and acceptance of chiropractic. Chiropractors should watch closely the stance that the AOA chooses in future years for its potential impact on chiropractic. Will osteopathy retain its distinctive characteristics and differences from orthodox medicine? Or will osteopathy become more and more "medical," perhaps differing only in name but not in substance from orthodox medicine? (For example, although Hahnemann Medical School in Philadelphia continues to bear the name of the founder of homeopathy, it is an orthodox medical school.) Is it possible that as chiropractors become better established within the health care system some osteopaths may develop a sense of kinship with chiropractors and seek professional alliance with them, perhaps in joint opposition to those policies and actions of the AMA that both groups oppose? Or will osteopaths resent

chiropractors even more than they have in the past because they now feel caught in the middle between chiropractic and medicine and left with so little room to maneuver between them?

The fate of naturopathy seems sealed. With only one very small school remaining (in Portland, Oregon) few new practitioners are entering the field, and several states that formerly licensed naturopaths no longer do so. Those chiropractic colleges that formerly taught naturopathy along with chiropractic (three of them as recently as 1948) no longer do so. Naturopathy apparently will soon disappear as a distinct therapeutic field, although logically the term (naturopathy) should have attracted popular support because of continuing interest in natural foods, natural living, cleaning up the environment, etc. Despite its cumbersome name, chiropractic now clearly dominates the drugless healing field.

Why did naturopathy lose out in competition with chiropractic? Although B. J. Palmer would give total credit to the greater effectiveness of straight chiropractic, it was probably B. J. himself who was most responsible for chiropractic's survival as a separate and distinct healing art. As the controversial leader of the profession, he and his school served as the focus of the field for over a half century no matter what version of straight chiropractic B. J. propounded at a particular time. Palmer's charismatic leadership, his ability to attract and retain a loyal group of followers, his organizational talents, and especially his skill in developing public and legislative support for separate chiropractic licensing laws and boards of examiners were decisive in perpetuating chiropractic as a separate drugless profession. Even the constant bickering between the straights (i.e., Palmer's supporters) and the mixers (i.e., all other chiropractors) did not weaken chiropractic but, on the contrary, strengthened it by motivating the members of the opposing groups to struggle for the causes they supported. Naturopathy lacked a specific theoretical focus comparable to the chiropractic adjustment as well as a charismatic leader such as B. J. Palmer around whom, or in opposition to whom, the field could mobilize.

Conclusion

There are five different possible outcomes that chiropractic could experience in the future:

1. One would be complete fusion with medicine, as happened with homeopathy and as seems to be on the horizon for osteopathy. Fusion could occur in one of two different ways: Either chiropractors could become essentially like M.D.'s, or M.D.'s could take over chiropractic and eliminate the need for chiropractors. Enough has been said already to rule out these alternatives and therefore this outcome.

2. The second possible outcome would be for chiropractors to practice under medical supervision, as physical therapists do. And there are two routes by which this outcome could occur: One would be for chiropractors to be willing to subordinate themselves to physician prescription, while the other would be for physical therapists to become, in effect, chiropractors, by expanding their scope of practice to include chiropractic. There is no likelihood for the former, but some possibility of the latter. Indeed, if M.D.'s should ever fully accept chiropractic, predictably they will want to control it by encouraging their physical therapy assistants to develop the skill to use it, though probably only for limited purposes. However, it is not likely that the combination of M.D.'s and physical therapists practicing chiropractic will happen to any significant degree.

3. The third possible outcome would be for chiropractic and chiropractors to disappear. There is almost no likelihood of this happening; it is mentioned only for the purpose of logical completeness.

4. The fourth possible outcome is for chiropractors to continue in their present status separate from orthodox medicine but "marginal" or "parallel" to it. One is reminded of the earlier "separate but equal" doctrine of the United States Supreme Court pertaining to relationships between blacks and whites, a doctrine reversed in 1954 when the Supreme Court decided that "separate" is not "equal." The opposite principle is, however, also valid—that is, being equal is incompatible with remaining separate. Whenever two groups attain economic, educational, and occupational equality, the artificial barriers that previously separated them tend to fall, and as in the case of blacks and whites, integration proceeds quite rapidly. Similarly, when a formerly marginal practitioner group such as osteopaths becomes so nearly equal to the dominant medical profession as to be parallel to it, the barriers between them come tumbling down and they tend to merge. However, even if chiropractic should become fully parallel to medicine, it would be much less likely than osteopathy ever to merge into medicine.

5. The fifth possible outcome is for chiropractic to become what has been called a limited medical profession—independent of medical supervision but limited in its scope of practice both in terms of the range of illnesses it treats and the range of therapies it employs. Although some chiropractors may disagree, there is no stigma associated with being a limited medical practitioner. Consider, for example, dentists, admittedly the most prestigious of that group, which also includes podiatrists, optometrists, and psychologists. Dentists are now so extensively the professional peers of M.D.'s that medical and dental schools frequently share the same faculty. Nevertheless, dentists clearly remain limited practitioners. They therefore can serve as prestigious role models for chiropractors.

Which of these outcomes is most likely? It would be crystal-ball gazing to try to answer the question, especially since chiropractic's future lies mainly within the conscious control of chiropractors themselves. The questions then become: What do chiropractors really want? Is there substantial agreement among them, or are there significant differences between subgroups of chiropractors? How many want to be physicians? Alternatively, how many would like to work under medical prescription? How many are well satisfied with the present situation?

How many want to follow the path of osteopathy and become parallel with medicine but try to remain separate from it? How many would feel that an independent but frankly limited status like that of dentists or optometrists would be best? Although chiropractors alone cannot determine their future, no other group—organized medicine included—can exert a greater influence on it. Only if chiropractors fully understand the various alternatives available to them and their advantages and disadvantages can they achieve the ultimate goals that they desire for chiropractic.

REFERENCES

American Medical News. March 21, 1977

Baum AZ: Who on earth goes to a chiropractor? Med Econ, July 19, 1971, p 89

Bruce E, et al.: Medical discipline: Part II. Constitutional considerations—the police power. J Am Med Assoc 233: 1427, 1975

Cichoke AJ, West HG Jr: Comparative low-back study of patients treated by a chiropractic physician and those treated by a medical physician. Dig Chiropr Econ 21:118, 1978

Duffy DJ: Public attitude toward chiropractic and patient satisfaction with chiropractic in the state of Wisconsin. ACA J Chiropr 16:19, 1979

Goldstein M (ed): The Research Status of Spinal Manipulative Therapy. NINCDS Monograph No. 15. U.S. Department of Health, Education, and Welfare, Washington DC, 1975

Harding R, et al.: CHP task force surveys chiropractic utilization in a Florida county. ACA J Chiropr 14:26, 1977

Judicial Committee, American Medical Association: Osteopathy. Special report to the house of delegates. JAMA 177:774, 1961

Mazzarelli JP: A closer look at the FACTS/HEW study of chiropractic. Int Rev Chiropr 32:8, 1978

New York State Chiropractic Association. Results of chiropractic opinion poll completed. NYSCA Newsletter. July 15, 1972, p. 10

Parker G, Tupling H: The chiropractic patient: Psychosocial aspects. Med J Aust 2:373, 1976

Sandoz R: A perspective for the chiropractic profession. ACA J Chiropr 15:25, 45, 1978

Shenk J C: Composite Student Profile (Fall 1972). Des Moines, ACA, 1973

Shenk JC: Report on Survey and Statistical Study. Des Moines, ACA, 1974

Sparlin E: Medical manual manipulators—A threat to chiropractic. Dig Chiropr Econ 21:107, 1978

Velie EC: Personal communication, 1979

Wardwell WI: A marginal professional role: The chiropractor. Soc Forc 30:339, 1952

Wardwell WI: Limited and marginal practitioners. In Freeman H, et al. (eds): Handbook of Medical Sociology. Englewood Cliffs, Prentice-Hall, 1979

White Paper, AOA–AMA Relationships, No. 2. Chicago, AOA, 1968

White Paper, Secretary's Report, Independent Practitioners under Medicare. American Chiropractic Association, International Chiropractors Association, Council of State Chiropractic Examining Boards, 1969

Wilk CA, et al.: Complaint #76C3777 filed October 12 in the U.S. District Court for the Northern District of Illinois, Eastern Division, 1976

SECTION TWO
Principles of Chiropractic

CHAPTER THREE

The Anatomy of the Intervertebral Foramen and the Mechanisms of Compression and Stretch of Nerve Roots

SYDNEY SUNDERLAND

In the second century Galen, in his *Methodus Medendi,* wrote that "the magnitude of a disease is in proportion to its deviation from the healthy state, and the extent of the deviation can be ascertained only by one who is perfectly acquainted with the healthy state."

In accord with Galen's dictum, attention will first be directed to those normal anatomical features of intervertebral foramina which constitute an essential background for the subsequent consideration of those pathophysiological mechanisms operating in this region which disturb spinal nerve and nerve root function.

Anatomical Considerations

Some Basic Components of Spinal Nerves and Nerve Roots

Certain terms used in this text need defining in order to avoid any misunderstanding or confusion that might arise when the pathophysiology of spinal nerve and nerve root dysfunction is being considered (Fig. 1).

A funiculus or fasciculus is a bundle of nerve fibers within a supporting framework of connective tissue called the endoneurium. The fine collagen fibrils of the endoneurium separate and encircle each nerve fiber to form its outer sheath which may be regarded as constituting the wall of an endoneurial tube enclosing the nerve fiber. This sheath has elasticity and tensile strength and resists an axonal pressure.

The perineurium is the thin lamellated sheath of specialized perineurial cells interspersed with fine collagen fibrils, which encircles each funiculus. Importantly this sheath:

1. Gives tensile strength and elasticity to a nerve;
2. Maintains and resists an intrafunicular pressure;
3. Functions as a diffusion barrier.

The epineurium is the areolar connective tissue separating the funiculi and forming an outer sheath for the nerve trunk. This tissue provides little tensile strength to the nerve but forms a protective packing for the funiculi which cushions them against compression.

Relevant Structural Features of an Intervertebral Foramen

Two structural features call for special comment:

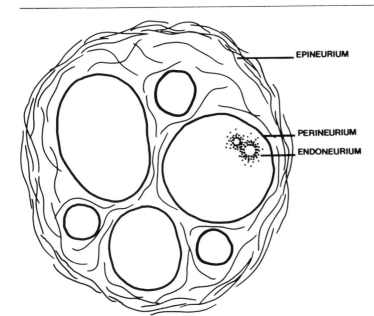

FIG. 1. **Transverse section of a nerve to illustrate the terminology used in naming certain histologic features.**

1. The margin of each foramen is normally smooth and has no significant attachments.
2. The manner in which the intervertebral disc and the apophyseal joint contribute to the formation of the foramen varies according to the vertebral level (Fig. 2).

Cervical Region. Here the apophyseal joint is situated posterosuperiorly, and the joint surfaces are so aligned that the vertebra above is prevented from moving forward on the vertebra below and in this way reducing the dimensions of the foramen. Anterosuperiorly the uncinate lip of one vertebral body overlaps the body of the vertebra above and approximates its pedicle, thereby all but excluding the intervertebral disc from taking any part in the formation of the foramen.

Thoracic Region. When the thoracic intervertebral foramina are studied from above downward, it will be seen that the apophyseal joint gradually moves down the posterior margin of the foramen from a superior position above to an inferior position below. As in the cervical region, the alignment of the apophyseal joint surfaces prevents the vertebra above from being displaced forward on the vertebra below. The intervertebral disc increases in thickness from above downward and comes to form more of the anterior margin of the foramen.

Lumbar Region. Here the greatly thickened intervertebral discs now form approximately the lower half of the anterior margin of the foramen. The apophyseal joints are located posteroinferiorly and, importantly, the opposing joint surfaces are so related that movement is possible in both vertical and anteroposterior directions. This arrangement is one which introduces an element of instability into the system.

*Effects of Vertebral
Movement on the Dimensions
of the Intervertebral Foramina*

The foramina are narrowed and widened during dorsal extension and ventroflexion of the spine, respectively (Turner and Oppenheimer 1936; Badley 1939, 1944, 1949; Frykholm 1951; Payne and Spillane 1957; Breig 1960).

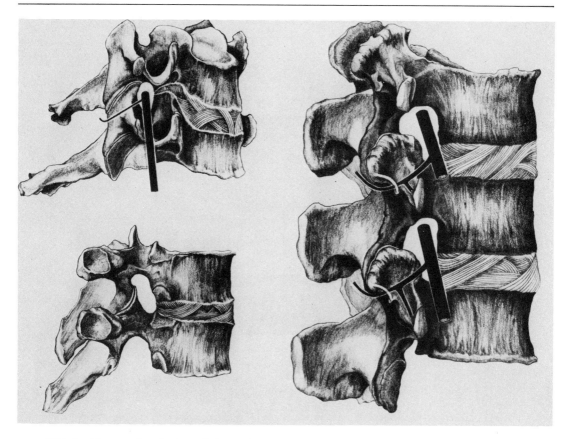

FIG. 2. **Form and articular relations of an intervertebral foramen in the lower cervical, mid thoracic and mid lumbar regions of the vertebral column. (Adapted from Sunderland 1975.)**

These changes are not sufficient to threaten the contents of the foramina.

The Contents of the Foramen

Corresponding anterior and posterior nerve roots and the posterior root ganglion come together in the foramen to form a spinal nerve. This conjunction of structures will, henceforth, be referred to as the neural complex.

The neural complex and its sheath account for 35 to 50 percent of the cross-sectional area of the foramen, the remaining space being occupied by areolar and adipose connective tissue, the spinal artery and its anterior and posterior branches, numerous veins, lymphatics, and a recurrent meningeal nerve (Sunderland 1974a, 1974b). Thus there is ample space to allow the complex to move freely in the foramen.

The Meningeal Relations of the Neural Complex

The essential meningeal relations of the complex are shown in Figure 3 from which it will be seen that:

1. Opposite the intervertebral foramen each pair of anterior and posterior nerve roots invaginates the dura and arachnoid to form a cone-shaped depression which is carried into the foramen. At the apex of this cone,

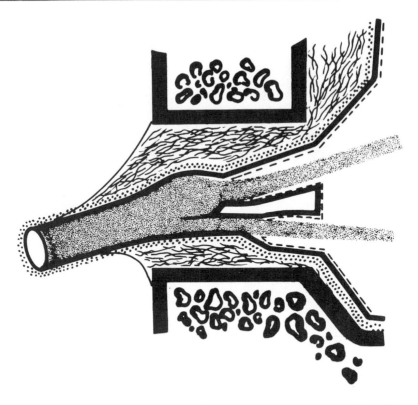

FIG. 3. Arrangement of the meninges in relation to the nerve root system in an intervertebral foramen. (———) dura, becoming the perineurium; (------) arachnoid; (::::) condensation of epidural connective tissue which becomes the epineurial tissue of the spinal nerve. (From Sunderland 1976a. Used with permission of the Elsevier/North Holland Biomedical Press.)

each nerve root perforates the meninges to form for itself a bilaminar sleeve of dura and arachnoid.

2. The dura is continued laterally to form the perineurial sheath of the spinal nerve, the looser epidural tissue becoming the epineurium.

3. The meninges have no attachment to the foramen.

4. The addition of the perineurial-epineurial connective tissue sheath to the spinal nerve increases its thickness so that its cross-sectional area is greater than the combined cross-sectional areas of the nerve roots which form it.

The Course Taken by Nerve Roots to Reach and Enter the Foramen

In the lower cervical and upper thoracic regions it is common for the nerve roots to descend intradurally to a level well below the foramen into which they are destined to pass (Fig. 4). After passing through the dura in the manner described above, they must then ascend acutely enclosed in their dural sleeves, to enter the foramen over the lower margin of which they are again angulated. Thus the nerve roots abruptly change direction at two points around which they may be deformed following traction on the corresponding spinal nerve.

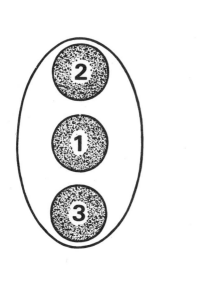

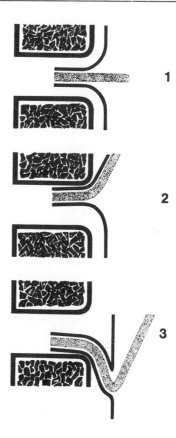

FIG. 4. **Variations in the course taken by nerve roots (represented by a single bundle) to reach the intervertebral foramen and the manner in which this influences their position in the foramen. (From Sunderland 1975.)**

The Mobility of the Neural Complex in the Intervertebral Foramen

The space occupied in the foramen by the neural complex and its sheath and the arrangement of the meninges means that the complex normally enjoys considerable freedom of movement in the foramen.

Ventroflexion of the neck tenses the nerve roots so that the neural complex is drawn inward and upward (Inman and Saunders 1942; O'Connell 1943, 1951, 1956; Frykholm 1951, 1952; Cave et al. 1955). With dorsal extension the complex returns to its original position. On the other hand, the traction on peripheral nerves which occurs during limb and trunk movements is transmitted to the spinal nerves. However, the relations of the meninges to the neural complex and to the foramen are such that lateral traction on a spinal nerve would draw the neural complex and its dural cone outward in the foramen. This means that during limb, trunk, and neck movements the neural complex is being continually displaced to and fro in the foramen in a piston-like manner.

The Structure of Nerve Roots

The nerve fibers constituting a nerve root are arranged in parallel bundles, the supporting framework of individual nerve fibers and nerve bundles being provided by endoneurial connec-

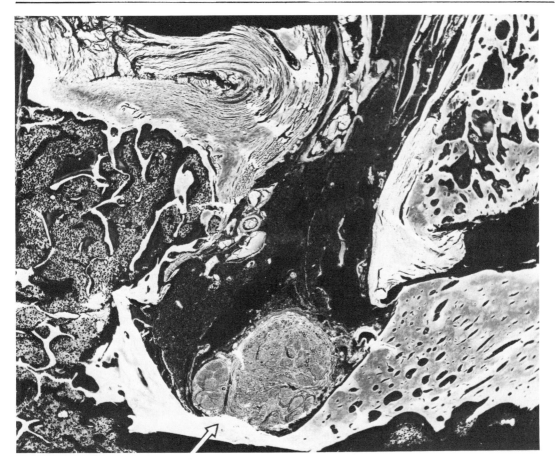

FIG. 5. **Lumbar nerve root system in the intervertebral foramen illustrating the relative sizes of the anterior and posterior nerve roots (arrow).**

tive tissue. Nerve roots lack the epineurial and perineurial tissue component of peripheral nerves.

The posterior nerve root is considerably thicker than the corresponding anterior root (Fig. 5).

The Structure of Spinal Nerves

Immediately distal to the posterior root ganglion the nerve fibers derived from the union of the two nerve roots are collected into a single funiculus in which the motor fibers are located anteroinferiorly (Fig. 6).

The funiculus is enclosed in a thin but strong perineurial sheath external to which is the areolar connective tissue constituting the epineurium. Within a few millimeters of its formation the single funiculus of the spinal nerve divides into several bundles which engage in plexus formations. These funicular plexus formations lead to a mixing of the motor and sensory fibers and to their repeated funicular redistribution within the nerve.

With the conversion of the monofunicular spinal nerve into a multifunicular structure, the epineurial tissue is increased in amount and forms a protective packing for the funiculi.

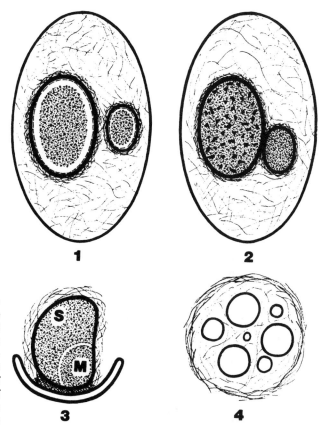

FIG. 6. **Transition from nerve roots, enclosed in their meningeal sheaths, to the formation of the spinal nerve composed initially of a single funiculus which soon divides into several funiculi. The only attachment of the nerve complex to bone is in the cervical region where the sheath of the spinal nerve is attached to the gutter of the transverse process. (S) sensory fibers; (M) motor fibers. (From Sunderland 1975.)**

Mechanisms Protecting Nerve Fibers of Spinal Nerves and Nerve Roots

Nerve trunks and nerve roots possess structural features and properties which ensure that, within normal limits, the nerve fibers constituting the conducting elements of the nerve trunk are protected from mechanical deformation.

The Course Pursued by a Peripheral Nerve and by the Nerve Fibers Within the Nerve. Peripheral nerves are subjected to tension during limb movements which is greater when the nerve crosses the extensor aspect of a joint. It is noteworthy that most nerves cross the flexor aspect of joints with, however, two notable exceptions, the ulnar nerve at the elbow and the sciatic nerve at the hip.

A nerve trunk runs an undulating course in its bed, its component funiculi an undulating course in the supporting epineurium, and the nerve fibers an undulating course inside the funiculi (Fig. 7).

Increasing traction on a nerve first eliminates the undulations in the nerve trunk, then the undulations in the funiculi, and finally the slack in the nerve fibers. It is only at the last point that the nerve fibers come under tension. This structural arrangement means that during limb movements the delicate conducting elements of the nerve trunk are normally protected from traction deformation.

The Cushioning Effect of the Epineurium. The epineurial connective tissue packing is greater in amount where a nerve trunk is composed of many funiculi as opposed to where it has a monofunicular structure. In the

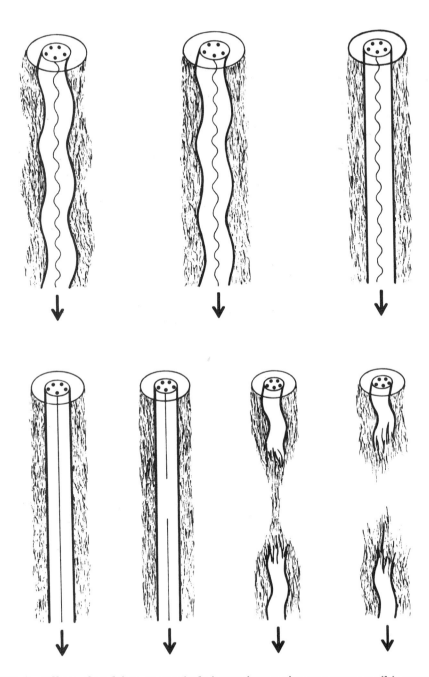

FIG. 7. **Effects of applying progressively increasing traction on a nerve until it ruptures.**

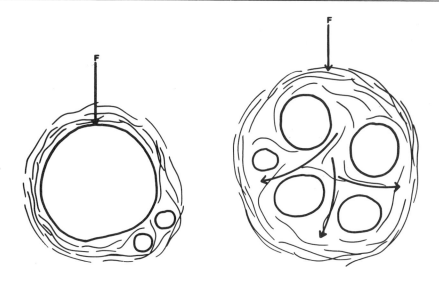

FIG. 8. **Impact of deforming forces on monofunicular structure.**

former, the effects of compression are minimized, deforming forces being cushioned and dispersed by the epineurial packing. In the latter, deforming forces would fall maximally on the funicular tissue and, therefore, nerve fibers (Fig. 8).

In this respect the spinal nerve is particularly at risk at its origin in the foramen where it is composed of a single funiculus. Here a deforming force would fall maximally on the funiculus and its contents whereas the same deforming force applied further laterally, where the nerve is composed of many funiculi, would be absorbed and dissipated through the supporting epineurial tissue.

The Elasticity of Nerves. Nerve trunks are elastic structures with considerable tensile strength. The principal component imparting these properties to the nerve is the perineurium.

When a nerve trunk is gradually stretched, a point is rapidly reached when the undulations in the nerve trunk and then in the funiculi are eliminated while the funicular tissue and, later, the nerve fibers begin to take load. Beyond this point there is a linear relationship between load

and elongation until the elastic limit is reached and structural failure occurs. The nerve trunk behaves as an elastic structure only as long as the perineurium remains intact. It should be noted that nerve fibers rupture inside the funiculi while the nerve trunk is still elongating as an elastic structure and before the point of structural failure of the nerve trunk is reached (see Fig. 7).

Data from tensile tests on nerves carried through to their destruction have given elongations within an elastic range of from 8 to 22 percent. However the range of elasticity is influenced by, inter alia, the rate of application of the load which, for the values given above, was 7.5 cm/minute (Sunderland 1978). Thus, both the time for which a deforming force operates, as well as its magnitude, determine the fate of nerve fibers when the nerve is being stretched and the production of traction lesions. Providing that the deforming forces are applied sufficiently slowly, a nerve can be stretched to a remarkable degree without any disturbance of function. On the other hand, with abrupt and violent stretching nerve fibers rapidly succumb, physiologically and then structurally.

Because the perineurium is absent in nerve

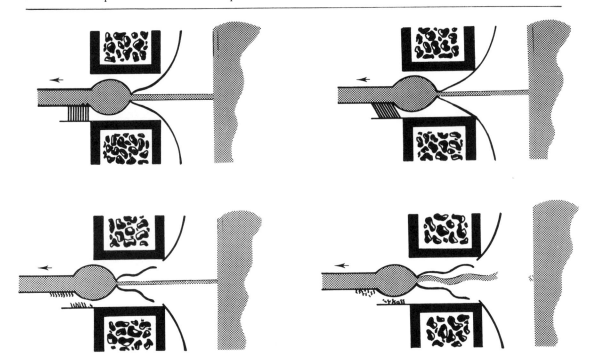

FIG. 9. **Effect of lateral traction on a spinal nerve. Displacement outwards of the nerve complex and tension on the nerve roots is limited by: (1) the attachments of the spinal nerve to the cervical transverse process and (2) the plugging action of the dural cone as it is drawn into the foramen at the foramina and elsewhere where no attachments exist. For simplification only one dorsal rootlet is shown. Traction forces may reach magnitudes which rupture the protective attachments to the cervical transverse process and the dural cone. The nerve roots, now left unprotected, are then avulsed from the spinal cord. (From Sunderland 1976a. Used with permission of the Elsevier/ North Holland Biomedical Press.)**

roots, the latter lack the tensile strength and elasticity of peripheral nerves. Nevertheless, what elasticity they do possess allows them to accommodate to the tension generated during the normal limb and trunk movements.

The Arrangement of the Dural Cone. As previously noted, lateral traction on a spinal nerve pulls the neural complex outwards in the foramen and tenses nerve roots. Thus fully flexing the hip and extending the knee generates forces which are transmitted from peripheral nerves to spinal nerves and on to the corresponding nerve roots. The latter, however, are prevented from being overstretched by a protective device (Fig. 9).

Reference has been made to the cone or fun-

nel of dura which is formed by the passage of the nerve roots into the foramen, the dura being continued beyond the apex of the cone to form the strong perineurial sheath of the spinal nerve. Traction on the nerve pulls the neural complex and its associated cone of dura laterally, but this displacement is finally checked as the apex of the dura funnel becomes wedged in the entrance to the foramen. In this way the transmitted effects of traction on the spinal nerve are curtailed and the nerve roots escape further deformation.

The Attachment of Certain Spinal Nerves to the Corresponding Vertebral Transverse Process. Of all the spinal nerves, those most subjected to traction forces are the fourth, fifth, sixth, and seventh cervical. This is because:

1. These spinal nerves, and the upper and middle trunks of the brachial plexus formed from them, are in direct line with the dependent forelimb.
2. The wide range of movements occurring at the cervical spine, shoulder girdle, and shoulder joint introduce additional forces which fall maximally on these particular nerves.

The eighth cervical and first thoracic spinal nerves, and the lower trunk of the plexus formed by their union are less exposed because they take a less direct course to the limb.

If the forces developed in this way were transmitted uninterruptedly to the corresponding short cervical nerve roots the latter could suffer traction damage. The roots, however, are normally protected from such injury because the fourth, fifth, sixth, and seventh cervical spinal nerves are securely attached to the vertebral column. Each, on leaving the foramen, is immediately lodged in the gutter of the transverse process to which it is securely bound by its sheath, by reflections of the prevertebral fascia, and by slips from the musculotendinous attachments to the transverse processes (Fig. 10). It is this secure attachment which prevents the forces generated in the brachial plexus from reaching the nerve roots and overstretching them.

The importance of this protective attachment is evidenced by the relative susceptibility to avulsion injury of the several nerve roots contributing to the brachial plexus. Clinical experience confirms that in severe traction injuries of the upper limb, the incidence of nerve root avulsion from the spinal cord is much higher for the lower spinal nerve roots which, anatomically, are at a greater risk. On the other hand, rupture of the spinal nerves at the vertebral transverse processes is more common in the upper part of the plexus (Sunderland 1974a,b, 1976a).

Such protective attachments to the vertebral column are not needed for the remaining spinal nerves since they are not, normally, subjected to the same deforming forces during movements of the trunk and limbs.

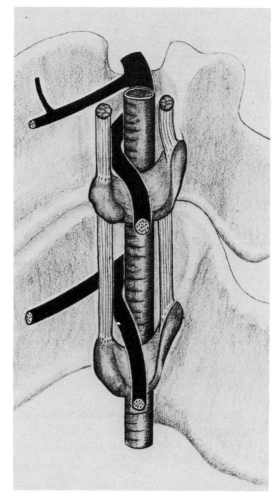

FIG. 10. **Relationship of the emerging spinal nerve to the cervical transverse process, to which it is securely attached, and to the vertebral artery. (From Sunderland 1975.)**

Pathophysiological Considerations

A Classification of Nerve Injury

Traumatic nerve injuries interrupting conduction may be classified in many ways. The classification used in this text is based on the histological structure of the nerve trunk and recognizes five degrees of injury, of increasing severity (Sunderland 1978; Fig. 11).

A *first degree injury* is one in which conduction is blocked but continuity of the axon is preserved. The nerve continues to conduct as far as and below the damaged segment but not across it. There is no Wallerian degeneration and the pathological changes are of minor nature from which the nerve rapidly recovers. After a latent period lasting from days to weeks conduction across the affected segment returns and function is fully restored.

In a *second degree injury* the endoneurial sheath of the nerve fibers is left intact but the axons are damaged to a degree which results in Wallerian degeneration. When regeneration commences, each regenerating axon is confined to the endoneurial tube which originally contained it—which means that the restored pattern of innervation is precisely the same as the original. Recovery is accordingly complete but takes place more slowly than after a first degree in-

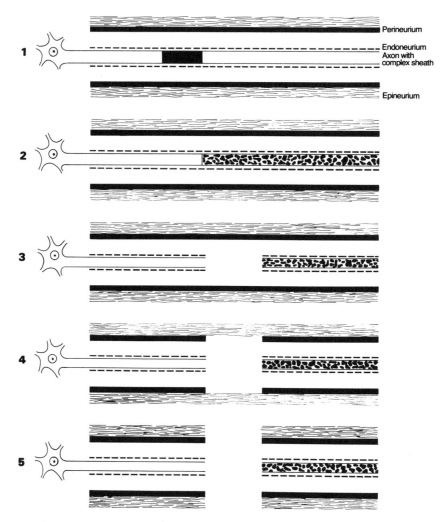

FIG. 11. **Classification of nerve injury based on the effects of trauma of increasing severity. (From Sunderland 1978. Used with permission of Churchill Livingstone.)**

jury because of the additional time taken for the restoration of axonal continuity with the periphery. Furthermore, the pattern of recovery is characterized by a serial order of reinnervation in which individual structures recover in the order in which they were originally innervated. This is not the case in first degree damage where the affected structures recover at or about the same time and without reference to their order of innervation. This is because recovery is not dependent on the restoration of axonal communications with the periphery.

With a *third degree injury* there is intrafunicular damage in which both axon and endoneurial sheath continuity is lost within an intact perineurial sheath. The funicular architecture of the nerve trunk is not disturbed. Regenerating axons which are not blocked by scar tissue are no longer confined to the endoneurial tubes that originally contained them but are free to enter foreign tubes which may direct them back to functionally unrelated structures. Regeneration is therefore both incomplete and imperfect.

In a *fourth degree injury* the funiculi are ruptured and disorganized by the injury, continuity of the nerve trunk being maintained by way of damaged disorganized tissue. The obstacles to useful regeneration in these cases are considerable and no useful recovery is to be expected.

Finally, in a *fifth degree injury* the nerve is severed, either cleanly or raggedly, with separation of the nerve ends. Though some regenerating axons may bridge the gap in the nerve, their chances of reaching the periphery and establishing useful connections there are negligible.

It should be noted that injuries may not be of uniform severity, either across or along the length of the nerve trunk. Partial and mixed lesions are produced in this way.

Compression, Stretch, and Chronic Irritation

Pathophysiological mechanisms causing spinal nerve and nerve root dysfunction and loss of conduction include compression, stretch, and chronic irritation.

While pathology in and about the foramen may reduce its dimensions and in this way compress the nerve, more likely causes of nerve involvement are friction over osseofibrous irregularities or traction on a nerve or nerve roots fixed in the foramen by adhesions.

Restrictive adhesions and fibrosis, which fix a nerve trunk in its bed and reduce its elasticity, lower the threshold at which traction begins to produce harmful effects.

Damaged nerve fibers are more susceptible to physical deformation and ischemia than normal fibers.

Latent toxic and metabolic neuropathies and some febrile conditions of viral or other origin render nerve fibers more vulnerable to traumatic or ischemic incidents.

Compression

The following generalizations should be kept in mind when considering the development of compression lesions in the foramen.

1. Though the intervertebral foramen represents a potential entrapment site, the space occupied by the neural complex and the fat containing connective tissue surrounding it normally protects it from being compressed, nor is the complex embarrassed by the narrowing of the foramen which occurs with dorsal extension of the spine.
2. Providing compression occurs sufficiently slowly and does not impair the blood supply to a nerve, the latter can tolerate remarkable degrees of deformation without any disturbance of function.
3. The nerve fibers of nerve roots are well protected in the spinal canal. However, the absence of a protective packing of epineurial tissue renders them more susceptible to direct compression than nerve trunks.
4. A study of compression lesions affecting the spinal nerves and nerve roots involves for consideration:
   a. the sources of compression,
   b. the mechanisms by which compression brings about its harmful effects, and
   c. the severity of compression lesions.

Sources of Nerve Compression. Paravertebral pathology leading to nerve compression includes:

1. Malignant and nonmalignant enlarging masses in the spinal canal and intervertebral foramen;
2. Destructive lesions of the vertebral bodies resulting in their collapse;
3. Thickening of the ligamentum flavum, the hypertrophic tissue encroaching on the foramen posteriorly;
4. Osteophytic enlargements which reduce the size of the foramen and compresses the neural complex;
5. Apophyseal joint swelling secondary to subluxation of the joint and trauma to the capsule could reduce the cross-sectional area of the foramen. Magnuson (1944) found that injecting saline into the joint capsule narrowed the foramen by 2 mm.
6. Intervertebral disc herniation and atrophy.

In disc herniation the herniated mass encroaches on the foramen anteriorly and directly compresses the nerve. It should be noted that, in the lumbar region, the nerve roots descend across the disc immediately above the foramen which they are to enter before leaving the spinal canal.

Atrophy and herniation of the disc both result in a narrowing of the intervertebral distance with effects on the intervertebral foramen which vary according to the vertebral level.

Cervical Region. Disc atrophy cannot result in any significant reduction in the overall dimensions of the intervertebral foramen (see Fig. 2) because:

1. The discs are thin and take little part in the formation of the foramen.

2. The proximity of the bony uncinate lip to the pedicle of the vertebra above on each side, and the form and position of the apophyseal joints prevent any reduction in the vertical diameter of the foramen.

Thoracic Region. From an examination of the thickness of the disc and the position and alignment of the joint surfaces of the apophyseal joints, it will be seen that narrowing of the disc will result in some reduction in the vertical diameter of the foramen but not enough to threaten its contents (see Fig. 2).

Lumbar Region. Here the thickness of the disc and the alignment of the apophyseal joint surfaces are such that when the disc atrophies, the intervertebral distance is significantly reduced by both the subluxation of the joints and the narrowing of the disc (Fig. 12). This may also cause the ligamentum flavum to bulge forward into the foramen.

The overall effect of these changes is a substantial reduction in the cross-sectional area of the foramen to which any apophyseal joint swelling would also contribute. With this reduction the veins would suffer first, and venous congestion originating in this way could impair the circulation through the neural complex to a degree that could be responsible for the earliest neurological signs and symptoms associated with the condition (see pp. 59–61).

Effects of Nerve Compression. Compression may be acute, chronic, transient, intermittent, stationary, progressive, reversible, or irreversible. Apart from these qualifications, compression produces its harmful effects on the nerve in two ways, direct and indirect, though there are compression lesions in which the two mechanisms have operated concurrently to produce the lesion.

Direct Effects. These are seen in cases of acute compression in which the characteristic feature of the lesion is the physical deformation of nerve fibers. This takes the form of a nodal intussusception at the margins of the compression in which the nodal region of a nerve fiber is telescoped into the adjacent part of the fiber, the direction of the telescoping being away from the zone of compression (Fig. 13; Ochoa et al. 1971, 1972). Associated with this structural deformation is a segmental demyelination. In extreme cases deformation progresses to the total destruction of the compressed section of the nerve.

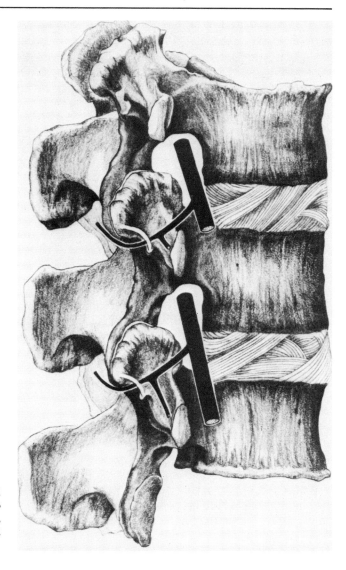

FIG. 12. **Relations of a lumbar spinal nerve and its posterior primary ramus to the intervertebral foramen, lumbar disc, and apophyseal joint. (From Sunderland 1975.)**

Indirect Effects. Here compression disturbs nerve conduction, not by physically deforming nerve fibers but by interfering with their blood supply (Sunderland 1976). This is the mechanism operating in chronic progressive compression and the manner in which it brings about its harmful effects can be illustrated by following the changes which develop in a nerve when it is subjected to slowly increasing pressure where it passes through a confined space with unyielding walls. The monofunicular spinal nerve in the intervertebral foramen which is, in fact, a short canal (Fig. 14).

Mechanisms of Nerve Compression. Capillaries are the only nutrient vessels present inside the funiculus. This endoneurial capillary network is fed by arterioles and drains to venules and veins all of which are in the epineurium; venous vessels outnumber the arterial. As the nutrient vessels pass through the perineurium they do so obliquely, the ar-

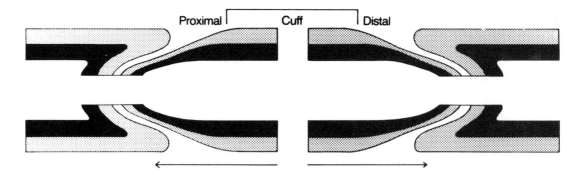

FIG. 13. **Manner in which a nerve fiber is physically deformed when acutely compressed by a force of considerable magnitude. (From Sunderland 1978. Used with permission of Churchill Livingstone.)**

rangement being one that leads to the closure of the vessels with any swelling of the funiculus.

There are at least five interrelated pressure systems in the foramen:

1. P^A is the pressure in the nutrient arteries in the epineurium.
2. P^C is the pressure in the endoneurial capillary network.
3. P^V is the pressure in the veins in the epineurium.
4. P^F is the intrafunicular pressure.
5. P^T is the pressure inside the foramen.

In order to insure an adequate blood supply for the nutrition of the nerve fibers, the pressure gradient within the foramen must be:

$$P^A > P^C > P^F > P^V > P^T$$

Should the pressure in the foramen, P^T, increase, such as occurs when the lumen of the foramen is reduced or its contents enlarge or swell, the first structures to feel the effects of this change will be the veins, pressure on which will obstruct the return of blood from the funiculus. The ensuing venous congestion and the impairment of the intrafunicular capillary circulation to which it gives rise, have far-reaching consequences which threaten the survival of nerve fibers. These will be followed through to the destruction of the nerve fibers.

The pathological features of the lesion, which are not necessarily uniform throughout the funiculus, will, for convenience, be described as developing in three stages.

Stage 1. Obstruction to the venous return from the funiculus slows the intrafunicular capillary circulation and leads to capillary congestion. Because of the unyielding properties of the perineurium these changes result in an increase in the pressure inside the funiculus which still further embarrasses the circulation. This slowing of the capillary circulation and the related increase in intrafunicular pressure impair the nutrition of the nerve fibers to a point where hypoxia renders them hyperexcitable and they commence to discharge spontaneously. In this respect the large myelinated fibers are known to be more susceptible than the fine fibers, and fiber dissociation originating in this way could be the basis of the pain associated with the lesion.

If the pressure on the nerve is relieved at this point, the circulation recovers and conduction in the nerve fibers is rapidly and completely restored.

Stage 2. With increasing compression the capillary circulation ultimately suffers to a degree where the resulting anoxia damages the capillary endothelium. Proteins then leak through the capillary wall and accumulate in

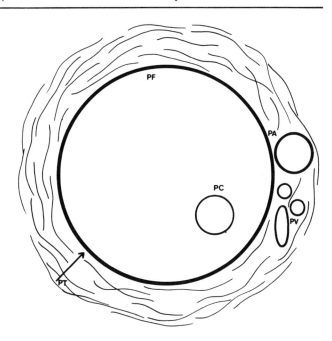

FIG. 14. **Key pressure systems operating in the intervertebral foramen in relation to the monofunicular spinal nerve and its accompanying vessels.**

the endoneurial tissues which become edematous. The diffusion barrier properties of the perineurium restrict the removal of this fluid from the funiculus and with increasing edema the intrafunicular pressure continues to rise. This and the related anoxia now threaten the survival of nerve fibers by:

1. Impairing their nutrition and metabolism;
2. Deforming them physically;
3. Promoting the proliferation of fibroblasts in the edematous endoneurial matrix which leads to the development of constrictive connective tissue.

Nerve fibers become thinner, some show segmental demyelination while structural damage proceeds to Wallerian degeneration in others. The most resistant fibers still conduct, the conduction velocity is reduced in others, some will have sustained a conduction block lesion, and yet another group will have been damaged to the point of undergoing Wallerian degeneration. In such a mixed lesion, motor and sensory functions will have suffered commensurately.

Providing that the deforming force subsides or is eliminated at this stage, the circulation improves, the edema resolves, and conditions inside the funiculus gradually return to normal. The manner in which motor and sensory functions are restored depends on whether individual nerve fibers have suffered first or second degree damage and the extent to which pathological changes are irreversible.

Stage 3. With continued unrelieved compression the nerve lesion takes on a permanent state. A stage is finally reached when the arterial supply to the nerve is severely impaired, and the lesion now takes on the features characteristic of ischemic damage. Fibroblasts have multiplied in the intrafunicular protein exudate and finally convert the affected segment of the funiculus into a relatively avascular fibrous cord in which only a few constricted nerve fibers persist. This pathology is irreversible.

The Severity of Nerve Compression Injuries. In terms of the classification of nerve injury outlined earlier, compression deformation may result in first, second, or third degree damage, with mixed and partial lesions comprising another group.

Stretch Injury of Spinal Nerves and Nerve Roots

Structural features of nerve trunks and anatomical arrangements protecting nerves and nerve roots from stretch injury have been outlined in an earlier section. At times traction forces reach levels which overcome these protective mechanisms and the nerve fibers then suffer traction damage of varying severity (see Fig. 7).

The sequence of changes caused by traction forces of gradually increasing severity is somewhat as follows. The mildest injury, which is a conduction block or first degree lesion, occurs soon after the undulations in the nerve fibers have been straightened out. With increasing traction a point is reached when the axons rupture inside the endoneurial tubes and second degree damage results.

With traction of still greater severity, nerve fibers and blood vessels rupture inside the funiculi though funicular continuity is fully preserved. This is a true intrafunicular third-degree lesion. It should be noted that as a funiculus is elongating under tension its cross-sectional area is also diminishing. This increases the intrafunicular pressure and introduces a compression-ischemic factor into the pathology of the lesion. With further stretching, funiculi rupture and, finally, continuity of the entire nerve trunk is lost.

During traction on the spinal nerves, the nerve roots remain protected as long as the dural cone, which has been pulled laterally and wedged into the foramen, does not rupture, and the attachments binding the spinal nerves to the cervical vertebral transverse processes do not fail.

In these stretch injuries the epineurial connective tissue is also affected, the resulting peri- and intraneural fibrosis contributing to the pathology of the lesion impairing nerve function.

With particularly severe traction injuries, which more commonly involve the forelimb, the spinal nerves are either ruptured at the intervertebral foramen or tears appear in the dural cone in which case the entire neural complex is pulled outward and the nerve roots, now no longer protected, are avulsed from the spinal cord (see Fig. 9). This represents the most severe stretch injury and from it there can be no recovery.

Chronic Irritation of the Neural Complex in the Foramen

Osteoarthritic changes may replace the smooth contour of the foramen with bony spurs and irregularities which irritate and traumatize the neural complex as it is repeatedly drawn to and fro in the foramen. Repeated trauma to the nerve originating in this way not only damages nerve fibers directly but is also together with the related inflammatory reaction, responsible for:

1. The development of an intra- and perineural fibrosis which imperils nerve fibers by constricting them and interfering with their blood supply;
2. The formation of adhesions which fix the neural complex in the foramen and by doing so aggravate the effects of traction on the spinal nerve.

Chronic trauma to the spinal nerve and nerve roots in the intervertebral foramen is a more potent cause of trouble than nerve compression.

The Lumbar Dorsal Rami in Relation to the Apophyseal Joints

This relationship, though somewhat out of context, is given special consideration because of its relevance to the symptoms associated with lumbar joint and disc pathology and, in particular, to low backache.

The dorsal ramus of each lumbar spinal nerve proceeds downward and backward across the lateral surface of the adjacent articular process from a point immediately above and anterior to the apophyseal joint, to which it gives twigs. It reaches and crosses the upper surface

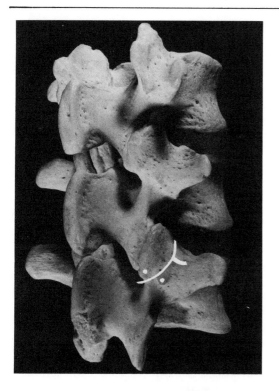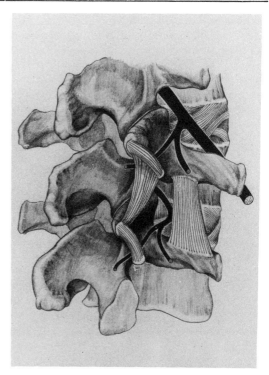

FIG. 15. Illustrations showing the course of the medial division of the posterior primary ramus in relation to the mammillary and accessory processes (white dots), the musculotendinous arcade arching between them, and the apophyseal joint. (From Sunderland 1975.)

of the base of the transverse process, where the ramus divides into medial and lateral divisions as do the accompanying vessels (Fig. 15; see also Fig. 12; Sunderland 1975).

The finer medial branch enters a groove between the accessory and mammillary processes of the vertebra beyond which it curves medially following the lower border of the apophyseal joint. In the groove and over this infraarticular section of its course the neurovascular bundle is covered and tightly bound to bone by exceedingly dense tissue formed by fibrous extensions from the capsule of the joint, the intertransverse ligament, and the tendinous attachments of the longissimus thoracis, multifidus, rotatores, and medial intertransverse muscles. In this infraarticular transverse section of its course within the tunnel, the medial branch sends twigs downward to the capsule of the

joint below as well as upward to the joint above.

After a course of about 1 cm in the tunnel, the nerve emerges to pass on to the lamina. It sends branches upward before turning downward to descend for some distance, branching as it does so, to combine with corresponding branches of neighboring rami to form an openly arranged plexus. The medial branch innervates ligaments and muscles medial to the line of the vertebral joints, while the joint itself is richly supplied by multiple articular twigs from both the parent ramus and its medial branch.

The intimate relationship of the medial branch of the lumbar dorsal ramus and its accompanying vessels to the capsule of the apophyseal joint, where it is confined within an osseofibrous tunnel, represents a potential site of fixation and deformation following pathological changes involving the joint. Any narrowing of the intervertebral disc, whatever the cause, results in the apophyseal facet of the vertebra above being forced downward over the corresponding apophyseal joint surface of the vertebra below (see Figs. 12 and 15). This displacement involves the neurovascular bundle in two ways:

1. Trauma to the joints results in an inflammatory reaction which entraps the nerve in the tunnel.
2. As the medial (superior) articular pedicle is displaced downward it stretches the capsule and comes to press directly on the nerve.

Reference to this nerve entrapment site has been included because, when reviewing the problem of low back pain, one should not concentrate exclusively on the intervertebral disc as the site of the offending lesion. The course of the medial branch of the lumbar dorsal rami and its associated vessels in an osseofibrous canal and the intimate relationship of this neurovascular bundle to the capsule of the apophyseal joint represents a potential site of fixation and entrapment which should not be overlooked.

REFERENCES

Breig A: Biomechanics of the Central Nervous System. Stockholm: Almqvist and Wiksell, 1960

Cave AJE, Griffiths JD, Whiteley MM: Osteoarthritis deformans of the Luschka joints. Lancet 1:176, 1955

Frykholm R: Cervical nerve root compression resulting from disc degeneration and root-sleeve fibrosis. A clinical investigation. Acta Chir Scand [Suppl] 160, 1951

Frykholm R: Lower cervical nerve roots and their investments. Acta Chir Scand 101:457, 1951

Frykholm R: The mechanism of cervical radicular lesions resulting from friction or forceful traction. Acta Chir Scand 102:93, 1952

Hadley LA: Anatomicoradiographic studies of the spine. NY State J Med 39:969, 1939

Hadley LA: Roentgenographic studies of the cervical spine. Am J Roentgenol 52:173, 1944

Hadley LA: Constriction of the intervertebral foramen. JAMA 140:473, 1949

Inman VT, Saunders JB de CM: The clinico-anatomical aspects of the lumbosacral region. Radiology 38:660, 1942

Magnuson PB: Differential diagnosis of causes of pain in the lower back accompanied by sciatic pain. Ann Surg 119:878, 1944

Ochoa J, Danta G, Fowler TJ, Gilliatt RW: Nature of the nerve lesion caused by a pneumatic tourniquet. Nature 233:265, 1971

Ochoa J, Fowler TJ, Gilliatt RW: Anatomical changes in peripheral nerves compressed by a pneumatic tourniquet. J Anat 113:433, 1972

O'Connell JEA: Sciatica and the mechanism of the production of the clinical syndrome in protrusions of the lumbar intervertebral discs. Br J Surg 30:315, 1943

O'Connell JEA: Protrusions of the lumbar intervertebral discs. J Bone Joint Surg 33B:8, 1951

O'Connell JEA: Discussion on cervical spondylosis. Proc R Soc Med 49:202, 1956

Payne EE, Spillane JD: The cervical spine. Anatomico-pathological study of 70 specimens (using a special technique) with particular reference to the problem of cervical spondylosis. Brain 80:571, 1957

Sunderland S: Meningeal-neural relations in the intervertebral foramen. J Neurosurg 40:756, 1974a

Sunderland S: Mechanisms of cervical nerve root avulsion in injuries of the neck and shoulder. J Neurosurg 41:705, 1974b

Sunderland S: Anatomical perivertebral influences on the intervertebral foramen. In Goldstein M (ed): The Research Status of Spinal Manipulative Therapy. NINCDS Monograph No. 15, U.S. Department of Health, Education, and Welfare. Washington DC, 1975

Sunderland S: Avulsion of nerve roots. In Vinken PJ, Bruyen GW (eds): Injuries of the Spine and Spinal Cord (Handbook of Clinical Neurology, vol 25). New York, North-Holland, 1976a

Sunderland S: Nerve lesion in the carpal tunnel syndrome. J Neurol Neurosurg Psychiatry 39:615, 1976b

Sunderland S: Nerves and Nerve Injuries, 2nd ed. Edinburgh, Churchill Livingstone, 1978

Turner, EL, Oppenheimer A: A common lesion of the cervical spine responsible for segmental neuritis. Ann Intern Med 10:427, 1936

CHAPTER FOUR
Compression Physiology: Nerves and Roots

MARVIN W. LUTTGES
and RICHARD A. GERREN

Knowledge of the effects of compression is a part of the life experience of most persons. This has been true for hundreds of years. We undoubtedly share with our ancestors the experience of having limbs "go to sleep" when allowed to remain in cramped, tortuous positions for excessive periods of time. Nevertheless, we seem as mystified now about the cause of such phenomena as were our ancestors. We have vague notions that circulatory and neurophysiological mechanisms are at the bottom of these and an ever-increasing list of related experiences originating from compression. We can cite many correlates of these experiences. And, we suspect that static or dynamic, irritative compressions result in a number of poorly recognized pathological conditions. To date, however, we can neither identify the exact causal factors for such conditions nor can we generate an exhaustive list of the consequences of such conditions. There is little doubt, however, that these problems constitute a challenge to the ingenuity of experimentalists and clinicians alike.

Physiological research, including functional anatomical, neurophysiological, neurochemical, and behavioral analyses, focused upon neural tissues, has exhibited exceedingly rapid advancements in the last two decades. The number of professional journals, in English alone, covering experimental and clinical studies of neural tissue physiology must certainly exceed a hundred, and new journals dealing with these subjects are appearing regularly. It would be presumptuous to consider that the treatment provided in this chapter gives an exhaustive account of all that literature germane to compression pathophysiology. Other writers will cover much of the physiology considered crucial to their presentations. Regardless, we must realize that only a great deal more work will finally show whether or not any of our current knowledge, theories, or guesses will ultimately have provided the kind of insight necessary to understanding compression physiology and its many consequences. This is part of the challenge and the excitement of our present efforts.

Compression

A Definition of the Proposed Independent Variable

For the purposes of all ensuing discussion, compression will be considered in a very broad sense. Compression will include the reduction of radial dimensions in neural cells, neural support elements, or any combination thereof. Compression will also include impingement depressions of such tissues, where the normal tissue morphologies are altered. Sufficient localized compression delivered to the side of a nerve, for example, can result in nerve tissue displacements. The compression effects in this case may be subtle but could be quantified. In special geometric situations, compression can produce both stretch and shear forces. Compression need not exhibit symmetry and, indeed, some of the pathologies associated with compression may be responses to material and/or force asymmetries. These possibilities will be discussed later.

Temporally, compression may be acute or chronic, lasting for fractions of a second or for years, respectively. The compression also may be continuous or intermittent. Further, it may occur once or many times. And finally, the amount or degree of compression may be quite large or extremely small.

Compression parameters, as outlined above, probably are not independent of each other. Although both experimentalists and clinicians suspect that degree of compression and duration of compression interact in producing observable consequences on neural physiology, no single consequence has been thoroughly examined to the point where the interaction could be clearly specified and quantified. The boundaries for such parameters are unknown. A colleague, for example, recently demonstrated (Sharpless 1975) that spinal roots are several times more sensitive to compression than peripheral nerves. Aside from some small errors associated with hysteresis, this study represented one of the few careful quantifications of degree of compression. Duration of compression was not studied especially in terms of the temporal ranges noted above. Experiments were terminated in relatively brief periods. Also, it was obvious that the demonstrable recovery of test tissue excitability following release from compression did not continue to occur when repeated compressions were attempted. We have noted similar compression interaction effects using a different compression methodology and a different experimental species (Luttges et al. 1976). The details of these studies will be discussed elsewhere, but it seems clear that any final description of compression physiology must deal with both the main parameters of compression as well as the interactions between these parameters.

Experimental Precision Versus Clinical Simulation

The study of compression as an independent variable capable of producing changes in many dependent variables can take two different forms. The first is that of experimental precision. Carefully applied compression must be accurately quantifiable in order to assure a precise relation between this causal factor and subsequent, measurable consequences. Controls must assure the unique importance of compression in the absence of other, possibly confounding, factors. Such controls and precision are unlikely to produce effects directly analogous to those with which the clinician is familiar. Experimental precision, including the examination of interaction effects, however, can provide the basis from which clinical observations can be synthesized.

In contrast, compression variables may be studied as clinical simulations. In these cases the precision of independent variable quantification is diminished and the search for identifiable clinical analogies is emphasized. Assumed compression is often the independent variable. Attempts at mechanical displacement of various facets of the spinal column with splints or at the implantation of mechanically irritative materials (Triano and Luttges 1978) fall into these classes of studies. Of course, a whole constellation of effects may arise and many of these effects may be reminiscent of clinical compressive disorders which are to be modeled. Unfortunately, knowledge of the unique causative value of the independent variable is lost. Usually, such studies revert to an attempt to quantify or at least understand the nature of the independent variable. Every clinician is familiar with this problem in that patients may often express the same general maladies but the causes for such maladies may differ quite significantly. Differential diagnosis, by any name and by any practitioner, is often the key to successful recognition of etiology and to effective application of treatment.

At present, there is inherent value in both of the above approaches. The experimental precision and clinical simulation approaches can be combined in animal models. Although these two approaches can be made to converge with a successful multidisciplinary focus upon a suitable model, no such model has been adopted for studies of compression. Such an enterprise

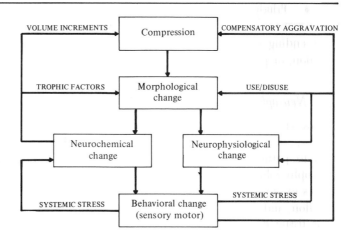

FIG. 1. **The possible intricacies of compression, in all forms, yielding clinically observable disorders. The correlates can interact as both causes and effects in compression disorders.**

is large, expensive, and difficult to coordinate. Until such studies are done, research will remain an eclectic endeavor with each experimentalist and clinician generating portions of the puzzle which ultimately may be placed together into a comprehensive understanding of compressive physiology (Fig. 1).

Compression Effects

Candidates for Clinically Related Disorders

The eclectic approaches described above can be subdivided into the effects of compression with which they are concerned. Experimentally, these effects may be an intermediate step in a chain of events leading to clinically recognized disorders or these effects may be a fractional portion of those, making up clinically recognized disorders. More likely, both are true. In any event the effects usually relate directly or indirectly to loss of control, loss of function, or pain.

Morphological Effects

Compression is known to produce morphological consequences in neural tissues or neural support tissues. This is, in fact, a portion of the

broad definition of compression. There is a good deal of suspicion that morphological alterations are neither necessary nor sufficient to produce loss of control, loss of function or pain (see Goldstein 1975; Korr 1978). Among the possibilities for crucial morphological alterations are many which have no particular significance for clinical correlates. There may be morphological correlates yet to be elucidated which best fit the definition of a causal factor. As improvements in tissue visualization occur, it is a near certainty that the appropriate alterations will be identified. Such visualization may be at the level where convergence between biological structure and function is reached.

From a different point of view it does seem certain that visualization techniques can provide information regarding possible pathological spatial relations between hard and soft tissues. The work of Sunderland and his colleagues (see Chapter 3, this volume) provides an excellent example of the analysis of such relationships. Knowledge of these relationships must be acquired for both normal and pathological conditions.

Unless tissue integrity is lost, tissue obstructions occur, or tissue deletions appear it is unlikely that morphology, except in the most reductionistic sense, will be found to be a direct cause of pathology. Rather, morphological alterations are more probably associated with a chain of events initiated by compression and finally ending with a loss of control, a loss of function, or pain.

Neurophysiological Effects

Those who concern themselves with the most likely candidates for compression effects which lead to pathologies, usually focus upon the neurophysiological functioning of the neural tissues in question. It seems clear that control, function, and pain are the business of the nervous tissue excitability, conduction, transmission, and integration. The problem with such postulated neurophysiological alterations is that there is presently no way to separate normal from aberrant messages within the range of neurophysiological functioning. The normal control mechanisms, functions, and pain mechanisms of the nervous system remain an enigma even in simplified studies with all but the rudimentary elements of model systems dissected away.

One can only hope that neurophysiological effects of compression will yield a clear pattern of normal versus pathological states. For example, we have long been able to recognize electroencephalographic patterns associated with epileptic foci in the brain, yet we cannot always identify the potential epileptic, and we do not understand the neurophysiological messages of the epileptic focus or the entrainment events which lead to a forthright seizure episode. Only if compression effects are gross does certainty of neurophysiologically-aided diagnosis result. More subtle compression effects have not been subjected to a thorough examination, but it is clear that the "either-or" appearance of simple neurophysiological indices will not suffice diagnostically.

Another problem associated with neurophysiological effects is that such effects may not represent a static endpoint of compression represented by a single disorder. Rather, such disorders, once initiated, may produce morphological alterations in neural tissues as well as support tissues, and these alterations can either reduce or exacerbate the original pathology. There is considerable evidence of these interactions in terms of trophic influences over other tissues as well as alterations induced in the neural tissue itself.

Chemical Effects

Although less generally considered a consequence of compression with direct clinical significance, chemical alterations in neural tissue are gaining an ever more prominent place in understanding the etiology of neural disorders. The phenomenon of Wallerian degeneration is being reexamined chemically and several new, far-reaching possibilities are being brought to the clinician. Focal demyelination remains a fertile area of exploration for chemical examinations and the impact of recently discovered endogenous polypeptides of the nervous system, such as enkephalin, is without comparison as a revolution for the clinical scientist.

The chemical steps resulting from compression were generally considered remote from clinical observations. Now, however, few people would challenge the direct role of the endorphins in at least one clinical reality, pain. The significance of neurotransmitters, of course, falls within a similar framework. Also, the overall systemic levels of hormones especially as related to the stress responses mediated by the pituitary-adrenal axis can no longer be overlooked. As will be seen later, compression effects on the dynamics of axoplasmic transport, for example, may bring new meaning to chemical correlates of compression physiology.

Behavioral Effects

Compression disorders are usually thought of in terms of the behavioral correlates. This is the basis for declaring losses of control, losses of function, and pain. The clinician relies upon these indices and directs therapeutic activities accordingly. Surprisingly, reliable quantification of these effects has not been forthcoming. There exist few diagnostic maneuvers readily quantified in the literature, and very few innovative attempts have been aimed at remedying the situation. Until such quantification occurs, it is unlikely that the relation between

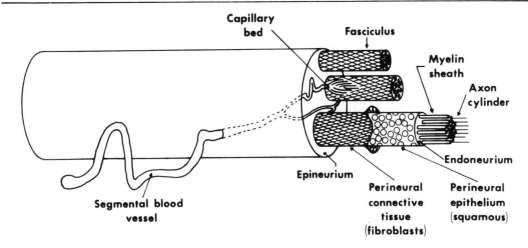

FIG. 2. **Summary of peripheral nerve structure. This summary includes the dual perineurium concept introduced by Shantha and Bourne (1968) which shows an outer connective layer with fibroblasts laced into the collagenous web and an inner epithelial layer made up of contiguous squamous cells with little connective web. Microvascular summary originates from the work of Sjöstrand et al. (1978). Larger vessels originating from nearby arteries and veins meander over the surface of the trunk to enter the epineurium and through numerous anastomoses communicate with the perineurium of each fasciculus where penetrating vessels of the endoneurium are primarily arranged in longitudinal capillary beds.**

compression and behavior will be thoroughly understood.

Degrees of control and function are quantified in other areas. Chemically, for example, the diabetic can be acquainted with sugar and ketone levels. Hearing losses are easily quantified as are vision problems. Yet, the characterization of behavioral effects remains, at best, qualitative. The establishment of agreed upon, reliable, and reproducible behavioral indices is crucial to the diagnosis, treatment, and study of compression disorders. Again, however, the normal behaviors must be quantified in order to establish a workable clinical measurement system.

Neural Tissue Morphology

Nerves

Peripheral nerves exhibit the general morphology as summarized (Fig. 2). Both the neural and supportive elements are noted. In addition, the

circulatory vessels are schematized. The overall nerve trunk possesses a facade of considerable collagen in a loose configuration. Fibroblasts, small amounts of elastic tissue, and fat cells are apparent. Blood vessels are sometimes seen to adhere to the epineurium before penetrating to the perineurium. The epineurium can be seen to separate fasciculi in multifascicular nerve trunks, but the epineurium in monofascicular nerves is fused together with the connective perineurium.

The perineurium appears to possess two different layers (Shantha and Bourne 1968), an outer collagen-rich connective layer and an inner, squamous cell dominated, epithelial layer. A capillary plexus is often sandwiched between layers prior to entry into the endoneurial spaces. The perineurium is the boundary of each fasciculus.

The endoneurium, likewise, possesses two distinct layers. The inner sheath is composed of a fine web of collagen fibers running outside the Schwann cell membrane around individual axon cylinders. These webs are disoriented in

TABLE 1. **Summary of Peripheral Nerve Fiber Types**

Type	Subtype	Input	Diameter (μ)	Myelination	Velocity (m/sec)
A efferent	α	Extrafusal muscle	9–20	yes	50–120
A efferent	β	Extra- and intrafusal muscle	9–15	yes	50–85
A efferent	γ	Intrafusal muscle	2–8	yes	10–40
A afferent	Ia	Primary intrafusal ending	9–22	yes	50–130
A afferent	Ib	Golgi tendon ending	9–22	yes	50–130
A afferent	II	Ruffini joint endings, secondary intrafusal, pacinian endings, paciniform endings, follicle endings	5–15	yes	25–90
A afferent	III	Thermoreceptors, nociceptors, vascular wall	1–7	yes	6–30
B efferent	Ach, EPI	Postganglionic	1–3	generally	3–15
C efferent	Ach	Smooth muscle, heart glands	0.2–1.5	no	0.4–2
C afferent	Somatic, visceral	Thermoreceptors, mechanoreceptors nociceptors (multimodal)	0.2–1.5	no	0.4–2

From Berthold (1978).

comparison to the outer endoneurial sheath which shows long, continuous collagen fibers running longitudinally with nerve fibers and which are devoid of irregularities at nodal regions in the underlying nerve fibers. The endoneurium also houses fibroblast-like cells, capillary beds, macrophages, and, in some instances, phagocytic Schwann cells.

Internal to the above layers are the Schwann cell outer cytoplasmic membranes and basement membranes with prominent Schwann cell nuclei. These membranes are continuous with and encapsulate the compressed, concentric Schwann cell membranes which are generally recognized as the myelin sheath. The most central element of course, is the nerve fiber and finally, the axon cylinder. The periaxonal space occurs between the inner Schwann cell compartment and the axonal membrane. The inner Schwann cell compartment is continuous with the much more compressed cytoplasmic space in the concentric myelinic wraps, referred to as the major dense line. The minor dense line of myelin consists of the outer surfaces of two successive wraps of Schwann cell membrane pressed together into normal, compact myelin.

The cytoplasmic surfaces contain more electron dense (major) material than the adjacent outer surfaces (minor).

A generally accepted classification of axons within nerve trunks is provided in Table 1 (Boyd and Davey 1968). The range of sizes varies from 0.2 μ in small, nonmyelinated (nociceptive) axons to 20 μ in large, myelinated motor axons. The axons vary from 1 cm to 1 m in length and often contain most of the total cell volume.

A good deal of the tubular (240 A) and filamentous (~ 100 A) material is prominent inside axons and probably relates to axonal transport phenomena. The smaller the axon, the more tubules there are compared to filaments (Friede and Samorajski 1970) since the number of filaments per axon varies while the number of tubules per axon does not. Both tubules and filaments are oriented longitudinally within the axon cylinders.

Associated nerve-fiber Schwann cells may or may not provide myelination. In nonmyelinated axons the association of Schwann cells with any given axon depends upon many factors and no simple stochastic values provide an accurate account of numbers of Schwann cells per unit length of axon or numbers of axons supported by any single Schwann cell (Eames and Gamble 1970). These normal variances discourage the global usefulness of Schwann cell–axon relationships for investigations of demyelinated axons in peripheral nerve disorders.

Myelinated axons show more stereotypic relations with Schwann cells. The distances between nodes of Ranvier depend primarily on axon diameter. Large A fibers may exhibit internodal distances of 2000 μ, while smaller A fibers typically exhibit 200–300 μ distances (Landon and Hall 1976). Since larger axons tend to have thicker myelin sheaths (up to 120–150 lamellae in Aα fibers) than small axons (10–20 lamellae in 1-2 μ axons), it seems that both internodal distances and myelin thickness are somehow determined by axonal size (Williams and Wendell-Smith 1971). In this context, however, we should be reminded that axon diameter (and shape) varies along the length of any given axon by as much as 25 percent in large fibers (Berthold 1978). The cross section of axons at nodes may be one-third to one-sixth the cross-sectional area of the same axon between nodes.

Roots

The spinal roots exhibit the general morphology summarized (Fig. 3). Being inside the meningeal membranes of the spinal cord, the roots are devoid of the elaborate epineural and perineural membranes characteristic of spinal and peripheral nerves. Upon gross dissection, both anterior and posterior roots exhibit a good deal of flaccidity or extra length as they typically collapse loosely to the lateral, anterior surface of the cord. Many of the metabolic needs of the roots are served by the cerebral spinal fluid which is replenished by exchange and transport functions from the often distant pial membranes. Also, fine capillaries invade the roots from locations in the immediate, superficial pial membrane and from adjacent spinal cord tracts proximally as well as from sites of the vascular complex converging upon the posterior root ganglion. Direct astrocytic end foot apposition

at the junction between Schwann and oligodendroglial myelination (Berthold 1978) may also play a role in supporting metabolism.

Notably, the roots are held together by only the fragile structures of the endoneurium continuous with pial membrane. The pia mater also forms the loose denticulate ligament between roots of different segmental levels. The endoneurium, itself, is more loosely organized than typically seen in nerves. It may be postulated that such organization favors better cerebrospinal fluid circulation but this organization also could permit more susceptibility to mechanical insult (Sunderland 1978).

As posterior roots approach within a few hundred microns of the cord, they reportedly (Berthold and Carlstedt 1977) begin to group according to respective diameters. The small, unmyelinated axons gather superficially at the anterolateral aspect of the fanning rootlets probably in preparation for superficial spinal gray terminations. The larger fibers remain in the posterior and core portions of the rootlet distribution. The meandering paths of the posterior root fibers prior to spinal cord entry are in considerable contrast to the small, organized bundles of fibers which exit the cord to form the anterior root. The meandering paths of posterior root fibers compared to relatively straighter paths of anterior root fibers may have significantly different consequences for stretch transmitted through the attached nerves. It would appear that the posterior roots could sustain more stretch.

Schwann cell to oligodendroglial myelination transitions which occur within the roots present several discontinuities. In large fibers the internodal distance to diameter ratios characteristic of peripheral nerves are exchanged for the smaller ratios typical of CNS myelin. Gaps of myelin occur in some instances and overlap occurs in others. In small fibers, nonmyelinated in the spinal and peripheral nerves, modest myelination often occurs at the PNS-CNS transition with 10–15 lamella and 10–40 μ internodal distances (Berthold 1978). Some of the CNS myelination at the transition is irregular along single fibers. The very small fibers (< 0.6–0.7 μ

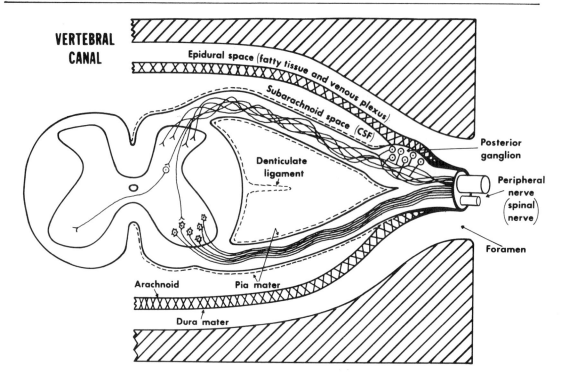

VERTEBRAL CANAL

Epidural space (fatty tissue and venous plexus)

Subarachnoid space (CSF)

Posterior ganglion

Peripheral nerve (spinal nerve)

Denticulate ligament

Foramen

Arachnoid

Pia mater

Dura mater

FIG. 3.   Diagrammatic representation of transverse view of the spinal roots and surrounding supportive tissues (adapted from Callander 1939). The loose endoneurium is bounded by the fragile pia mater which provides a capillary plexus. The subarachnoid space containing cerebrospinal fluid (CSF) extends to the arachnoid and the tough, superficial dura mater which contains large amounts of compact collagen. The two membranes slide readily against each other and a considerable cavity often develops between the two. The epidural space contains fatty tissues and venous plexuses through which the dura is attached by adhesions to anterior and posterior walls of the vertebral canal.

dia.) often join together into tight bundles prior to CNS entry and show only astrocytic contacts with no evidence of myelination. These bundles branch and separate only within the spinal cord.

The transition of PNS to CNS occurs at a "transitional node" for most PNS myelinated axons (Gamble 1976). Where such nodes do not exist, the typical oligodendroglia sheath of the CNS extends peripherally and is covered by the Schwann sheath of the PNS. The diameter of any one axon generally does not vary from one side of the transitional node to the other. Only small axons occasionally appear to decrease in diameter when projecting through the transi-

tional node into the CNS (Berthold 1978). As the PNS fibers approach the transitional node, however, they often exhibit as much as a 25 percent decrease in diameter.

Neurophysiology

Nerves

The excitability of axons has received so much attention in various systems that it is somewhat surprising how little is known about the neurophysiology of human or even mammalian nerves. Rather succinct summaries of excitable

PATCH OF MEMBRANE

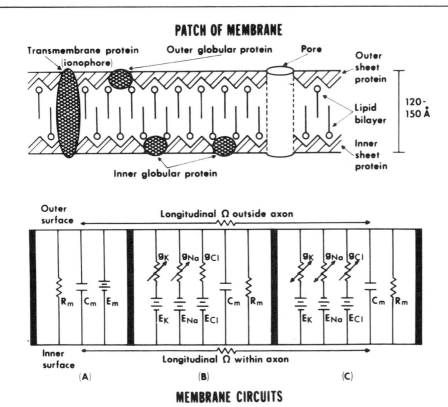

MEMBRANE CIRCUITS

FIG. 4. Schematic diagram of a patch of membrane (above) and of several different membrane circuits (below). The simplified diagram of the patch reveals two polar sheets consisting of proteins and phospholipids separated by a nonpolar environment of hydrocarbon lipid tails. The patch is penetrated from one side to the other by large, transmembrane proteins, and functional pores. No active membrane sites dependent upon energy utilization are depicted. Such a patch of membrane can be represented by numerous equivalent circuits as seen below. (A) The patch is passive with a total transmembrane capacitance (C_m), resistance (R_m), and potential (E_m). (B) The patch has active possibilities as indicated by the variable conductance for potassium (g_K) in series with the Nernst potential for potassium (E_K). Sodium is also shown with an associated variable conductance (g_{Na}), and Nernst potential (E_{Na}). The chloride conductance is fixed (g_{Cl}) together with the Nernst potential (E_{Cl}). Total membrane values (C_m and R_m) are paralleled to the ionic mechanisms. The final circuit (C) represents two-way, variable conductances. In all circuits the values for longitudinal resistance inside and outside the cell are crucial.

membrane qualities are available (e.g., Tasaki 1975; Grundfest 1975; Keynes 1975). Simplistic ideas of nerve fiber activity including resting potential, action potential, and refractory periods prescribed by the Hodgkin and Huxley equations appear unsatisfactory, however, for a comprehensive description of peripheral nerve activity.

The ionic and electrical factors known to influence membrane excitability are summarized by schematized equivalent circuits (Fig. 4). The first circuit (A) represents the overall electrical characteristics of an inexcitable membrane. Since ionic gradients exist across virtually all membranes as a residual consequence of ionic movements used in energy-dependent regulation of cell volume and, since most membranes show considerable leakage encouraged by such gradients, virtually all membranes exhibit a transmembrane potential (E_m). Since most membrane structure is relatively impermeable to ions due to the hydrophobic barrier posed by the hydrocarbon tails of the lipid constituents, leakage must occur at transmembrane pores or functional equivalents thereof. The conductivity of the pores, the concentration of such pores per unit area of membrane, and the total area of membrane operate together to determine membrane resistance (R_m). The outer and inner surfaces of a membrane exhibit polar characteristics and interact with the electrically conductive fluids nearby. These surfaces are quite close together with a reasonably good dielectric material between them. The resulting membrane capacitance (C_m) is considerable and stores transmembrane charges in accord with the imposed transmembrane potential and the area of the involved membranes (size of capacitor plates). Across the membrane the electrical factors must be in equilibrium with the ionic factors and both must be in equilibrium with osmotic or hydrostatic forces in order for the membrane to maintain structural and functional integrity.

The maintenance of equilibrium is only temporarily sacrificed in electrically excitable membranes (Fig. 4, circuit B). The equivalent circuit reflects the changing interactions between the ionic potentials as determined by the Nernst equation and the transmembrane conductance for each ionic species at different times during the excitation cycle. The schematic representation of an electrical potentiometer suggests the increased transmembrane conductance from outside to inside for sodium ions (g_{Na}) during the rapid rise of an action potential followed by increased conductance from inside to outside for potassium ions (g_K) during the rapid fall of the action potential. The conductance for chloride ions (g_{Cl}) remains unchanged. Such a rapid change in transmembrane potential must interact with the time constant ($R_m \times C_m$) of the patch of membrane involved. The completion of the crucial circuit must involve both the longitudinal resistance inside and outside the membrane of the excitable cell. These latter factors, of course, determine whether or not the excitability of one portion of the membrane will be conducted to the next.

The last schematic (Fig. 4, circuit C) summarizes some general trends in neurophysiological work suggesting that the conductance for crucial ions may both increase and decrease from the values maintained in the resting cell membrane. In some systems, the chloride ion has been demonstrated to exhibit increases in transmembrane conductance. The interactions between ions, therefore, may be more complicated than previously imagined.

In nerves, changes in the relations between each of the above factors yield potent functional consequences. To date most of these consequences relate to simple geometric changes in nerves but it is fair to assume that the relations between ionic gradients, membrane-bound, ion-selective pores and intraaxonal compartmentalizations will prove to be reasonably complex.

Some of the electrical characteristics of large and small medullated fibers as well as small nonmedullated fibers are given in Table 2. This summary accounts for the combined factors noted above and covers a good deal of geometric information (Paintal 1978). The conduction velocity is linearly related to axon diameter in normal axons but many associated factors must behave to assure such a relationship. The axon spike must have a predictable duration based upon spike rise time (from capacitive current Ic, change in sodium conductance Δg_{Na}, and resulting total membrane current I_m) as well as spike fall time (return in Δg_{Na}, increase in Δg_K, and restoration of Ic). The refractory periods (absolute and relative) must be sufficiently short to assure conduction velocity without either total spike blockade (absolute refractory period) or slowing of spike production (relative refractory period). The interactive geometry is such that during temperature shifts (and other abnormal situations) myelinated axons with predetermined active membrane dimensions (internode distances, etc.) are blocked before nonmyelinated axons.

In terms of simple interactions the nondimensional ratio between conduction velocity

TABLE 2. **Action Potential Characteristics of Myelinated and Nonmyelinated Nerve Fibers**

	A Fibers (20–31 μ diam)	C Fibers
Characteristics (37C)		
Conduction velocity (m/sec)	120–124.5	3.0–0.5
Spike duration (msec)	0.3–1.6	1.1–2.8
Rise time (msec)	0.07–0.4	0.2–0.5
Fall time (msec)	0.23–1.2	0.8–2.4
Absolute refractory period (msec)	0.45–3.2	1.1–2.8
Low temperature block (C)	7.6	4.3–2.7
Interactions		
Conduction velocity/axon diameter	5.7–6.0	4.5
Internodal length/axon diameter	100	
Internodal conduction time (μsec)	16–20	
Axon diameter/fiber diameter	0.6–0.7	
Safety factor $\left(\dfrac{\text{available current}}{\text{current used}}\right)$	5–7	
Internodal excitation (%)*	22–29	

Note: Typical interactions between fiber dimensions and excitability characteristics are provided for myelinated fibers.

$$* \frac{\text{nodal dwell time}}{\text{nodal rise time}} = \frac{(L \div D)/(CV \div D)}{\text{nodal rise time}}$$

and nerve diameter is approximately 6 for myelinated and 4.5 for nonmyelinated fibers. The simplicity of these relations is questionable when one considers the known variance of diameter along the length of many axons (Sunderland 1968; Waxman 1978). Nodal constrictions of myelinated axons also raise some interesting questions of electrical perturbations. Even the proportionality between internodal length and axon diameter is an assumption underlying conduction velocity, since many factors are known to influence internodal length. And finally, there is a relatively constant relation between axon diameter and total fiber diameter of about 0.65 assumed for most myelinated fibers (Ruston 1951). And again, many factors can influence this relation.

For each of the above relations to hold, internodal conduction times must be relatively constant, as indeed they are at approximately 16–20 μsec durations regardless of internodal lengths. If conduction velocity is large, the dwell time at any node must be but a fraction of the rise time of a spike generated at that node.

From Table 2, for example, the nodal rise time for large fibers is approximately 70 μsec but the nodal dwell time is only 16 μsec. Only a little over 22 percent of the nodal current (I_m) must be required to maintain internodal excitation and ongoing axonal conduction. The residual 78 percent of the nodal current is often considered a "safety" factor. Accordingly, longer nodal rise times coupled with the comparatively short nodal dwell times characteristic of smaller fibers can yield residual nodal currents of greater than 90 percent. A greater safety factor is ensured for continued nodal excitation and axon conduction in smaller fibers.

The compound evoked potentials obtained from complex facets of either monofascicular or multifascicular nerves are even more difficult to analyze. The interactions are certain to exist but elude easy identification and characterization. Morphological, ionic, electrical, and metabolic interactions have been reported. Some of the morphological interactions have received attention in terms of experimental demyelination (McDonald 1963). It has long been known that ionic and electrical phenomena interact to produce both negative and positive afterpotentials following the spike potential in normal mono- or multifascicular nerves (Gasser and Grundfest 1936). We have shown the importance of triethyl tin toxicity to ionic interactions (Gerren et al. 1976) and electrical interactions (Jones and Luttges 1977). Metabolic interactions are less well known but the work by Hydén and his colleagues (1962) opened up numerous possibilities.

Roots

Aside from assumption of common neurophysiological functions, the work on spinal root excitability is quite limited. Experimentally, spinal roots are either ignored in preference for the more accessible, longer peripheral and spinal nerves or they are exposed for use in stimulating and recording specific spinal cord responses. In any event, the neurophysiology of roots is mostly derived from extrapolations of findings in other tissues. A few general points should be recognized in accord with the above discussion.

The roots exhibit a continuity of axon cylinder membrane with that of the spinal and peripheral nerves. There is no a priori reason to suspect that these membranes differ in the molecular components supporting excitability. The glial surround, however, does vary appreciably. As noted earlier, the transition from PSN to CNS is marked by the substitution of oligodendroglia for Schwann cells often with an intervening area with astrocytic end feet. In general, the single Schwann cell regularity of myelination is sacrificed to the less regular nodal organization and the multiple myelination chores of the oligodendrocyte. Many of the geometric considerations are altered at this point. In addition, the bifurcation of posterior root axon cylinders at the posterior root ganglion must have special implications for these fibers which find a low-resistance current sink inserted within the path of conduction (cf. Kirk 1974; Howe et al. 1977).

The loose association of perineurium and the meandering paths of the root fibers organizing into various fiber size groups or into various fasciculi leads to a more "open" mechanical configuration than observed in nerves. Accordingly, the ionic and electrical assumptions of classical neurophysiologic mechanisms probably are better satisfied by root morphology than by nerve morphology.

The general lack of knowledge concerning root function creates difficulties for the interpretation of experimental compression results as we will see later.

Neurochemistry

Nerves

The chemistry of nerves does not differ, in the main, from that of other highly differentiated eukaryotic cells. All major intracellular organelles exist in nerve cells and all major intracellular functions find counterparts in these cells (Fig. 5). It is the nerve cell specializations, however, which make them distinctly interesting. These cells represent some of the longest, finest processes of the body with small cell bodies providing synthetic products for the maintenance of processes several feet in length. The same cells often refuse to show proliferation or multiplication electing to persist a lifetime or to degenerate without hope of replacement. Also, these cells exploit both transmembrane differences in ionic concentrations to support intracellular conduction and synthetic machinery to support intercellular transmission. Most of these functions are achieved with the aid of poorly understood trophic and metabolic interactions with nearby glial cells.

Many of the structural elements of nerves and nerve components can be envisioned by dissociation and subsequent separation with high resolution chemical systems. The protein components of nerve and nerve components are shown (Fig. 6). From whole nerves it is obvious that, quantitatively, myelin components dominate the majority of the structural proteins. A major glycosylated protein (GX) is the signature of PNS, Schwann cell myelin. Be-

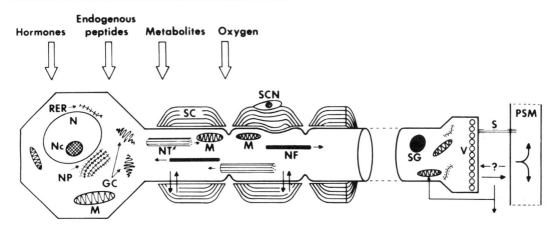

FIG. 5. **Schematized view of the major neurochemical components of an axon, associated cell body, and axonal presynaptic terminal. The transcriptional products originate within the nucleus (N) and nucleolus (Nc) to direct translation in the nearby nucleoproteins (NP) of the rough endoplasmic reticulum (RER). These processes are dependent upon the oxidative energy production of the somal mitochondria (M). Lipid membrane subunits synthesized in the Golgi complex (GC) combine with proteins to form a number of products for transport by neurotubules (NT) and/or neurofilaments (NF). Some of these products may interact across the axonal membrane with surrounding Schwann cells (SC). Some products are rapidly transported to the axon terminal as transmitter storage granules (SG) and/or transmitter vesicles (V). Localized energy production and synthesis occurs in the ending. Some products reach the postsynaptic membrane (PSM) and are taken into it while others are subject to reuptake or loss. Attached to the pre- and postsynaptic membrane is a tubule-like structure consisting of synapsin (S) a protein much like tubulin. Various functions of the system are responsive to hormones, endogenous peptides, metabolite concentrations, and oxygen availability.**

tween this and the major basic proteins (BP_{S1}, BP_{S2}, BP_{F1}, BP_{F2}) of myelin almost 50 percent of the structural proteins are accounted for. Blood components are also quite evident as albumin (TMS) and erythrocyte membrane protein (RBC). The structural proteins of neurofilaments and neurotubules are apparent in the form of actin ($\sim TN_2$) and myosin-like proteins or as tubulin (TN_1, TN_2), respectively. The remaining identified protein bands are the large structural proteins A, C, D, and E (E_1 is postulated to be collagen), the nuclear histones (h_1, h_2, h_3, and h_4) and nerve cylinder proteins (N_1, N_2). All of these proteins have been carefully quantified for normal adult nerves, normal nerve development (Groswald and Luttges 1979) and nerve degeneration (Luttges et al. 1976).

The transport of these and other proteins throughout the length of nerves has received considerable attention (Ochs 1978; Droz 1975). It appears that the transport of synthetic products and countertransport of metabolites depend upon neurotubule integrity since disruption of such structures with vinca alkaloids simultaneously disrupts transport. Excitability is not altered, in the short term, by such treatments although synaptic transmission is severely affected. Transport rates have been reported to vary from a few millimeters per day (slow axoplasmic transport) to several hundred per day (fast axoplasmic transport). Various intracellular components have been reported to move at various intermediate rates (Lasek 1970) and at rates as high as 2000 mm/day. The dependence of axoplasmic transport on energy production within the cell is well known (Droz 1975), and slow transport is not so sensitive as fast transport which is known to be more energy-dependent than cell excitability.

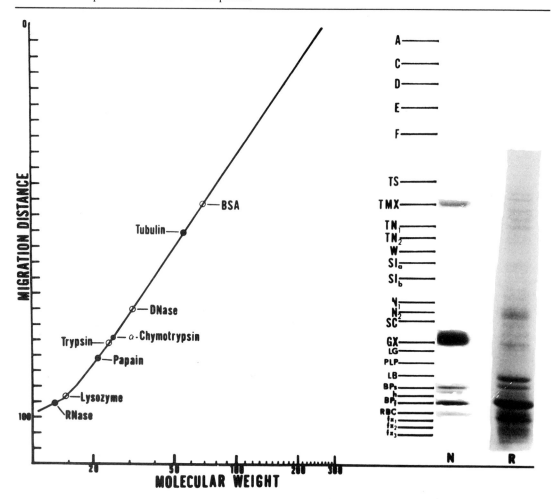

FIG. 6. **Summary of nerve specific proteins separated by polyacrylamide gel electrophoresis.**

The overall diameter of a nerve apparently does not affect the pattern of axoplasmic transport. Transport speed does not vary systematically with the diameter of individual nerve fibers or with the fact that individual fibers may or may not be myelinated. Complete cold block of transport appears to require less cooling (11 C) than necessary to achieve conduction block (7 C), an observation which seems related to the cold-induced dissociation of neurotubules. It also appears that most of the transport involves particulates since it has been demonstrated that less than 15 percent of the total fast trans-

ported, radioisotopic label is recoverable in a soluble form (Sabri and Ochs 1973). The fate of all transported material is not known but it is certain that isotopic label is moved transsynaptically to other nerve cells since whole neural pathways have been mapped in this fashion (Grafstein 1973). Some of the anterograde transport may return to the cell soma by retrograde transport documented to travel at approximately half the outward rate (LaVail and LaVail 1974). It is interesting that anoxic blockade of axoplasmic transport has been reported as reversible for periods up to approximately 7 hours, after which axoplasmic transport does not recover and Wallerian degeneration begins (Leone and Ochs 1973). Such a correlation, however, suggests that retrograde flow dynamics of uninjured, proximal nerve fibers may be quite complicated. In all of these studies it is curious that selective denial of membrane ATPase systems has not been exploited through the clever use of a membrane ATPase inhibitor such as ouabain. The recent studies using sodium influx inhibitors tetrodotoxin (TTX) and saxitoxin (STX) are apparently without consequence for axoplasmic transport whereas the batrachotoxin (BTX)-induced opening of sodium pores readily blocks fast axoplasmic transport (Ochs and Worth 1975). Large amounts of sodium resulting from BTX may result in Na–K pump stimulation and consequent competition for membrane-bound ATPase which is crucial to fast axoplasmic transport. Large amounts of sodium adjacent to the inside of membranes may also show competitive inhibitory interactions with intracellular calcium which is known to be critical for axoplasmic transport (Ochs et al. 1977).

The cell body production of neurotransmitters is another characteristic to be considered in nerve chemistry. Assuming that transport mechanisms are intact, the regulation of transmitter synthesis remains an enigma. Also, once synthesized, stored in vesicles or granules and made available at the synapse, the mechanisms of use and reuse are unclear. The production of anterograde trophic substances is known (Thesleff 1960) but the regulation of production is not (Drachman 1974). Chromatolytic alterations in the nucleoproteins of the soma are well known but the regulatory mechanisms for this phenomenon remain elusive. Even the crucial intercellular communication between axons and supporting myelinic cells has escaped effective chemical characterization. Unfortunately, the possible interactions abound. One is reminded, for example, that some transmitter biosynthetic pathways begin with substrates which must be shared for other cellular functions and the disruption of one of these linked functions is bound to alter the other. A classical example is the collection of problems which

arise from a genetic error in phenylalanine metabolism where tyrosine and tryptophan pools are altered and even cellular protein synthesis machinery is inhibited. A large number of disorders occur and all are accommodated under the one general heading of phenylketonuria (cf., Gerren and Luttges 1978), a well-known but poorly understood disorder.

Among the more recent far-reaching discoveries in the area of chemistry are those related to the endogenous peptides of the CNS (cf. Snyder 1977). These substances are capable of major cellular and synaptic actions including those important to the mediation of "pain." Although much of the work is quite recent and necessarily sparse, it appears that the peptide, enkephalin, has morphine-like properties both in the brain (Snyder 1977) and, possibly, in the spinal cord. The control mechanisms for enkephalin concentrations within the nervous system are unknown but interactions with prostaglandins and aspirin are suspected. In any event, these peptide studies deserve special attention in the future, especially by those people concerned with the inherent capacities of the body during both healthy and unhealthy states.

Roots

The structural building blocks of roots are different from those of nerves in two major ways. First, with the prevalence of Schwann cell myelin, GX is diminished due to the substitution of oligodendroglial myelination. And secondly, the appearance of large structural proteins, including collagen, is lessened. Wolfgram and proteolipid proteins typical of CNS myelin begin to appear (Kelly and Luttges 1976). Fewer blood proteins (RBC and TMS) appear among the structural proteins.

Transport phenomena have not been studied in spinal roots per se. However, the continuity of transport from anterior horn cells or posterior ganglion cells following introduction of radioisotopic labels is well documented (Ochs and Worth 1978). The fact that transported, synthetic products from the posterior ganglion cells must divide into both peripherally and centrally directed flow has received little attention. Also, the axon terminal prevalence of amino acid transmitters in posterior roots as compared to the more easily metabolized adrenergic and cholinergic transmitters in anterior roots has found no remarkable functional correlates.

Behavior

As stated above, there is a tacit assumption that behavior, the most outward sign of nervous system function, is clearly understood in relation to nerve and root disorders. This, of course, has not been the case. Only a few yeas ago, Tinbergen (1974) in his acceptance of the Nobel prize noted that many neuromuscular disorders have not been systematically observed or quantified behaviorally. These comments come from a man dedicated to the study of behavior of various animals in appropriate natural habitats. Such study, commonly called ethology, results in a systematic characterization of the complete behavioral repertoire of an organism, and the characterization often forms the basis for subsequent reductionistic explorations: anatomical, neurophysiological, or chemical. In essence, Tinbergen has pointed out that behavioral analysis remains a fruitful area of exploration in the study of humans. This point of view has been advocated by clinicians as well (Janda 1978).

It is unreasonable to expect that experimentalists or clinicians can afford the time to develop complete "ethograms" for their subjects or patients, respectively. However, nerves and roots play a major role in affect input and effect output. Both are amenable to systematic tests through behavioral studies. To some extent, portions of a complete neurological examination satisfy the criterion of systematic testing but the results are invariably qualitative. Quantification is necessary to provide useful diagnostic information and treatment efficacy feedback to the clinician. Quantification is necessary also for the experimentalist who wishes to relate experimental models of nerve or root insult to behavioral alterations typical of the clinical experience.

Systematic tests do exist and many are readily quantified (Fitts 1964; Adams 1967). Only recently, some of these tests have been exploited in the evaluation of pain mediation devices (Jones and Luttges 1978; Jones and Luttges 1979). It has been possible to use skin sensitivity and motor control sensitivity tests to quantify the effects of such devices. Motor response speed and accuracy tests also provide reliable, quantifiable data. While such tests may not reveal the basis of sensory or motor deficits, they can play an important role in the systematic quantification of such deficits during differential treatment regimens.

Physiological Basis for Compression Disorders

Having reviewed some of the general characteristics of nerves and roots, one can more easily determine what information is or is not available regarding compression effects.

Compression

The methods of producing experimental compression have ranged widely among all possibilities. Early studies (e.g., Mitchell 1872) focused primarily upon the use of a tourniquet in human work and upon the use of weighted, pliant bags for direct nerve compression in animals. The tourniquet methods have been used more recently in studies of nerve compression (Denny-Brown and Brenner 1944; Lewis et al. 1931; Bentley and Schlapp 1943), and in studies of motor control mechanisms (Kelso 1977). The use of a pressurized, pliant compression device has been modified for carefully calibrated studies of compression block in the nerves and roots of both cats and rats (Sharpless 1975). A variety of nerve constriction devices also have been used to produce compression. Spring clips have been applied (Denny-Brown and Brenner 1944) or clamps have been used to produce nerve crush (Kline et al. 1969; Luttges et al. 1976). Simple mechanical reduction of nerve diameter has been employed to study conduction block (Luttges et al. 1976; Aguayo et al. 1971) as well as structural alterations in nerves. The work of Weiss and his colleagues (Weiss and Davis 1943; Weiss and Hiscoe 1948) used pliant arteriole sleeves to reduce nerve diameter, but these arterioles remained sensitive to circulating levels of epinephrine, thus yielding variable amounts of compression. Beginning with the use of a pressure-membrane held at the outer circumference by rigid walls and allowed to compress a nerve passing through the center (Meek and Leaper 1911), little improvement has been made in the application of uniform radial pressure to nerves. Classical studies on large fiber conduction block using compression delivered by such an apparatus are well known (Gasser and Erlanger 1929), and the more recent work using a similar, radial compression device in intact nerves (Bentley and Schlapp, 1943) generally corroborates the earlier work. Many of these and other methods have been reviewed elsewhere (Sharpless 1975; Haldeman and Drum 1971).

Two things become obvious from a cursory review of the above procedures: first, acute and chronic compression methods vary and, second, few compression variables have been measured with any degree of accuracy and without the confounding influences of variables not attended. Perhaps an example of such shortcomings will help in the evaluation of such criticism. The Meek and Leaper (1911) paradigm used by Gasser and Erlanger (1929) permits an accurate measure of applied radial pressure but the nerves were sectioned prior to testing. Also, the rheological properties of the membrane were not specified so a certain amount of hysteresis unaccounted for remained. Most critically, the distribution of pressure radially was not corroborated by any independent means. The pressure may have been applied uniformly to the length of nerve enclosed in the device. But, membrane end-effects could have decreased or increased the pressure on the nerve near containment boundaries compared to the center of the test section of the nerve.

Even now, it is not possible to relate the compression pressures to the duration of compression in a quantitative manner. Although, it seems clear that both variables interact in the production of large fiber conduction block (Sharpless 1975). Of course, the duration variable is known to be critical for the blockade of axoplasmic transport (Leone and Ochs 1973) as well as ischemia (Sjöstrand et al. 1978).

As the major independent variable in experimental work and a major etiological postulate in clinical work, compression has evaded rigorous characterization and independent corroboration. When the compression is used for long or chronic periods, the underlying fact that dynamic tissue physiology may adapt or be exacerbated must be considered, characterized, or quantified. These goals have not been achieved.

Morphological Changes

The effects of experimental compression on nerve and root morphology falls into two categories: (1) gross alterations in the spatial relations among different tissues and (2) alterations in the tissue-specific cytoarchitecture (Fig. 7).

Acute compression studies generally have not been a source of gross morphological observations since the compression by definition is of short duration. The fact that functional alterations do occur has not inspired many researchers to investigate any changes in morphology. Presumably, tissues could be rapidly frozen or fixed (Causey and Palmer 1949) during the course of acute compression to aid such studies, but apparently these studies and associated technical difficulties have attracted little attention by researchers.

Acute compression studies are similarly lacking in detailed information regarding immediate cytoarchitectural changes. Causey and Palmer (1949) demonstrated a selective reduction in the diameter of large fibers when they were fixed during compression at comparatively high pressures. Rather rapid changes, also, have been reported in vascular components of nerves during and following acute compression (Lundborg 1970; Lundborg 1975; Sjöstrand et al. 1978). And, in terms of "recovered" neurophysiological function it appears that acute compression may cause a modest amount of displacement of the nodes of Ranvier (Fowler et al. 1972). It is crucial to recog-

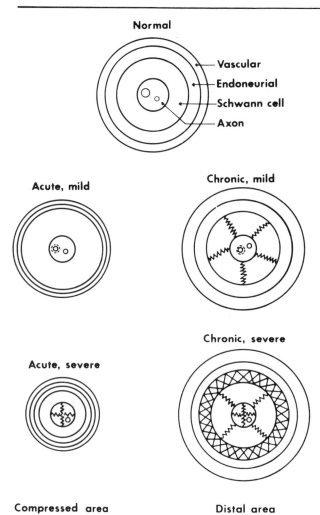

Normal

- Vascular
- Endoneurial
- Schwann cell
- Axon

Acute, mild

Chronic, mild

Acute, severe

Chronic, severe

Compressed area

Distal area

FIG. 7. **Schematic representation of the changes in relative tissue space produced by different degrees and duration of radial compression. The spaces are limited to endoneurial components: vascular space, endoneurial extracellular fluid space, Schwann cell space, and axon space (in which a large and small axon are represented). The sawtooth lines indicate massive destruction and/or large changes in tissue morphology.**

nize that acute compression is realized in reduction of axon diameter and not in changes in the myelinic components of the nerve fibers (Weiss and Hiscoe 1948), and continued modest compression of the radial dimension of nerves must be applied for up to 48 hours before a steady-state reduction in axon cylinder diameter together wtih longitudinal ballooning (displaced axoplasm) occurs. Most studies, nevertheless, employ acute compressions for investigations of rapidly occurring neurophysiological and neurochemical changes.

General speculations regarding morphological and cytoarchitectural changes can be of-

fered but require experimental verification. Fascicular alterations probably do not explain acute compression conduction blocks. Large fibers are more sensitive than small fibers to compression (Gasser and Erlanger 1929; Haldeman and Meyer 1970; Luttges et al. 1976) yet small fiber conduction is more sensitive to anoxia (Wilcox 1975) and ion imbalances (Jones and Luttges 1977). At least partial dissociation of ischemia and conduction block has been noted in several studies (Sharpless 1975; Lundborg 1970). It is also notable that anoxia alone readily produces focal demyelination (Raine and Schaumburg 1977), a consequence not evident in acute compression studies which lead to conduction block. The selective compression-induced reduction in large fiber diameter (Causey and Palmer 1949; Weiss and Hiscoe 1948) can be modeled analytically (MacGregor et al. 1975) and physically (Luttges et al. 1974; Weiss and Hiscoe 1948). Such changes in fiber geometry are known to have immediate conduction effects based upon alterations in several crucial electrical variables (Waxman 1978; Rall 1960). These factors will be considered in more detail later.

Long-term changes in morphology and cytoarchitecture are known to result from both acute, harsh compression and chronic, moderate compression. In these cases, however, the independent variable, compression, is often poorly described.

Perhaps the most exhaustive studies of compression on nerve morphology are those summarized by Weiss and Hiscoe (1948) using arteriole sleeves in regenerating nerves. As noted above, modest experimental constriction requires a good deal of time before axon diameters are reduced to steady dimensions and the connected longitudinal cylinder sections exhibit ballooning along adjacent unconstricted lengths. These observations indicate that the epineurium and/or perineurium initially buffer the endoneurium from the constrictive effects. With larger amounts of compression, of course, the effects are more rapid (Causey and Palmer 1949). The compressive effects soon result in a wide range of membrane permeability changes (Lundborg 1975) which can change the structural proximity of all elements within the endoneurium and perineurium. Such changes are more noticeable when compression is released (Lundburg and Rydevik 1973) and edema appears. Taken together, these observations indicate that compression yields variable pressure gradients within a nerve initially and the transition to chronic effects depends upon the uniform transmission of these pressures throughout the microstructure of a nerve. Pressure evidently collapses vascular space and, perhaps, endoneurial-perineurial fluid spaces followed by the slower collapse of axon cylinders filled with highly viscous axoplasm containing tubules and filaments. When the viscous axoplasm is finally displaced, it is possible for vascular supplies to return, in part, and sustain those nerve elements that survive the reduction in diameter. Such small and reduced-diameter axons have been noted to survive experimental nerve constriction (Weiss and Hiscoe 1948).

Both Wallerian degeneration and connective tissue proliferation are known to occur with more chronic compression (Luttges et al. 1976; Weisl and Osborne 1964; Aguayo et al. 1971). Morphological alterations are most evident in the vascularized spaces where considerable enlargement occurs (Weisl and Osborne 1964). By weight this enlargement can almost double the mass per unit length of the nerve, and it has been shown that such enlargement does not decrease the proportional protein content per unit length (Luttges et al. 1976). Thus, cell invasion and/or proliferation coupled with proteins in exudate must make up much of the increased nerve dimensions following compression. Cellular proliferation has been identified by the rapid accumulation of nuclear histones in quantified nerve proteins (Luttges et al. 1976), and the protein-laden exudate has been identified by Evans blue binding with nerve albumin (Triano and Luttges 1978). If compression is maintained for long periods, fibrotic collagen accumulations occur (Sunderland 1968).

If compression is sufficiently radical the consequences are identical to experimental nerve crush. The axons and associated myelin are physically parted and displaced from beneath the constricted area (Haftek and Thomas 1968). In these instances, there is no evidence of recovery when compression is released. Nevertheless, Schwann cell basal lamina and endoneurial collagen remain intact.

Constrictive siliconized rubber tubing tied around the nerves of immature rabbits was shown to produce progressive nerve damage as the rabbits matured and the nerves increased in size (Aguayo et al. 1971). In these cases it was clear that segmental or focal demyelination occurred in the absence of more extensive demyelinative damage. On either side of the compressed area, fiber diameters remain normal and when the rubber tubing size was sufficiently large to avoid compression of full-size adult rabbit nerves there was no evidence of fiber diameter or conduction velocity alterations. It is interesting that no long-term irritative effects were reported in these studies despite the continued presence of the rubber tubing.

Experimental compression studies concerned with nerve root morphology are almost nonexistent. Recent surgical studies, however, offer some suggestion of morphological changes which occur in roots following disruption (Meier and Sollmann 1978). It appears that astroglia cell bundles invade the proximal roots from the spinal cord during regeneration and that these bundles provide a barrier which promotes the outgrowth of oligodendroglial myelination into roots previously myelinated by Schwann cells. Such outgrowth occurs almost exclusively in posterior roots (Meier and Sollmann 1977). These extensions of the transition between PNS and CNS myelination further into spinal roots have been demonstrated as glial domes or islands in experimental research with rats (Fraher 1974). The significance of the preferential outward growth of CNS myelin into posterior roots remains to be examined. However, the changes known to occur at the transition zones of normal tissue due to shorter internodal distances, fewer lamellae, etc. are likely to be more pronounced in the tissues with more extensive transition zones. It should be pointed out that some fibers retain normal transition sites within the roots whereas others show the previously noted transitions located further from the spinal cord. The effect of such morphological changes on temporal coding of afferent input could be profound (Waxman 1978).

Changes in the arrangement of neurotubules and neurofilaments within axoplasm is a well-known consequence of compression (Ochs and Worth 1978), and blocked bulk transport by axoplasmic flow has been demonstrated in a wide range of compression (ligation) studies (Dahlstrom 1971; Weiss and Hiscoe 1948).

Neurophysiological Changes

The preferential blockade of large as opposed to small fiber conduction by acute compression (Gasser and Erlanger 1929; Causey and Palmer 1949; Luttges et al. 1976; cf. Haldeman and Drum 1971) had been an enticing observation to theorists (Noordenbos 1959; Melzack and Wall 1965) but remains to be explained. The physical deformations endured by large fibers, as seen above, are greater than those experienced by small fibers. From the discussion of general neurophysiological mechanisms, there are several explanations of acute compression blockade which immediately present themselves (Fig. 8).

Since small fibers have a larger safety factor than large fibers, conduction could be expected to persist in these fibers preferentially. Acute compression does not alter the internodal distances in large fibers but does decrease axon cylinder dimensions as well as endoneurial space. Translated to consequences for an equivalent electrical circuit, the longitudinal resistance both inside (decreased axon diameter) and outside (decreased endoneurial space) would increase as would the transmembrane capacitance, C_m. The overall internodal conduction velocity, including the nodal I_C, would be slower and smaller. Conduction could fail at this point since current leakage, I_L, could be unchanged or increased while the depolarizing current was only marginally adequate. Consistent with this view is the fact that acute compression does result in modest decreases in conduction velocities or total blockade (Gasser and Erlanger 1929; Granit et al. 1944). The analytic work reported by Goldstein (1978) in considering nonmyelinated fibers showed that conduction would not be expected to fail as a constriction of axon diameter was approached by an action potential but would be expected to fail as a larger diameter was approached. It seems, therefore, that neurophysiological measures at the points of compression block are necessary before these puzzles are resolved.

Other neurophysiological consequences of acute compression cannot be summarily ruled out. At nodes, sufficient distortion of the membrane can change g_{Na}, g_K, g_{Cl} or any combination thereof, resulting in a mechanically induced discharge and subsequent polarization block. The preferential distortion of large fibers may also result in a severe enough distortion of the membrane to distort the manner in which I_C

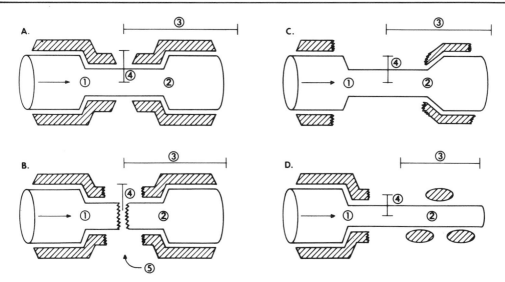

FIG. 8. **Geometric changes important for equivalent circuits of axons and associated myelinic cells when subjected to different degrees and durations of radial compression. (A) Represents acute, mild compression, (B) acute, severe compression, (C) chronic, mild compression, and (D) chronic, severe compression. The numbers identify significant geometric alterations and the arrow represents normal orthodromic conduction direction. 1) Site of cylinder narrowing, 2) site of cylinder widening, 3) internodal length, 4) cylinder diameter, nodal C_m, R_m and g_{ion} values, and 5) extracellular influences especially in disrupted tissues.**

usually alters the g_{Na}. Or, the mechanical deformation may reduce transmembrane resistance, R_m, such that a significant amount of I_C is lost across the membrane without discharging the C_m. A number of internodal C_m and R_m may be postulated also. As noted earlier, a number of candidates exist for explaining acute compression conduction blocks, but a considerable amount of empirical data must be obtained before the appropriate explanations can be selected.

Acute compression that results in irreversible losses of nerve and root excitability is not any more clearly understood than the reversible blockades discussed above. Usually, current leakage associated with the loss of membrane integrity results in a high-frequency, repetitive volley with progressively slower and smaller discharges. This activity is followed by quiescent periods where only strong stimuli are effective in eliciting a response. It is known that after a postinjury period of approximately 3 hours, sensory but not motor fibers begin to exhibit spontaneous activity (Wall and Gutnick 1974;

Wall et al. 1974). The source of these spontaneous spikes remains a matter of conjecture.

Available evidence suggests that acute conduction block in nerve roots mimics that of nerves (Sharpless 1975) except that compression block pressures are generally four to five times smaller in exposed roots than nerves. These experiments suggest that the mechanisms responsible for conduction block reside in the endoneurial morphology since roots possess neither the peri- or epineurium of nerves.

A special set of morphological and functional considerations arise in considering compression and mechanical deformations of posterior roots. Prior to the transition from PNS to CNS myelination, large fibers are known to show up to 25 percent decreases in axon diameter and numbers of myelin layers (Berthold and Carlstedt 1977) and these zones appear to be excellent sites for focal or ectopic spike generation if further decreases are sustained (Goldstein 1978). The substantially slowed spike would simply persist for a period longer than the refractoriness of the more rapidly conducting adjacent node. A similar situation could exist at the junction of posterior root bifurcations into the soma of the ganglion and, indeed, evidence for spikes originating in these cell bodies has been presented (Howe et al. 1976). The interpretation is somewhat more complex, however, since subsequent work by the same researchers (Howe et al. 1977) demonstrates that maintained mechanical deformation of posterior ganglia results in the production of sustained trains of spike discharges. Experimental demonstration of impulses arising from posterior root ganglia disconnected from peripheral influences had been reported previously (Kirk 1974). As noted earlier, spontaneous activity appears in acutely injured sensory fibers within a few hours of separation from peripheral input (Wall and Gutnick 1974).

Chronic compression of nerves and roots results in a large number of morphological and cytoarchitectural changes. In Wallerian degeneration, gross nerve morphology is characterized by both degenerative and proliferative changes in cell populations, collagen fibers, and basement membranes. Vascular changes are pronounced. Even the original elements may show profound alterations in geometry (Raine 1978; Weiss and Hiscoe 1948; Aguayo et al. 1971; Gerren et al. 1976; Luttges et al. 1976). Virtually every alteration in associated neurophysiological function has been reported for these changes. Some of the more fascinating alterations in function appear to originate in regenerating elements of nerves, including sprouting ends of nerves whether normal or participating in the formation of neuromas. Many such phenomena have been the subject of a recent review by Rasminsky (1978).

Chronic compression can produce severe or relatively mild demyelinative lesions resulting in complete (Mayer and Denny-Brown 1964) blockade or in decreased conduction velocity (McDonald 1963), respectively. These two demyelinative effects are derived from a combination of underlying changes in membrane excitability as demonstrated by Rasminsky and Sears (1972). Using demyelinated spinal root preparations, these investigators showed that even in the absence of myelin, nodal saltatory conduction often persists in some fibers while continuous conduction is exhibited by others. Previously myelinated fibers which persist in saltatory conduction are easily blocked while those which revert to continuous conduction typically show only conduction velocity changes. In focally demyelinated axons showing saltatory conduction, an increase in refractoriness is quite evident lengthening from the normal 0.5–1.0 msec to over 4.0 msec (McDonald and Sears 1970). Trains of stimuli result in irregular "following" responses or intermittent responses more typical of normal roots (Raymond and Pangaro 1977). With sustained stimuli at frequencies of 10 Hz or more, profound post-tetanic depression occurs (Davis 1972) in pressure-disrupted nerves. Also, demyelinated nerves are easily blocked by temperature increases within physiologically acceptable ranges for normal fibers (Davis et al. 1976), a condition not fully exploited clinically. These temperature blocks are reportedly more complete in the presence of anoxia (Rasminsky 1973). Some of these demyelinative changes are reproduced with triethyl tin toxicity and have behavioral correlates (Gerren et al. 1976).

Neurochemical

Compression effects on the chemical structure of nerves has been limited primarily to Wallerian degeneration and disruption of axoplasmic transport (Labinska 1975). To a lesser extent the chemical consequences of vascular constriction and the chemical mediation of neurophysiological alterations have also received attention (Fig. 9).

Using constrictive Teflon cuffs, ligations, crush and cut insults to peripheral nerve, Luttges and his colleagues (1976) examined the changes in whole nerve proteins throughout the course of degeneration and regeneration. Much of this work answered questions raised about changes in specific nerve components (cf., Wood and Dawson 1974; Adams et al. 1971). The compression produced by constrictive cuffs (approximately one-third to one-half reduction in nerve diameter) was found to produce degenerative effects different from, but as

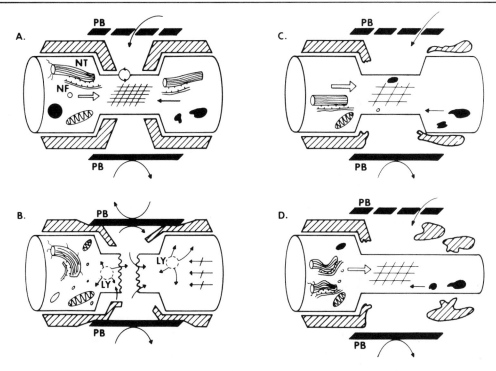

FIG. 9. **Biochemical changes in compressed nerve fibers following different degrees and durations of compression. A, B, C, and D are the same as in Fig. 8. Compression alters the permeability barriers (PB) to extrafiber influences. Tubule and filament (NT, NF) systems are disrupted to varying degrees. Organelles and vesicles show reduced transport (///). In some instances, intra- and extracellular enzymes (LY) promote further fiber insult.**

profound as, those produced by nerve section. The most rapid alterations in nerve structure occurred in myelin proteins. Within a day both the Schwann cell specific glycoprotein, GX, and the basic myelin proteins exhibited decreased nerve concentrations. In nerve sections proximal to the damaged segment, changes appeared later and were much more modest. After two weeks of continuous compression all evidence of myelin protein was absent from the nerve segment distal to the damaged site and there was little evidence of residual metabolites in the nerves. This observation has been interpreted as evidence for rampant phagocytic activity within the degenerating nerve segment. Since these proteins begin to disappear quite rapidly and since such proteins were not inherently more sensitive to enzymatic digestion than

other proteins, it has been hypothesized that Schwann cells themselves could be responsible for the rapid degradation of attached myelinic components (Groswald and Luttges 1977). The proliferation of cells in the damaged and degenerating segment, however, leaves open the possibility of phagocytosis by invading monocytes. The overall size and weight increases in degenerating nerve segments (Luttges et al. 1976) suggested that, had the degenerating segments been bounded by rigid walls, the internal cellular proliferation could have produced added exacerbation of the initial compressive effect.

Quantification of structural proteins in nerves allowed to regenerate following compressive damage suggests that Schwann cell myelination regenerated but involves a larger number of cell nuclei (Groswald and Luttges 1976). This observation is consistent with the shorter internodal distances typical of regenerated nerve segments (Vizoso and Young 1948; Ochoa et al. 1972). All other major structural proteins in regenerated nerves returned to concentrations typical of undamaged nerves. It is curious that the proximal segments of nerve also exhibited a long-term increase in proteins associated with cell nuclei.

Compression and ligation have both been used to reduce axoplasmic transport (Ochs and Worth 1978). If the compression variable is severe, axoplasmic organization including neurotubular and filamentous orientation is disrupted. Within a short period the synthetic products necessary to support synaptic transmission diminish (Ochs 1975) and distal segments of large fibers may begin to exhibit "dying back" pathologies (cf., Sumner 1978). Chromatolysis may be a consequence of disrupted axoplasmic retrograde transport but this possibility requires a substantial amount of investigation. Similar possibilities for transmitter substances, peptides, precursors, organelles, vesicles, and other products remain to be examined in regard to compression effects. Ischemia appears to be but one of many means available for inhibiting transport (Sjostrand et al. 1978).

Behavior

Compression effects on behavior were inherent to early work with tourniquets (Denny-Brown and Brenner 1944) and with direct pressure on nerves (Meek and Leaper 1911). These studies on muscle responsivity opened many possibilities for more comprehensive, quantitative work. Such work was not forthcoming. As noted earlier, compression studies on behavior have been limited to those studies concerned with motor performance and control systems. Compression is simply used as a tool for the partial separation of sensory and motor functions in short-term experiments. Subjects in motor tasks are apparently capable of relatively sophisticated motor responses without benefit of much sensory feedback (Kelso 1977). Even

this assumption, however, has come into question. This remains an area ripe for technically modest experimentation.

Summary of Effects

Both normal and compression-treated nerves and roots have been reviewed. These effects can be synthesized into a variety of experimental or clinical scenarios. As it happens, a scenario of this type has appeared quite recently (Wall and Devor 1978). The problem for these researchers was to relate nerve injury, regeneration, and neuroma formation to alterations in sensations. One of the major sensations of interest was pain as observed in a clinical situation. The point of the review was to demonstrate that PNS mechanisms may be largely responsible for the mediation of painful sensations. The authors admit that CNS mechanisms are important but demonstrate that currently information is not adequate to separate the roles of PNS and CNS mechanisms. In particular, 12 factors are developed as candidates for PNS mechanisms crucial to pain sensation. It should be instructive to mention these candidates. One can imagine that the problems of nerve and root compression cover similar grounds.

1. Modification of receptor sensitivity may occur.
2. Reinnervation of tissue may be abnormal even for appropriate types of nerves.
3. Reinnervation of tissue may be abnormal due to presence of the wrong type of nerve.
4. Afferent activity may originate at any of several nonreceptor mechanisms of the nerve.
5. Sympathetic efferents may initiate activity chemically or electrically in sensory fibers.
6. Change in axon dimensions and in the temporal patterning of input.
7. Selective loss of certain fibers or cells can yield differential sensory inputs.
8. Differential sprouting may favor the production of neuromas and single fiber sizes.
9. Changes in major or minor fiber projections to the spinal cord may occur.

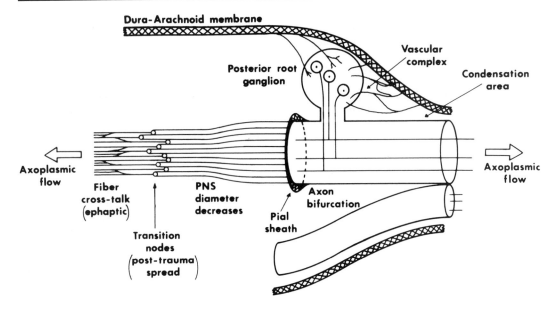

FIG. 10. **Schematic summary of the physiological susceptibility of the posterior root and posterior root ganglion to disrupt and/or abberant function (see text for details.)**

10. Changes in nearby afferents can alter sensory input.
11. Changes in spinal cord cells may occur because of altered input.
12. Schwann cells or other supporting tissue may exhibit altered functions.

Wall and Devor note that until these comparatively more simple consequences of nerve injury are fully understood, it may not be helpful to search for alterations in the CNS which mediate pain sensation. By the same argument a good deal of simple compression work remains to be done in both nerves and spinal roots.

Since a good deal of emphasis is often accorded spinal root disorders, the most susceptible portions of the posterior roots are summarized (Fig. 10). Most of the summary derives from partial evidence reviewed above, however, it appears that closer and more direct examinations of spinal root responses to compression may yield exciting new insight into currently enigmatic disorders seen by the clinician.

Acknowledgments

This work was supported, in part, by a National Institute of Health grant NINCDS, NS-12226, by Stanley Aviation Corporation, and by the International Chiropractors Association. The authors wish to thank D. Jones and D. Groswald for their help and J. Button and W. Bank for their technical assistance.

REFERENCES

Adams JA: Human Memory. New York, McGraw-Hill, 1967

Adams CWM, Csejtey J, Hallpike JF, Bayliss OB: Histochemistry of myelin, XV. Changes in myelin proteins of the peripheral nerve undergoing Wallerian degeneration. Electrophoretic and microdensitometric observations. J Neurochem 19:2043, 1972

Aguayo A, Nair CPV, Midgley R: Experimental progressive compression neuropathy in the rabbit. Arch Neurol 24:358, 1971

Bentley FA, Schlapp W: Experiments on the blood supply of nerves. J Physiol 102:72, 1943

Berthold CH: Morphology of normal peripheral axons. In Waxman SG (ed): Physiology and Pathobiology of Axons. New York, Raven Press, 1978

Berthold C-H, Carlstedt T: Observations of the morphology at the transition between the peripheral and the central nervous system in the cat. II. General organization of the transition region in S₁ dorsal rootlets. Acta Physiol Scand [Supp] 446:23, 1977

Boyd IA, Davey MR: Composition of Peripheral Nerves. Edinburgh, Livingstone, 1968

Causey G, Palmer E: The effect of pressure on nerve conduction and nerve-fiber size. J Physiol 109:220, 1949

Dahlstrom A: Axoplasmic transport with particular respect to adrenergic neurons. Philos Trans R Soc B 261:325, 1971

Davis FA: Impairment of repetitive impulse conduction in experimentally demyelinated and pressure injured nerves. J Neurol Neurosurg Psychiatr 35:537, 1972

Davis FA, Schuaf CL, Reed BJ, and Kesler RL: Experimental studies of the effects of extrinsic factors on conduction in normal and demyelinated nerve. 1. Temperature. J Neurol Neurosurg Psychiatr 39:442, 1976

Denny-Brown D, Brenner C: Paralysis of nerve induced by direct pressure and by tourniquet. Arch Neur Psychol 51:1, 1944

Drachman DB: Trophic functions of the neuron. Ann NY Acad Sci 228:1, 1974

Droz B: Synthetic machinery and axoplasmic transport: maintenance of neuronal connectivity. In Tower DB (ed) The Basic Neurosciences, vol 1. New York, Raven Press, 1975

Eames RA, Gamble HJ: Schwann cell relationship in normal human cutaneous nerves. J Anat 106:417, 1970

Fitts PM: Perceptual-motor skill learning. In Melton (ed) Categories of Human Learning. New York, Academic Press, 1964

Fowler RJ, Danta G, Gilliat RW: Recovery of nerve conduction after a pneumatic tourniquet: observations on the hind limb of the baboon. J Neurol Neurosurg Psychiatr 35:638, 1972

Fraher JP: Probable glial islands in a rat spinal nerve root. A longitudinal study. J Neuropath Exp Neurol 33:552, 1974

Friede RL, Samorajski T: Axon caliber related to neurofilaments and microtubules in sciatic nerve fibers of rats and mice. Anat Rec 167:379, 1970

Gamble HJ: Spinal and cranial nerve roots. In Landon DN (ed) The Peripheral Nerve. London, Chapman and Hall, 1976

Gasser H, Erlanger J: The role of fiber size in the establishment of a nerve block by pressure or cocaine. Am J. Physiol 88:581, 1929

Gasser HS, Grundfest H: Action and excitability in mammalian A fibers. Am J Physiol 117:113, 1936

Gerren RA, Groswald DE, Luttges MW: Triethyltin toxicity as a model for degenerative disorders. Pharmacol Biochem Behav 5:299, 1976

Gerren RA, Luttges MW: The effects of α-methylphenylalanine upon nervous system development and function: a model of phenylketonuria. Paper presented at the Ninth Annual Biomechanics Conference on the Spine, Atlanta, 1978

Goldstein SS: Models of conduction in nonuniform axons. In Waxman SG (ed): Physiology and Pathobiology of Axons. New York, Raven Press, 1978

Grafstein B: Axonal transport: the intracellular traffic of the neuron. In Kandel (ed): The Handbook of the Nervous System, Vol. 1. Cellular Biology of Neurones. Washington, DC, Am Physiol Soc, 1975

Granit R, Leksell L, Skoglund CR: Fibre interaction in injured or compressed region of nerve. Brain 67:125, 1944

Groswald DE, Luttges MW: Changes in sciatic nerve protein composition during postnatal development of mice. Dev Neurochem 2:51, 1979

Grundfest H: Physiology of electrogenic excitable membranes. In Tower DB (ed) The Basic Neurosciences, vol. 1. New York, Raven Press, 1975

Haldeman S: Interruption of normal peripheral nerve function. ACA J Chiropr, 16, 8:16, 1973

Haldeman S, Drum D: The compression subluxation. J Clin Chiropr, Arch Ed 1:10, 1971

Haldeman S, Meyer BJ: The effect of constriction on the action potential of the sciatic nerve. S Afr Med J 44:903, 1970

Howe JF, Calvin WH, Loeser, JD: Impulses reflected from dorsal root ganglia and from focal nerve injuries. Brain Res 116:139, 1976

Howe JF, Loeser JD, Calvin WH: Mechanosensitivity of dorsal root ganglia and chronically injured axons: a physiological basis for the radicular pain of nerve root compression. Pain 3:25, 1977

Hydén H: A molecular basis of neuron-glia interaction. In Schmitt FO (ed): Macromolecular Specificity and Biological Memory. Cambridge, MIT Press, 1962

Janda V: Muscles, central nervous motor regulation and back problems. In Korr IM (ed): The Neurobiologic Mechanisms in Manipulative Therapy. New York, Plenum Press, 1978

Jones DN, Luttges MW: Alterations in passive electrical parameters of nervous tissue and their relation to conduction block. AAAS, Southwestern and Rocky Mountain Abstract 180, 1977

Jones DN, Luttges MW: Transcutaneous electrical nerve stimulation effects upon reaction time responses of varying complexity. Paper presented at the Ninth Annual Biomechanics Conference on the Spine, Atlanta, 1978

Jones DN, Luttges MW: Transcutaneous electrical nerve stimulation influences on somatosensory and motor functions. Unpublished

Kelly PT, Luttges MW: Mouse brain protein composition during postnatal development: an electrophoretic analysis. J Neurochem 27:1163, 1976

Kelso JAS: Motor control mechanisms underlying human movement reproduction. J Exp Psychol: Human Perception and Performance, 3:529, 1977

Keynes RD: Organization of the ionic channels in nerve membranes. In Tower (ed) The Basic Neurosciences, vol. 1. New York, Raven Press, 1975

Kirk EJ: Impulses in dorsal spine nerve rootlets in cats and rabbits arising from dorsal root ganglia isolated from the periphery. J Comp Neurol 155:165, 1974

Kline DG, Hackett ER, May PR: Evaluation of nerve injuries by evoked potentials and electromyography. J Neurosurg 31:128, 1969

Korr IM: Sustained sympathicotonia as a factor in disease. In Korr (ed): The Neurobiologic Mechanisms in Manipulative Theapy. New York, Plenum Press, 1978

Labinska L: On axoplasmic flow. Int Rev Neurobiol 17:241, 1975

Landon DN, Hall S: The myelinated nerve fiber. In Landon (ed): The Peripheral Nerve. London, Chapman and Hall, 1976

Lasek RJ: Protein transport in neurons. Int Rev Neurobiol 13:289, 1970

LaVail JH, LaVail MM: Intra-axonal transport of horseradish peroxidase following intravitreal injections in chicks. Soc Neurosci Abstr 4:299, 1974

Leone J, Ochs S: Reversibility of fast axoplasmic transport following differing durations of anoxic block *in vitro* and *in vivo*. Soc Neurosci Abstr 3:147, 1973

Lewis T, Pickering GW, Rothschild P: Centripetal paralysis arising out of arrested blood flow to the limb, including notes on a form of tingling. Heart 16:1, 1931

Lundborg G: Structure and function of the intraneural microvessels as related to trauma, edema formation and nerve function. J Bone Joint Surg 57:938, 1975

Lundborg G: Ischemic nerve injury. Experimental studies on intraneural microvascular pathophysiology and nerve function in a limb subjected to temporary circulatory arrest. Scand J Plast Reconstr Surg [Suppl. 6], 1970

Lundborg G, Rydevik B: Effects of stretching the tibial nerve of the rabbit. J Bone Joint Surg 55B:390, 1973

Luttges MW, Kelly PT, Gerren, RA: Degenerative changes in mouse sciatic nerves: electrophoretic and electrophysiologic characterizations. Exp Neurol 50:706, 1976

MacGregor R, Sharpless S, Luttges MW: A hoop stress model for nerve compression. J Neurol Sci 11:312, 1975

Mayer RF, Denny-Brown D: Conduction velocity in peripheral nerve during experimental demyelination in the cat. Neurology (MN) 14:714, 1964

McDonald WI, Sears, TA: The effects of experimental demyelination on conduction in the central nervous system. Brain 93:583, 1970

Meek WJ, Leaper WE: Effects of pressure on conductivity in nerve and muscle. Am J Physiol 27:308, 1911

Meier C, Sollmann H: Glial outgrowth and central-type myelination of regenerating axons in spinal nerve roots following transection and suture: light and electron microscopic study in the pig. Neuropathol Appl Neurobiol 4:21, 1978

Melzack R, Wall PD: Pain mechanisms: a new theory. Science 150:971, 1965

Mitchell SW: Injuries of Nerves and Their Consequences. Philadelphia, Lippincott, 1872

Noordembos W: Pain Amsterdam, Elsevier Press, 1959

Ochoa J, Fowler TJ, Gilliatt RW: Anatomical changes in peripheral nerves compressed by a pneumatic tourniquet. J Anat 113:433, 1972

Ochs S: Retention and redistribution of proteins in mammalian nerve fibers by axoplasmic transport. J Physiol (Lond.) 253:459, 1975

Ochs S, Chan S-Y, Worth R: Calcium and the mechanism of axoplasmic transport. In Korr IM (ed): The Neurobiologic Mechanisms in Manipulative Therapy. New York, Plenum Press, 1978

Ochs S, Worth R: Batrachotoxin block of fast axoplasmic transport in mammalian nerve fibers. Science 187:1087, 1975

Ochs S, Worth RM: Axoplasmic transport in normal and pathological systems. In Waxman SG (ed): Physiology and Pathobiology of Axons. New York, Raven Press, 1978

Ochs S, Worth R, Chan SY: Dependence of axoplasmic transport on calcium shown in the desheathed peroneal nerve. Soc Neurosci Abstr 3:31, 1977

Pantal AS: Conduction properties of normal peripheral mammalian axons. In Waxman SG (ed): Physiology and Pathobiology of Axons. New York, Raven Press, 1978

Raine CS: Pathology of demyelination. In Waxman SG (ed): Physiology and Pathobiology of Axons. New York, Raven Press, 1978

Raine CS, Schaumberg HH: The neuropathology of the diseases of myelin. In Morell P (ed): Myelin. New York, Plenum Press, 1977

Rasminsky M: The effects of temperature on conduction in demyelinated single nerve fibers. Arch Neurol 28:287, 1973

Rasminsky M: Physiology of conduction in demyelinated axons. In Waxman SG (ed): Physiology and Pathobiology of Axons. New York, Raven Press, 1978

Rasminsky M, Sears TA: Internodal conduction in undissected demyelinated nerve fibers. J Physiol (Lond.) 277:323, 1972

Raymond SA, Pangaro P: Mediation of impulse conduction in axons by threshold changes. Neurosci Abstr. 1:609, 1975

Ruston WAH: A theory of the effects of fiber size in medullated nerve. J Physiol (Lond.) 115:101, 1951

Sabri MI, Ochs S: Characterization of fast and slow transported proteins in dorsal root and sciatic nerve of cat. J Neurobiol 4:145, 1973

Shantha TR, Bourne GH: The perineural epithelium—a new concept. In Bourne (ed) The Structure and Function of Nervous Tissue, vol. I. New York, Academic Press, 1968

Sharpless S: Compression of spinal roots. In Goldstein M (ed): The Research Status of Spinal Manipulative Therapy. Bethesda MD, NINCDS #15, 1975

Sjöstrand J, Rydevik B, Lundborg G, McLean WG: Impairment of intraneural microcirculation, blood–nerve barrier and axonal transport in experimental nerve ischemia and compression. In Korr IM (ed): The Neurobiologic Mechanisms in Manipulative Therapy. New York, Plenum Press, 1978

Snyder S: The brain's own morphine. Sci Am, 1977

Sumner A: Physiology of dying-back neuropathies. In Waxman SG (ed): Physiology and Pathobiology of Axons. New York, Raven Press, 1978

Sunderland S: Nerves and Nerve Injuries. Edinburgh, Livingstone, 1968

Sunderland S: Traumatized nerves, roots and ganglia: musculoskeletal factors and neuropathological consequences. In Korr IM (ed): The Neurobiologic Mechanisms in Manipulative Therapy. New York, Plenum Press, 1978

Tasaki I: Evolution of theories of nerve excitation. In Tower DB (ed): The Basic Neurosciences. New York, Raven Press, 1975

Thesleff S: Physiological effects of denervation of muscle. In Drachman (ed): Trophic Functions of the Neuron. Ann NY Acad Sci 228:89, 1974

Timbergen N: Ethology and stress diseases. Science 185:20, 1974

Triano JJ, Luttges MW: Subtle, intermittent mechanical irritation of sciatic nerves of mice. Paper presented at the Ninth Annual Biomechanics Conference on the Spine, Atlanta, 1978

Vizoso AD, Young JZ: Internode length and fiber diameter in developing and regenerating nerves. J Anat 82:110, 1948

Wall PD, Devor M: Physiology of sensation after peripheral nerve injury, regeneration and neuroma formation. In Waxman SG (ed): Physiology and Pathobiology of Axons. New York, Raven Press, 1978

Wall PD, Gutnick M: Properties of afferent nerve impulses originating from a neuroma. Nature (Lond.) 248:740, 1974

Wall PD, Waxman S, Basbaum AI: Ongoing activity in peripheral nerve: Injury discharge. Exp Neurol 45:576, 1974

Waxman SG: Variations in axonal morphology and their functional significance. In Waxman SG (ed): Physiology and Pathobiology of Axons. New York, Raven Press, 1978

Weisl H, Osborne GV: The pathological changes in rat's nerves subject to moderate compression. J Bone Joint Surg 46B:297, 1964

Weiss P, Davis H: Pressure block in nerves provided with arterial sleeves. J Neurophysiol 6:269, 1943

Weiss P, Hiscoe H: Experiments on the mechanism of nerve growth. J Exp Zool 107:315, 1948

Wilcox GL: Doctoral dissertation. University of Colorado, 1975

Williams PL, Wendell-Smith CP: Some additional parametric variations between peripheral nerve fiber populations. J Anat 109:505, 1971

Wood JG, Dawson RMC: Lipid and protein changes in sciatic nerve during Wallerian degeneration. J. Neurochem 22:631, 1974

CHAPTER FIVE
Physiological Studies of the Somatoautonomic Reflexes

AKIO SATO

The effects of somatic afferent nerves on the various autonomic functions were extensively studied around 1900 by physiologists while observing the functions of visceral organs. However, analysis of the neural mechanisms of these somatoautonomic reflexes had to wait until electrophysiological techniques were developed. Then, when the technique of electrophysiology progressed in the early 1930s many physiologists seemed to have forgotten, or became disinterested in, the study of the somatoautonomic reflexes with these new electrophysiological techniques.

There are various reasons for the delay of electrophysiological analysis of somatoautonomic reflexes:

1. The somatoautonomic reflexes are much less consistent than the somatosomatic reflexes.
2. The autonomic nerve fibers are much thinner than somatic motor nerve fibers, so it is more difficult to record the electrical activity or the action potentials of the autonomic nerves, especially those of a single fiber.
3. The autonomic nerves usually have tonic activity, even in a resting condition, so that a quantitative analysis of the somatoautonomic reflexes is much more difficult than a similar analysis of the somatosomatic reflexes.

Within the last ten years an averaging technique for analysis of mass activity of the sympathetic reflex discharges and a poststimulus-time histogram technique for analysis of unitary activity of sympathetic nerves with a minicomputer were introduced. Since then there has been a great deal of new evidence relative to the somatosympathetic reflexes, including the central reflex pathway, somatic afferent characteristics, excitatory and inhibitory reflex characteristics, generalized and segmental organizations in the central nervous system, and more.

Sato and Schmidt (1971) stimulated various spinal afferent nerves at different spinal levels and recorded the mass reflex discharge activity from the lumbar sympathetic preganglionic fibers in anesthetized cats (Fig. 1). Parts B through J are averaged recordings of 10 individuals, which make it possible to measure the magnitude of reflex responses quantitatively. Figure 1 first demonstrates that there are two different reflex components: (1) an early spinal reflex with a short latency and (2) a late supraspinal (medullary) reflex with a long latency. The figure also shows that the large early reflex is elicited only by stimulation of the spinal nerves that enter the cord at the same or a nearby segment from which the sympathetic white ramus, which is used for recording, emerges, whereas the large late reflex can be elicited by stimulation of any spinal nerve. This indicates that the spinal reflex component of the somatosympathetic reflex response has a strong segmental organization, whereas the supraspinal (medullary) reflex component has a generalized character. These segmental and generalized characters of the somatosympathe-

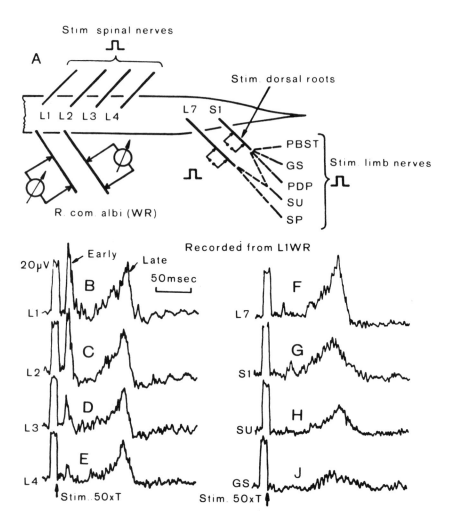

FIG. 1. (A) Schematic diagram of the arrangement of the stimulation and recording electrodes when recording sympathetic mass reflex discharges from the lumbar white ramus (WR) in cat. The stimuli were delivered to the spinal nerves L1–L4, the dorsal roots L7–S1, and also to cutaneous and muscle hindlimb nerves. (B–J) Sympathetic reflexes recorded from L1 WR. Single stimuli (indicated by arrows) were given at the end of the calibration pulses to the spinal nerves L1,2,3,4,7 and S1 (B–G) and to the (J) limb cutaneous nerve (sural nerve or SU) and (H) muscle nerve (gastrocnemius and soleus nerve or GS) with 50 times threshold (50 × T) intensity at a repetition rate of one per 4 sec. Each specimen is the average of ten individual reflexes. *Early* means an early spinal reflex component. *Late* means a late supraspinal reflex component. (From Sato and Schmidt 1971.)

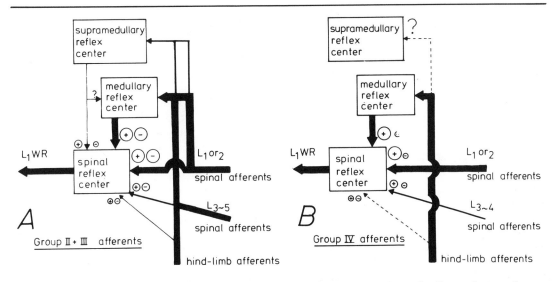

FIG. 2. Central reflex pathways of somatosympathetic reflexes. (A) Central reflex pathways of those reflexes induced by myelinated (groups II and III) somatic afferents. (B) Corresponding pathways for unmyelinated (group IV) afferents. Thickness of various pathways is a measure of their potency. Excitatory or inhibitory effects are indicated by + and −, respectively. Sizes of signs provide a rough measure of effectiveness of excitatory or inhibitory action. (From Sato and Schmidt 1973.)

tic reflex response might be useful for explaining regional and general (or massive) reactions in sympathetic nerve functions.

Classification of the Various Somatoautonomic Reflex Discharges

As shown in Figure 2, Sato and Schmidt (1973) summarized the functions of reflex pathways in the central nervous system for the somatosympathetic reflex response based on the results of averaged responses of sympathetic mass reflex discharges (Sato and Schmidt 1971; Sato 1972a, 1973); the results of unitary sympathetic discharge activity innervating the skin (Jänig et al. 1972), the skeletal muscles (Koizumi and Sato 1972), or the white ramus (Sato 1972b); and the results of the excitability test of mass reflex responses by using double shocks to the afferent nerves (Sato 1972c).

The central reflex pathways from various spinal input levels to a white ramus at the first lumbar level are represented (Fig. 2). The results in A are for the excitation of the myelinated (groups II and III) somatic afferent nerve fibers. Stimulation of the group I myelinated somatic afferents was ineffective. In A, stimulation of the same or nearby segmental spinal somatic afferent nerve produces strong spinal and supraspinal excitatory and inhibitory sympathetic reflexes, whereas stimulation of the distal spinal afferent nerve produces weak spinal, though strong supraspinal sympathetic reflexes.

The results in B are for the excitation of the nonmyelinated (group IV) somatic afferent nerve fibers. In B, the reflex inhibition is weak in contrast to the reflex excitation. The spinal reflex component is present when stimulation is given to spinal afferent nerves at the same or a nearby spinal segment, but the supraspinal reflex component is absent. However, the dominant supraspinal reflex component is present when distal spinal afferent nerves are stimulated.

In summary, the stimulation of myelinated or unmyelinated spinal afferent nerves can produce sympathetic reflex responses in sympathetic efferent nerve fibers.

Somatocardiac Reflexes

For a long time, it has been well known through clinical studies that the heart rate can be changed by somatic stimulation, but we have not had a clear physiological explanation for its neural mechanisms. Electrophysiological study of this subject was started by Schaefer's group (Sell et al. 1958) that first found that the central reflex pathway for the somatocardiac reflex discharges recorded from the cardiac sympathetic nerve to electrical stimulation of the limb afferent nerves was supraspinal. These studies were continued by Coote and Downman (1966) who found spinal reflex components in cardiac sympathetic nerves by stimulation of the thoracic spinal somatic afferents in addition to the supraspinal reflex component. There are also sporadic and short reports from other laboratories addressing themselves directly to this subject (Kumagai et al. 1975; Norman and Whitwam 1973a, b). These reports definitely indicate that somatic afferent activity does induce reflex changes in the sympathetic outflow to the heart which can clearly be separated from effects induced either by: (1) alterations of the vagal outflow, (2) humoral effects, or (3) more indirect reflex actions via baro- or chemoreceptor afferents.

This discussion describes, in some detail, the direct neural reflex effects of somatosensory input on the heart rate in anesthetized cats (Kaufman et al. 1977; Sato et al. 1977, 1979).

Cutaneocardiac Reflexes

Mechanical Stimulation. The effects of cutaneous stimulation on heart rate are summarized (Fig. 3). In the majority of anesthetized cats

(Kaufman et al. 1977) as well as in rats (Sato et al. 1976) at normal body temperature, a reflex increase in heart rate is elicited after natural stimuli such as pinching (noxious mechanical stimulation) (Fig. 3A–D) or rubbing (nonnoxious mechanical stimulation) were applied to the skin of the neck, chest, abdomen, or perineum. It was proved from the results of the denervation of cardiac nerves (Fig. 3E–H, J–M) and the recording of cardiac efferent nerve activities (not shown in Fig. 3) that this cutaneocardiac acceleration reflex was produced mainly by a reflex increase in the discharge rate of the cardiac sympathetic efferent nerves. On the other hand, in spinal animals (Fig. 3N–R), only stimulation of the chest skin produced a small reflex increase in heart rate (Fig. 3P). A possible explanation of this difference between animals with intact central nervous systems and spinal animals is that a spinal, segmentally organized component of the cutaneocardiac acceleration reflex is dominated by a supraspinal, diffusely distributed component in central nervous system intact animals.

Thermal Stimulation. A reflex increase in heart rate occurs after applying thermal stimulation at various temperatures to the skin (Kaufman et al. 1977). It is interesting that different thermal stimuli; i.e., either nonnoxious warm (< 45 C) or cool (> 10 C), or noxious warm (> 45 C) or cool (< 10 C) all cause a reflex increase in heart rate.

Electrical Stimulation of the Cutaneous Afferents. When electrical stimuli are repetitively delivered to cutaneous afferents, heart rate also increases by reflex. It has been shown that stimulation of the group III and IV cutaneous afferents of the hindlimb usually produces the reflex responses (Sato et al. 1979).

Musculocardiac Reflexes: Electrical and Chemical Stimulation of Muscle Afferents

Electrical stimulation of group III and IV muscle afferents of the hindlimb produces

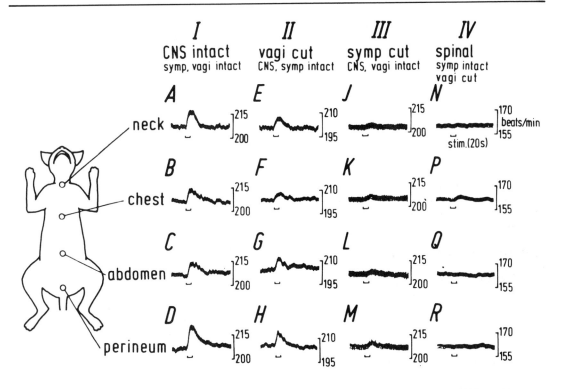

FIG. 3. The effect on heart rate of pinching various skin areas under different conditions. For sample recordings of heart rate in I (A–D), II (E–H), III (J–M) and IV (N–R), the animal's condition is indicated above the respective recordings. Pinching for 20-sec periods (indicated by a horizontal bar) was applied to the skin of the neck (A, E, J, N), chest (B, F, K, P), abdomen (C, G, L, Q), and perineum (D, H, M, R). The horizontal bar indicating pinching can also be used for time calibration. (From Kaufman et al. 1977.)

monophasic increases in heart rate in most experiments even when the vagus nerves and main baroreceptor afferent nerves are intact (Fig. 4A). In about 10 percent of experiments, stimulation of muscle afferents produces an initial decrease in heart rate followed by a marked increase. In such experiments the biphasic responses change to normal monophasic responses after bilateral vagotomy at the cervical level. From the results of sectioning the cardiac nerves and of recordings from the cardiac efferent nerves, it is concluded that an increase in heart rate is mainly caused by reflex increase of sympathetic efferent activity (Sato et al. 1977).

Heart rate reflex responses can also be ob-

tained when muscle afferent nerves are stimulated indirectly by injecting chemicals such as KCl and bradykinin into a muscle artery of the hindlimb (Fig. 4B) (Sato et al. 1977). Bradykinin and KCl are known to excite the thin myelinated group III and unmyelinated group IV muscle afferents (Mense and Schmidt 1974; Franz and Mense 1975; Hiss and Mense 1976; Fock and Mense 1976; Mense 1977) and to cause painful sensations, judging from the animals' behavior (Taira et al. 1968).

To summarize, in anesthetized animals with the central nervous system intact, we observed somatocardiac acceleration reflex responses produced by noxious or nonnoxious stimula-

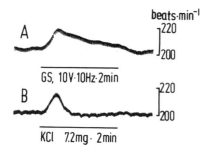

FIG. 4. **Effects on the heart rate of stimulation of muscle afferents. (A) Gastrocnemius-soleus muscle nerve was stimulated by electrical square pulses (10 V, 10 Hz, 0.5 msec). Period of stimulation for 2 min is indicated by an underbar. (B) KCl (7.2 mg) was injected into arteria articularis genu suprema within 2–3 sec just after occlusion of femoral artery and vein. Occlusion period of these vessels (2 min) is indicated by an underbar. (From Sato et al. 1977.)**

tion, and found two reflex characteristics: (1) a generalized one in the animals with intact central neuraxis, and (2) a segmental one in acute spinal animals. It was shown that a reflex increase in tonic efferent activity of a sympathetic cardiac nerve was mainly responsible for the somatocardiac acceleration reflex response. Noxious stimulation is more effective than nonnoxious stimulation in causing the acceleration reflex response. This summary is shown diagramatically in Figure 5.

Somatogastric Reflexes

A somatogastric reflex is well known clinically, and it has been reported that gastrointestinal motility is influenced by somatic afferent stimulation in dogs (Lehman 1913; Babkin and Kite 1950; Kehl 1974), in cats (Hodes 1940; Jansson 1969a, b), in monkeys (Patterson and Rubright 1934) and in humans (Ruhmann 1927; Freude 1927). But quantitative analysis of the reflex response and electrophysiological analysis of the reflex mechanisms have only recently been systematically performed. The following are some

of the results of recent studies on the somatogastric reflexes in anesthetized rats (Sato et al. 1975a; Kametani et al. 1978, 1979).

When balloon pressure inside the antrum is increased from zero to about 100–130 mm H_2O by expanding the volume of the balloon with water, rhythmic contraction waves of 5–6/min corresponding to peristaltic movements can be observed and continuously recorded (Fig. 6). Parts A through F show specimen records of gastric motility reflex responses elicited by pinching the various skin areas indicated in G. The responses in A, B, E, and F represent reflex facilitation; those in C and D represent reflex inhibition. G and H illustrate the results of pinching different skin areas. Pinching skin areas of the abdomen, the middle and caudal ventral, and the dorsal thorax inhibits gastric motility and/or reduces muscle tonus in the stomach, while pinching of the skin of nose, face, ears, neck, arms, legs, paws, sacral area, and tail facilitates gastric motility and/or increases muscle tonus (Kametani et al. 1978).

The neural mechanisms involved in both re-

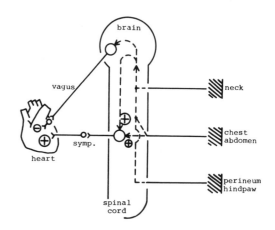

FIG. 5. **Schematic diagram of somatocardiac reflexes. Excitatory or inhibitory effects are indicated by + and − signs, respectively. Sizes of signs provide a rough measure of effectiveness of excitatory or inhibitory action on neuron and effector. Continuous lines indicate afferent and efferent reflex pathways; dashed lines indicate reflex pathways inside the spinal cord and brain.**

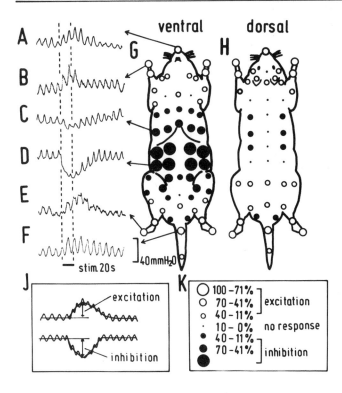

FIG. 6. **Effect on gastric motility of pinching various skin areas in rats. (A–F) Specimen records of gastric motility response. Pinching of 20-sec duration is shown by the bar and vertical dotted lines. (G and H) Schematic diagrams relating the skin areas pinched to the reflex changes in gastric motility. (J) Model illustrating the method of estimating the magnitude of the reflex response. A midline for each wave was drawn and the maximum shift of this line from the prestimulus level gave the magnitude of the reflex response. The largest mean absolute value in each rat was taken as 100 percent and all other mean reflex responses in the same rat were expressed as a percent of this value. (K) Open circles indicate excitation; filled circles indicate inhibition; circle size indicates magnitude. (From Kametani et al. 1978)**

flex facilitation and inhibition of gastric motility when stimulating different skin areas have been determined (Figs. 7 and 8). The hindpaw and abdominal skin areas are representative sites for the production of reflex facilitation and inhibition of gastric motility. Hindpaw stimulation markedly increases efferent discharge activity of the gastric vagal nerve (Fig. 7B) whereas it only slightly increases gastric sympathetic efferent activity (Fig. 8B). Abdominal skin stimulation greatly increases gastric sympathetic efferent activity (Fig. 8A) without affecting gastric vagal efferent activity (Fig. 7A). Thus, the increase in gastric vagal efferent activity is responsible for the reflex facilitation of gastric motility produced by hindpaw stimulation, and the increase in gastric sympathetic efferent activity results in the reflex inhibition of gastric motility produced by abdominal skin stimulation.

The facilitatory reflex responses of gastric motility abolishes or reverses to inhibitory reflex after spinal transection. This indicates that the facilitatory somatogastric reflex pathway is supraspinal. On the other hand, the inhibitory responses are almost identical in the spinalized or nonspinalized conditions (Kametani et al. 1979). This evidence means that there is a strong segmental organization of the somatogastric inhibitory reflex response regardless of the extent of central neural control. This is quite different from the twofold character (spinal and supraspinal) observed in the somatocardiac reflexes.

In summary, it has been concluded that the supraspinal reflex increase in the gastric vagal efferent activity is responsible for the reflex facilitation of gastric motility produced by pinching the skin, for example, the paws. Also, the spinal reflex increase in the gastric sympathetic efferent activity is responsible for the reflex inhibition of gastric motility produced by pinching the abdominal skin areas. This summary is shown diagramatically in Figure 9.

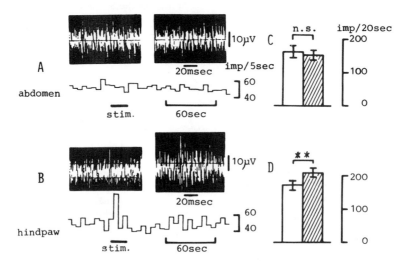

FIG. 7. Evoked vagal reflex activity. Gastric vagal efferent activity and responses to pinching abdominal skin (A and C) and hindpaw (B and D). (A and B) Specimens of activity (upper) and rate (lower) of gastric vagal efferent volleys. Upper records of each set record activity during control (left) and pinching of skin (right). Noise levels are less than 10 μ V peak to peak. (Lower record of each set) imp/5 sec. (Under bars) 20-sec pinch. (D and C) Mean ± S.E. of total vagal impulses discharged for 20 sec before stimulation (control, white) and during 20-sec stimulation (responses, shaded) for 10 trials. (Upper bars in C and D) paired t test significant difference; **P < 0.01; n.s. P > 0.05. (From Kametani et al. 1979.)

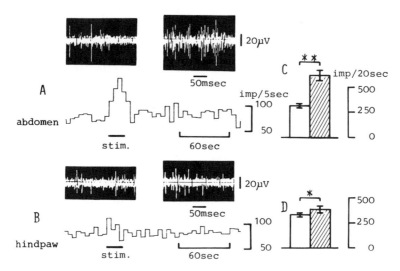

FIG. 8. Evoked splanchnic reflex activity. Gastric splanchnic efferent activity and response to pinching abdominal skin (A and C) and hindpaw (B and D). (A and B) Specimens of activity (upper) and discharge rate (lower) of gastric postganglionic sympathetic branch of coeliac ganglion. Upper records of each set activity during control (left) and pinching of skin (right). Noise levels were less than 10 μV peak to peak. Lower record of each set registers impulses per 5 sec; underbars, 20-sec pinch. (C and D) Mean ± S.E. of sympathetic discharges for 20 sec before pinch (controls, white) and 20 sec during pinch (responses, shaded) for 10 trials. Upper bars in C and D show paired t-test significant difference; **P < 0.01; *P < 0.05. (From Kametani et al. 1979.)

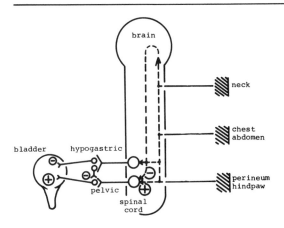

FIG. 9. **Schematic diagram of somatogastric reflexes. See Figure 5 for legend.**

Somatovesical Reflex

It is well known that cutaneous stimulation of the perineal area evokes micturition in chronic spinal patients and animals (Barrington 1914; Denny-Brown and Robertson 1933; McPherson 1966; De Groat and Ryall 1969). This cutaneovesical excitatory reflex response, however, has only recently been studied systematically in animals with intact spinal cords. It has been found that stimulation of the perineal skin of rats with intact central nervous systems (Sato et al. 1975b) and cats (Sato et al. 1977), whose bladders were not considerably expanded, evoked vesical contraction. Electrophysiological studies of the expanded bladder in cats (De Groat and Ryall 1969; De Groat 1975; Sato et al. 1977), in dogs (Okada and Yamane 1973, 1976) and in rats (Sato et al. 1975b) showed that stimulation of perineal skin usually inhibited the large rhythmic micturition contractions of the bladder. The following is a summary of results of recent studies on the somatovesical reflex response in anesthetized cats (Sato et al. 1977; Sato et al. 1977).

Cutaneovesical Reflex

Mechanical Stimulation. When the urinary bladder is not expanded enough the bladder has a quiescent or small, rapidly fluctuating tonus (Fig. 10, recording I). Nonnoxious (touch) or noxious (pinch) mechanical stimulation of the perineal skin of a central neuraxis intact animal produces a reflex increase in vesical tonus due to a reflex increase in efferent discharges of the vesical branch of the pelvic nerve. Hypogastric nerves do not seem to be essential for this vesical reflex response. Only perineal stimulation is able to produce this vesical excitatory reflex response (Fig. 10A–D) regardless of whether the spinal cord is intact or transected above the sacral level. This indicates that there is a very strong segmental organization for this cutaneovesical excitatory reflex response.

When the urinary bladder is expanded above a certain volume with an intravesical balloon, large, slow, rhythmic micturition contractions, driven by burst discharges of the pelvic efferent nerve, are initiated (Fig. 10, II and III). Noxious stimulation of perineal, abdominal, or chest skin produces reflex inhibition of micturition contractions in this order of effectiveness (Fig. 10F–H) as a result of reflex inhibition of burst discharges of the pelvic efferent activity. Hypogastric nerves do not seem to be essential for producing this cutaneovesical inhibitory reflex response.

Thermal Stimulation. Thermal stimulation applied at various temperatures to the perineal skin shows that nonnoxious warm (< 45 C) and cool (> 10 C), or noxious warm (> 45 C) and cool (< 10 C) stimuli all cause the cutaneovesical reflex responses.

Electrical Stimulation of Cutaneous Afferents. Electrical stimulation of group III and IV cutaneous afferents of the hindlimb produces an excitatory or inhibitory cutaneovesical reflex which depends on the vesical resting conditions.

Musculovesical Reflex: Electrical and Chemical Stimulation of Muscle Afferents

When the bladder has large, rhythmic micturition contractions, electrical stimulation of muscle afferent nerves of the hindlimb inhibits these contractions (Fig. 11A). When stimulus intensity is increased gradually, the inhibitory

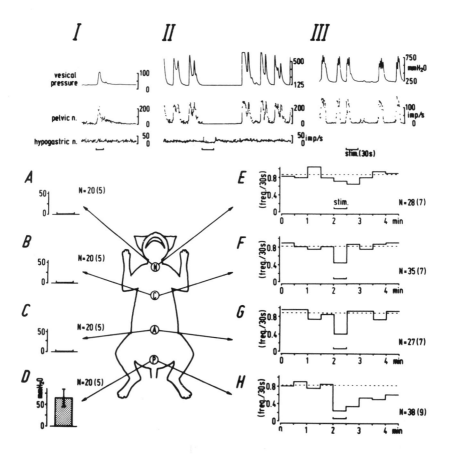

FIG. 10. The effect of pinching the skin on vesical pressure and vesical autonomic efferent nerve activity. Results in I, II, and III show simultaneous recordings of intravesical pressure, pelvic efferent nerve activity, hypogastric efferent nerve activity, pinching for 20 sec in I, and pinching for 30 sec in II and III. A part of the high vesical pressure in recording II was clipped by the polygraph pen limitation. The conditions for recording and counting nerve discharge rate were identical during I and II. (A–H) Effect on the bladder of pinching various areas of the skin; (A and E) neck stimulation; (B and F) chest stimulation; (C and G) abdominal stimulation; (D and H) perineal stimulation. (A–D) Reflex changes in the peak amplitude of vesical pressure after pinching the skin while the bladder was quiescent. The shadowed column and vertical line are the mean and ± S.D., respectively. The number of trials is indicated by N, and the number of animals used is in parentheses. (E–H) Poststimulus-time histograms of the large, rhythmic micturition contractions, compiled from N trials. (Abscissae) time in minutes. (Ordinates) frequencies of the onset of large micturition contractions per 30 sec for each trial. The horizontal dashed lines show the mean frequency during the 2-min period before stimulation. A contraction was added to the histograms only if its amplitude was 33 percent or more of the 4–5 control amplitudes of the prestimulus contractions. The 30 sec of stimulation are indicated by a horizontal bar in each histogram. (Modified from Sato et al. 1977.)

effect which the stimulation has on micturition contractions appears at the range in which the thin myelinated (group III) afferents are excited and becomes very dominant in the range in which the nonmyelinated (group IV) afferents are stimulated. On the other hand, when the bladder is quiescent, the effect of stimulation on the bladder is excitatory.

Inhibition of the micturition contractions of the bladder are also produced reflexly when muscle afferent nerves of the hindlimb are stimulated indirectly by injecting certain algesic chemical substances into a hindlimb muscle artery locally. A reflex inhibition of the vesical micturition contractions is produced by KCl (Fig. 11B). In some instances the inhibition is followed by increased contractions. Bradykinin applied locally to the hindlimb muscle also causes inhibition of micturition contractions. On the other hand, when the bladder is quiescent, the effect of algesic chemical stimulation to the hindlimb muscles on the vesical tonus is excitatory.

In anesthetized animals, somatovesical reflex responses are produced by noxious or nonnoxious stimulation. When the bladder is quiescent, the following stimuli may result in a reflex increase in the tonus of the bladder: (1) mechanical or thermal stimulation of the perineal skin,

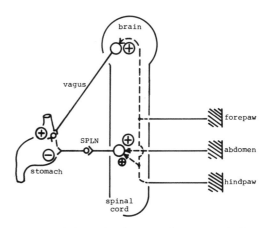

FIG. 12. **Schematic diagram of somatovesical reflexes. See Figure 5 for legend.**

(2) electrical stimulation of cutaneous as well as muscle afferents of the hindlimb, (3) algesic chemical stimulation of the hindlimb muscles. This somatovesical excitatory reflex is a spinal reflex with its efferent arc in the pelvic nerves. When there are spontaneous, large, rhythmic micturition contractions of the bladder, these contractions are inhibited by: (1) mechanical or thermal stimulation of the skin of the perineum, abdomen, or chest, (2) electrical stimulation of cutaneous or muscle afferents of the hindlimb, and (3) algesic chemical stimulation of the hindlimb muscles. The efferent arc for this reflex inhibition of large micturition contractions is also in the pelvic nerves. For both the excitatory and the inhibitory somatovesical reflex responses, noxious stimulation is much more effective than nonnoxious stimulation. This summary is shown diagramatically in Figure 12. This diagram also shows the inhibitory action on the bladder and postganglionic fibers of the pelvic nerve mediating the hypogastric nerve (De Groat 1975).

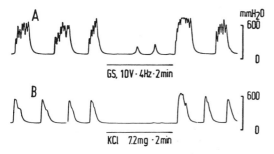

FIG. 11. **Effects on the rhythmic micturition contractions of the bladder by stimulation of the muscle afferents. (A) Gastrocnemius-soleus afferent nerve stimulated by electrical square pulses (10 V, 4 Hz, 0.5 msec). Period of stimulation for 2 min is indicated by an underbar. (B) KCl (7.2 mg) injected into arteria articularis genu suprema within 2–3 sec just after occlusion of femoral artery and vein. Occlusion period of these vessels (2 min) is indicated by an underbar. (From Sato et al. 1977.)**

Conclusion

Some results of recent studies of the somatosympathetic reflex as well as studies by Sato et al. of the somatovisceral reflex responses of the heart, stomach, and urinary bladder in anesthetized animals have been briefly introduced. The effects on various visceral organ functions of noxious and nonnoxious somatic stimulation at various spinal segmental levels have also been emphasized. If a suitable kind of stimulation of the skin or muscle at the proper spinal segmental level is selected, all these visceral organ functions can be reflexly affected by cutaneous or muscle stimulation. Contributions of the sympathetic and parasympathetic nerves for the somatovisceral reflexes are dependent on the organ. The effects of various kinds of stimulation of the spine on different visceral organs have not yet been systematically studied, but this kind of study could be carried on as an extension of the previously noted fundamental studies of the somatovisceral reflexes.

It can be foreseen that basic research into reflex clinical treatment of disorders of various visceral organs by somatic afferent stimulation will progress rapidly in the near future. Furthermore, somatoautonomic reflex responses resulting from the stimulation of skin and muscle cannot be ignored. Further basic investigation of these phenomena should have considerable significance for spinal manipulative therapy.

References

Babkin BP, Kite WC Jr: Central and reflex regulation of motility of pyloric antrum. J Neurophysiol 13:321, 1950

Barrington FJF: The nervous mechanism of micturition, Q J Exp Physiol 8:33, 1914

Coote JH, Downman CBB: Central pathways of some autonomic reflex discharges. J Physiol (Lond) 183:714, 1966

De Groat WC: Nervous control of the urinary bladder of the cat. Brain Res 87:201, 1975

De Groat WC, Ryall RW: Reflexes to sacral parasympathetic neurons concerned with micturition in the cat, J Physiol (Lond) 200:87, 1969

Denny-Brown D, Robertson EG: The state of the bladder and its sphincters in complete transverse lesions of the spinal cord and cauda equina. Brain 56:397, 1933

Fock S, Mense S: Excitatory effects of 5-hydroxytryptamine, histamine and potassium ions on muscular group IV afferent units: A comparison with bradykinin. Brain Res 105:459, 1976

Franz M, Mense S: Muscle receptors with group IV afferent fibers responding to application of bradykinin, Brain Res 92:369, 1975

Freude VE: Der experimentelle Nachweis des thermischen Haut-Eingeweidereflexes. Münch Med Wochenschr 52:2211, 1927

Hiss E, Mense S: Evidence for the existence of different receptor sites for algesic agents at the endings of muscular group IV afferent units. Pfluegers Arch 362:141, 1976

Hodes R: Reciprocal innervation in the small intestine. Am J Physiol 130:642, 1940

Jänig WA, Sato A, Schmidt RF: Reflexes in postganglionic cutaneous fibers by stimulation of group I to group IV somatic afferents. Pfluegers Arch 331:244, 1972

Jansson G: Extrinsic nervous control of gastric motility. Acta Physiol Scand [Suppl] 326:1, 1969a

Jansson G: Effect of reflexes of somatic afferents on the adrenergic outflow to the stomach in the cat. Acta Physiol Scand 77:17, 1969b

Kametani H, Sato A, Sato Y, Simpson A: Neural mechanisms of reflex facilitation and inhibition of gastric motility due to stimulation of various skin areas in rats, J Physiol (Lond) 294:407, 1979

Kametani H, Sato A, Sato Y, Ueki K: Reflex facilitation and inhibition of gastric motility from various skin areas in rats. In Ito M (ed): Integrative Control Functions of the Brain, Vol 1. Tokyo, Kodansha Scientific, 1978

Kaufman A, Sato A, Sato Y, Sugimoto H: Reflex changes in heart rate after mechanical and thermal stimulation of the skin at various segmental levels in cats. Neuroscience 2:103, 1977

Kehl H: Studies of reflex communications between dermatomes and jejunum. J Am Osteopath Assoc 74:667, 1975

Koizumi K, Sato A: Reflex activity of single sympathetic fibers to skeletal muscle produced by electrical stimulation of somatic and vagodepressor afferent nerves. Pfluegers Arch 332:283, 1972

Kumagai Y, Norman J, Whitwam JG: The sympathetic contribution to increase in heart rate evoked by cutaneous nerve stimulation in the dog. J Physiol (Lond) 252:36P, 1975

Lehman AV: Studien über reflektorische Darmbewegungen beim Hunde. Pfluegers Arch 149:413, 1913

Mense S: Nervous outflow from skeletal muscle following chemical noxious stimulation. J Physiol (Lond) 267:75, 1977

Mense S, Schmidt RF: Activation of group IV afferent units from muscle by algesic agents. Brain Res 72:305, 1974

McPherson A: The effects of somatic stimuli on the bladder in the cat. J Physiol (Lond) 185:185, 1966

Norman J, Whitwam JG: The effect of stimulation of somatic afferent nerves on sympathetic nerve activity, heart rate, and blood pressure in dogs. J Physiol (Lond) 231:76P, 1973a

Norman J, Whitwam JG: The vagal contribution to changes in heart rate evoked by stimulation of cutaneous nerves in the dog. J Physiol (Lond) 234:89P, 1973b

Okada H, Yamane M: Nervous control of the bladder [in Japanese]. Clin Physiol 3:366, 1973

Okada H, Yamane M: Effects of cutaneous stimulation on the parasympathetic outflow to the bladder in the dog. Autonom Nerv Syst 13:57, 1976

Patterson TL, Rubright LW: The influence of tonal conditions on the muscular response of the monkey's stomach. Q J Exp Physiol 24:3, 1934

Ruhmann W: Örtliche Hautreizbehandlung des Magens und ihre physiologischen Grundlagen. Arch Verdau-Krungskr 41:336, 1927

Sato A: Somato-sympathetic reflex discharges evoked through supramedullary pathways. Pfluegers Arch 332:117, 1972a

Sato A: The relative involvement of different reflex pathways in somato-sympathetic reflexes, analyzed in spontaneously active single preganglionic sympathetic units. Pfluegers Arch 333:70, 1972b

Sato A: Spinal and supraspinal inhibition of somato-sympathetic reflexes by conditioning afferent volleys, Pfluegers Arch 336:121, 1972c

Sato A: Spinal and medullary reflex components of the somatosympathetic reflex discharges evoked by stimulation of the group IV somatic afferents. Brain Res 51:307, 1973

Sato A, Sato Y, Schmidt RF: Autonomic reflexes elicited by stimulation of muscle afferent nerves in the cat. Proc 18th Int Congr Neuroveg Res, 1977

Sato A, Sato Y, Schmidt RF: The effect of somatic afferent activity on the heart rate. In Brooks CM, Koizumi K, Sato A (eds): Integrative Functions of the Autonomic Nervous System. Tokyo, University of Tokyo Press and Amsterdam, Elsevier/North Holland Biomedical Press, 1979

Sato A, Sato Y, Shimada F, Torigata Y: Changes in gastric motility produced by nociceptive stimulation of the skin in rats. Brain Res 87:151, 1975a

Sato A, Sato Y, Shimada F. Torigata Y: Changes in vesical function produced by cutaneous stimulation in rats. Brain Res 94:465, 1975b

Sato A, Sato Y, Shimada F, Torigata Y: Varying changes in heart rate produced by nociceptive stimulation of the skin in rats at different temperatures. Brain Res 110:301, 1976

Sato A, Sato Y, Sugimoto H, Terui N: Reflex changes in the urinary bladder after mechanical and thermal stimulation of the skin at various segmental levels in cats, Neuroscience 2:111, 1977

Sato A, Schmidt RF: Spinal and supraspinal components of the reflex discharges into lumbar and thoracic white rami, J Physiol (Lond) 212:839, 1971

Sato A, Schmidt RF: Somatosympathetic reflexes: afferent fibers, central pathways, discharge characteristics, Physiol Rev 53:916, 1973

Sell R, Erdelyi A, Schaefer H: Untersuchungen über den Einfluß peripherer Nervenreizung auf die sympathische Aktivität. Pfluegers Arch 267:566, 1958

Taira N, Nakayama K, Hashimoto K: Vocalization response of puppies to intraarterial administration of bradykinin and other algesic agents, and mode of actions of blocking agents. Tohoku J Exp Med 96:365, 1968

CHAPTER SIX
Central Organization of Somatosympathetic Reflexes

J. H. COOTE

The activity of autonomic effectors may be increased or decreased by a variety of stimuli in the external or internal environment. For example, the heart rate increases in response to painful stimulation of the skin or to increased musculoskeletal activity, and it decreases in response to a raised arterial pressure. Blood vessels may constrict or dilate in response to different stimuli, whereas movements of the gastrointestinal tract are decreased by cutaneous afferent stimulation or by irritation of the tract wall. Sweat gland activity is influenced by changes in core temperature and by thermal and mechanical cutaneous stimuli. There are numerous other examples we could give (Korr 1978) and all are responses mediated via the sympathetic nervous system. In order for these motor nerves to perform their role they must receive a sensory input from a variety of sources. The organization of the sympathetic reflex arc is therefore central to our understanding of both normal and abnormal body functions. We shall begin by looking at the anatomical relationships of the various components involved in the sympathetic reflex arc and proceed by describing the physiology of these components. A more detailed picture is given in a recent review (Coote 1978).

The Sympathetic Preganglionic Motor Nuclei

The final common outflow of the sympathetic nerves from the central nervous system is via the preganglionic neuron situated in the gray matter of the segments T_1–L_2. These are small cells, 15–40 μm in diameter lying concentrated in a triangular region of the lateral border of the gray matter, between the dorsal and ventral horn, called the intermediolateral cell column. There are also a few cells scattered in the adjacent white matter of the lateral funiculus and in the medial gray matter—the nucleus intercalatus (Fig. 1). The groupings of motoneurons do not take the form of rounded nuclei but of longitudinal columns within the lateral gray matter. These columns can be imagined to form the sides of a ladder extending throughout the thoracic lumbar cord with the cells of the nucleus intercalatus forming the rungs (Petras and Cummings 1972).

The cell bodies of preganglionic neurons are smaller (15–40 μm) on average than somatic neurons of the ventral horn but larger than cells of the dorsal horn. They may be round or elongated with the majority of cells having dendrites orientated in the longitudinal (rostrocaudal) direction (Rethelyi 1972; Schramm et al. 1976; Fig. 2). The significance of this may lie in the degree of overlap that can occur between dendritic fields in different segments of the spinal cord and also in the ability of the neuron to "collect" input *en passant* from longitudinally running fibers; i.e., from bulbospinal pathways rather than from the segmental input.

The axons of the preganglionic neurons pass out ventrally, with no sign of collateral branches, to enter the ventral root (Petras and Cummings 1972; Rethelyi 1972). After joining

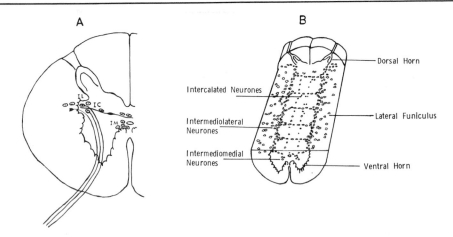

FIG. 1.   Diagrams illustrating the location in the thoracolumbar spinal cord of sympathetic preganglionic neurons. (A) Principal cell groupings; IL, intermediolateral neurons; IC, intercalated neurons; IM, intermediomedial autonomic interneurons. (B) Ladderlike arrangement of the autonomic cell groups. (Modified from Petras and Cummings 1972.)

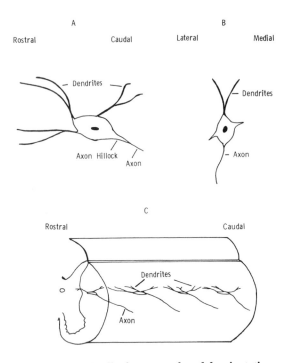

FIG. 2.   Longitudinal or rostralcaudal orientation of sympathetic preganglionic neurons. (A) Lateral view. (B) Transverse view. (C) View into spinal cord segment to show limited overlap of the dendritic tree of each neuron. (Based on results of Schramm et al. 1976)

the spinal nerve for a short distance the preganglionic fibers which may be myelinated B fibers (CV 2.5–15 msec) or unmyelinated C fibers (CV < 2.5 msec) separate to form the white rami communicantes. These fibers then synapse in the ganglia of the sympathetic trunk or in peripheral ganglia (Fig. 3).

Synaptic Connections

Peripheral Input

Segmental afferent fibers make synaptic contact with sympathetic preganglionic neurons via interneurons situated in the dorsal horn and also with neurons just ventral and lateral to the central canal. This latter group of interneurons is called the intermediomedial sympathetic nucleus (Petras and Cummings 1972; Bok 1928; Poljack 1924). Anatomical evidence suggests the possibility therefore of a four-neuron reflex arc (see Fig. 3). Thus dorsal root fibers synapse either with dorsal horn cells or with cells of the intermediomedial nucleus. Axons from these cells synapse on the intercalated or intermediolateral neurons whose axons synapse on postganglionic sympathetic neurons in sympathetic ganglia.

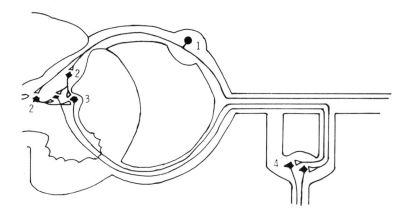

FIG. 3. The segmental sympathetic reflex arc: 1, afferent nerve cell; 2, autonomic interneurons; 3, sympathetic preganglionic neuron; 4, postganglionic neurons. (Redrawn from Wurster 1977.)

Central Input

Sympathoexcitatory and inhibitory fibers from the hypothalamus and lower brainstem descend mainly in the lateral funiculus of the spinal cord (Smith 1965; Illert and Gabriel 1972; Coote and Macleod 1974; Saper et al. 1976; Loewy and Burton 1978). The presynaptic fiber bundles which are part of these bulbospinal inputs to the preganglionic neurons enter the gray matter mainly from its lateral border and separate into individual fibers (Fig. 4). These fibers run longitudinally, parallel and in close proximity to the dendrites and cell body of the inter-mediolateral cells forming primarily en passant synapses (Rethelyi 1972; Fig. 4A).

Axon terminals may be classified into three groups: (1) those containing clear spherical vesicles exclusively, (2) those containing dense core vesicles which may indicate that these are the terminals of monoaminergic neurons descending from the medulla, and (3) those containing clear flattened vesicles which suggests this synapse could be inhibitory (Uchizono 1975; Fig. 4B,C,D).

Each sympathetic preganglionic neuron therefore receives a number of fiber terminals (Fig. 5). Some of these are part of the segmental and propriospinal input from dorsal horn cells or intermediomedial cells. The chemical transmitter at these synapses is unknown. Other fibers are part of the central input from bulbospinal pathways. Some of these synapses are

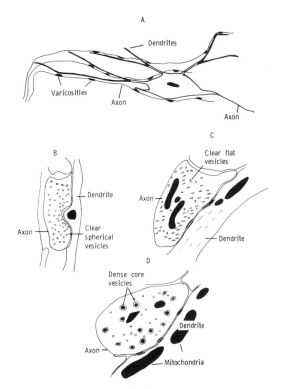

FIG. 4. Synaptic connections of sympathetic preganglionic neurons. (A) Presynaptic fibers converging on a preganglionic neuron making repeated contacts with dendrites and cell body via varicosities. (B) Synapse with clear spherical vesicles. (C) Synapse with clear flat vesicles. (D) Synapse with dense core vesicles. (Based on electronmicrographs in Rethelyi 1972.)

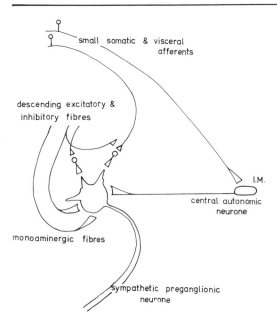

small somatic & visceral
afferents

descending excitatory &
inhibitory fibres

I.M.

central autonomic
neurone

monoaminergic fibres

Sympathetic preganglionic
neurone

FIG. 5. Diagram based on anatomical and neurophysiological evidence illustrating the connections of peripheral and central inputs to a sympathetic preganglionic neuron: IM, Intermediomedial nucleus.

monoaminergic; one releases noradrenaline and another 5-hydroxytryptamine (Dahlstrom and Fuxe 1965; Konishi 1968; Coote and Macleod 1974, 1977).

Physiology of the Sympathetic Preganglionic Neuron

Most of our knowledge of synaptic activity of cells in the central nervous system has come from studies inserting microelectrodes into the soma of the large motoneurons in the anterior horn of the cat spinal cord and recording the electrical events that follow stimulation of excitatory and inhibitory inputs to these cells.

There are only a limited number of intracellular recordings that have been made from sympathetic preganglionic neurons so that our knowledge of their properties is sparse (Fer-

nandez de Molena et al. 1965; Coote 1979; Coote and Westbury 1979). These cells have membrane potentials in the region of −60 mV and this shows short-duration increases and decreases of 2–3 mV occurring in an apparently random fashion. The duration of these postsynaptic potentials lies between 20 and 40 msec. This is interesting because it shows that the membrane is not displaying slow DC shifts lasting 0.5 sec or more of the sort seen in respiratory motoneurons (Sears 1964). Hence the critical period for the summation of additional postsynaptic potentials will be short. This process is illustrated schematically in Figure 6. The membrane potential of −60 mV is shown with small depolarization of 1 mV lasting 40 msec. Each arrow indicates the arrival of a single presynaptic action potential which results in a 1 mV depolarization of the postsynaptic membrane. (This is purely theoretical; we have no idea as yet whether this value is correct.) The threshold value of an EPSP sufficient to generate an action potential is about 5 mV (> 4 mV; Fig. 7B) in these neurons so therefore we would need at least five presynaptic action potentials to occur, providing they occur close to the peak of each depolarization. A second presynaptic action potential occurring at (2) 40 msec after (1) would not summate, unlike the situation shown by the dotted line where the membrane potential slowly depolarizes and repolarizes. This means that there has to be a high degree of synchronicity of the inputs in order to discharge the cell (Coote 1979; Coote and Westbury 1979). It is therefore not surprising that many—40 percent—sympathetic preganglionic neurons under "resting" conditions do not discharge action potentials. As a consequence there is a high potential for recruitment of neurons by facilitatory inputs.

The action potential of sympathetic preganglionic neurons is similar in shape and duration (Fig. 7) to that of other neurons in the central nervous system (Coote and Westbury 1979) although action potentials of up to 7 msec duration have been reported. After hyperpolarization ranges from 30 to 100 msec in duration but is limited in amplitude. It is doubtful

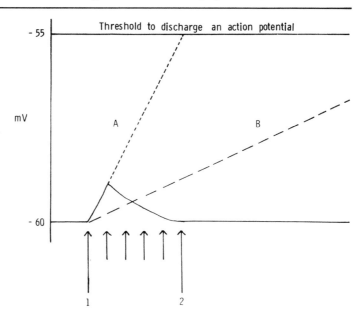

FIG. 6. **The continuous line shows the amplitude and time course of a single EPSP with the characteristics observed in intracellular records, elicited at time denoted by arrow 1. The upper dotted line running to a threshold value for discharging an action potential would be produced by synaptic inputs arriving precisely at the arrows between 1 and 2. A synaptic input at arrow 2 would not summate with the initial depolarization if there are no intervening synaptic inputs. The lower dotted line is a hypothetical slow depolarization which if it occurred following input 1 would allow summation of input 2.**

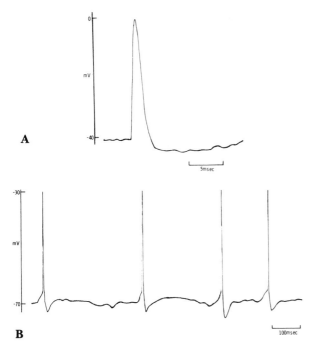

FIG. 7. **Intracellular potentials generated in a sympathetic preganglionic neuron. (A) Following antidromic stimulation. (B) A cell 'spontaneously' discharging following synaptic inputs.**

if this plays any important functional role in influencing the firing rate of the neurons. There is electrophysiological evidence (Gebber and Barman 1979; Lebedev et al. 1978) that there are axonal collaterals in a few preganglionic neurons by which interneurons are excited leading to a recurrent inhibition of the sympathetic cells similar to that produced by the Renshaw cell associated with inhibition of motoneurons in the ventral horn (Fig. 8). However, there is as yet no anatomical evidence for axon collaterals.

Under resting conditions some 60 percent of the population of preganglionic neurons discharge action potentials at a rate of 1 to 2 per second (Polosa 1968; Seller 1973). The pattern of activity is mainly determined by the interaction of excitatory and inhibitory inputs descending from the brainstem. These inputs are also influencing the excitability of the population of neurons that are not discharging (Lipski et al. 1977). Some rhythmic drive is generated in the spinal cord as is shown by the fact that ongoing activity of lower frequency can be recorded in the preganglionic neurons in the isolated spinal cord (Polosa 1968).

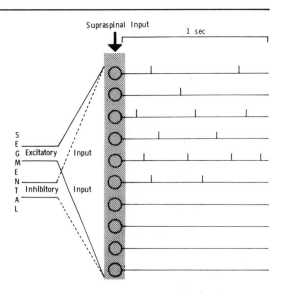

FIG. 9. **Segmental excitatory and inhibitory afferent fibers converge onto both "active" and "silent" sympathetic preganglionic neurons. All the cells are subject to a descending excitatory and inhibitory influence which is illustrated by the stipling. This leads to different rates of firing of the cells indicated schematically by the spikes on the right-hand horizontal lines emerging from each cell.**

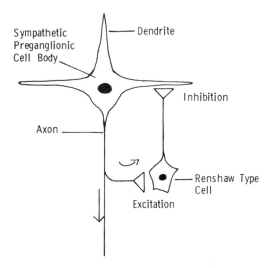

FIG. 8. **Diagram showing the sort of pathway that would be involved in recurrent inhibition of a sympathetic preganglionic neuron.**

It is on this background that the influence of somatic afferent fibers is superimposed (Fig. 9).

Reflex Pathways Onto Sympathetic Preganglionic Neurons

Stimulation of spinal afferent nerve fibers conducting below 40 m/sec (Koizumi and Brooks 1972; Sato and Schmidt 1973) causes a change in the activity of sympathetic neurons, mediated over several central pathways. These are illustrated diagrammatically in Figure 10.

Afferent nerves from muscle, joints, skin, and viscera can excite sympathetic preganglionic neurons over a spinal segmental pathway which is polysynaptic having a central delay of 6–15 msec (Beachan and Perl 1964;

Coote and Downman 1966; Coote et al. 1969; see Fig. 10). Preganglionic neurons can also be excited from adjacent or remote segmental inputs via propriospinal pathways (Beacham and Perl 1964; Sato 1971; see Fig. 10). It is generally true that as fewer neurons are discharged the farther away the afferent input becomes until at more than six segments distance no effect can be demonstrated over the propriospinal pathway (Sato 1971; Fig. 11). There is a third route the afferent volley can take, and that is to ascend to the brainstem to activate descending excitatory pathways to the preganglionic neurons to the suprasegmental reflex pathway (see Fig. 10). The size of the excitatory response elicited over this pathway is independent of the location of the stimulus (see Fig. 11).

Some examples of the central pathways by which functionally different preganglionic neurons are influenced by inputs from different types of receptor are illustrated in Figure

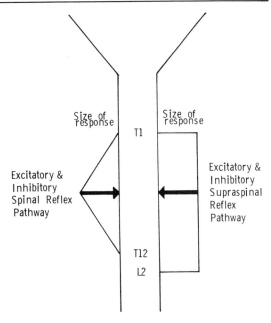

FIG. 11. **Diagram contrasting the effects of spinal and supraspinal pathways on the sympathetic neuron pool. The proporation of the neuron pool excited or inhibited by a segmental afferent input over the spinal and propriospinal pathway (left) and over a supraspinal pathway (right).**

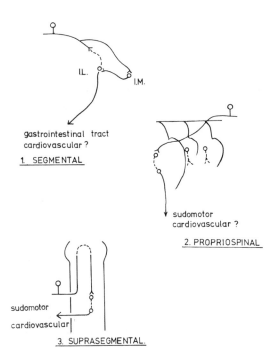

FIG. 10. **The three pathways that can be involved in somatosympathetic reflexes.**

12. The somatic afferent input from anywhere in the body to cardiovascular neurons favors a suprasegmental pathway as does that to pilomotor neurons. On the other hand, the input to neurons supplying the gastrointestinal tract favors a segmental pathway and its influence is localized to receptors in the thorax and abdomen. Sudomotor neurons may be influenced either very specifically by powerful propriospinal pathways or more generally by inputs from all over the body utilizing a suprasegmental pathway (Coote 1978).

Only a small proportion of neurons discharge an action potential in response to a single afferent input. Increasing the number of active afferent fibers or the frequency of action potentials in a single input may produce sufficient summation of EPSPs to discharge the cell. In this way, quite marked facilitation of somatosympathetic reflexes can be produced. This facilita-

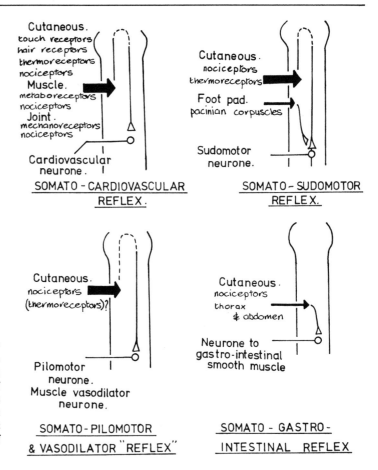

FIG. 12. Central pathways by which different sympathetic pre-ganglionic neurons are influenced by inputs from different types of receptors. Thick arrow represents afferent input from anywhere on body; the thin arrow, input localized to a specific region of body.

tion results in an increase in the number of neurons firing and also in their rate of firing.

Facilitation is absent or very weak when the descending excitatory influences have been removed by transection of the spinal cord. As a consequence fewer sympathetic preganglionic neurons can be discharged by somatic afferent fibers. We have learned that the firing of many sympathetic preganglionic neurons is dependent on the number and synchronicity of arriving excitatory inputs and therefore removal of some of these will result in fewer neurons being discharged by somatic afferent fibers. With time the excitability of the neurons increases and the efficiency of somatic afferent

fibers is improved. However, the somatic afferent input onto some preganglionic neurons; e.g., those supplying smooth muscle of the gastrointestinal tract, have a high synaptic potency and are little affected by removal of descending excitatory pathways (Sato et al. 1975; Sato and Terui 1976).

Stimulation of somatic afferent fibers can inhibit sympathetic activity via spinal and supraspinal pathways similar to those described for the excitatory effects. The supraspinal pathway mediates the most powerful inhibition affecting neurons equally at all segmental levels, whereas the spinal and propriospinal pathway is organized in such a fashion that the most pronounced inhibitory effects are at the level of the somatic afferent input (Sato 1972; see Fig. 11).

Differential Effects of the Sensory Input

Examination of the range of response that can be elicited by different peripheral receptors indicates a degree of complexity in the central organization of somatosympathetic reflexes which heretofore has not been dealt with. Stimulation of a single type of receptor may lead to excitation of one group of sympathetic neurons and yet inhibition of another group (Fig. 13). This is not seen in the spinal animal where a receptor produces either excitation or sympathetic neurons of all types or inhibition (Janig 1975).

How then is the differential response to a single type of input brought about? It is probably dependent on the pattern of activation of descending bulbospinal pathways which converge onto sympathetic preganglionic neurons. This pattern is triggered by the arrival of the afferent volley which has been long circuited to the brainstem. It is therefore only a feature of the suprasegmental reflexes. The evidence for this is illustrated in Figure 13 for a suprasegmental cardiovascular reflex. A cutaneous nociceptive input excites both cutaneous vasoconstrictor neurons and muscle vasoconstrictor neurons if descending pathways are removed (spinal condition), but differential effects on these two pools of neurons are produced when the descending pathways are present. Note how anaesthesia reverses the response seen in intact conscious animals. Another example is shown for hair follicle receptor input (Horeyseck and Janig 1974).

Although we are a long way from understanding or even describing all the events which underlie the pattern of response of sympathetic preganglionic neurons we can perhaps simplify the picture that emerges from the story so far.

First, how is it that the afferent volley gets long circuited to the brainstem when a perfectly

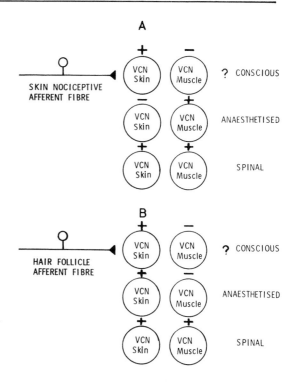

FIG. 13. **Diagram illustrating the changes in effect of specific receptors on two groups of cardiovascular neurons in different animal preparations—conscious, anaesthetized, and spinal: VCN, vasoconstrictor neurons. (Based in part on results of Horeyseck and Janig 1974)**

good segmental pathway exists, as shown by the response of the preganglionic neurons in the spinal animal? It is because, in this case, the segmental pathway is tonically inhibited by a supraspinal descending inhibitory pathway (Coote and Sato 1978; Fig. 14).

Second, the afferent volley activates a particular region of the brain which is able to elaborate a pattern of activity in descending excitatory and inhibitory fibers (i.e., a neuronal program appropriate to the quality and quantity of the stimulus). In the example illustrated in Fig. 13A, a nociceptive stimulus activates the defense region of the brainstem and among other changes this region promotes increased activity in ex-

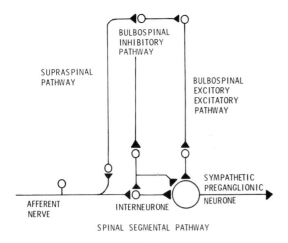

FIG. 14. **Postulated pathways involved in control of segmental reflex arc and suprasegmental reflex.**

citatory fibers to cutaneous vasoconstrictor neurons (with perhaps decreased inhibition of these neurons) and also increased activity in inhibitory fibers to muscle vasoconstrictor neurons (with perhaps decreased excitatory drive).

Summary

The neuronal elements that form part of the sympathetic reflex arc have been described. Both segmental and intersegmental polysynaptic connections exist. Cells of the intermediomedial nucleus of the thoracolumbar cord are interneurons in the sympathetic reflex arc, but we cannot identify with certainty other interneurons by which somatic afferent fibers make contact with preganglionic cells. Electrophysiological experiments show that shorter and more powerful pathways converge on some sympathetic neurons from adjacent or even more remote segments than do from the same segment. These pathways provide the basic circuit for strong functional connections between specific receptors and functionally discrete preganglionic neurons.

Descending inhibitory and excitatory pathways from various regions of the brainstem converge onto sympathetic preganglionic neurons or nearby interneurons and profoundly influence the excitability of somatosympathetic reflex pathways.

As well as these spinal reflex pathways, sympathetic neurons may be reflexly influenced by afferent fibers ascending to and descending from the brainstem.

Not all sympathetic preganglonic neurons are similarly affected by stimulation of somatic afferent nerves or by natural stimulation of specific receptors. Many cells do not discharge in response to synaptic input because there is insufficient summation illustrating a different synaptic potency among the cell population. Sympathetic preganglionic neurons can be inhibited or excited over both spinal and supraspinal pathways. The extent to which one is favored may be determined by the dominance of supraspinal excitatory or inhibitory influence. For those neurons supplying the smooth muscle of the gastrointestinal tract the segmental pathway is the more powerful, whereas for cardiovascular and sudomotor neurons often the suprasegmental pathway is preferred. Even so, specific spinal reflexes can be elicited in these neurons by stimulation of particular receptors. Where somatosympathetic reflexes are very specific and they do not disturb whole body homeostasis they are mediated over spinal pathways; otherwise the supraspinal pathway is favored. In this case the afferent volley which is long circuited to medullary or supramedullary regions enables the elaboration of a pattern of sympathetic response appropriate to the quality and intensity of the stimulus. In this case the response of sympathetic preganglionic neurons may be the opposite to that elicited through the segmental reflex pathway. There is, therefore, a specific organization of the sympathetic nervous system at different levels of the neuraxis. The magnitude of influence of neurons in these different regions on the sympathetic preganglionic neuron can change leading to altered autonomic motor response.

REFERENCES

Beacham WS, Perl ER: Background and reflex discharge of sympathetic preganglionic neurones in the spinal cat. J Physiol 172:400, 1964

Beacham WS, Perl ER: Characteristics of a spinal sympathetic reflex. J Physiol 173:431, 1964

Bok ST: Das Rückenmark. In von Mollendorf W (ed): Handbuch der mikroscopischen Anatomie des Menschen, vol. 4. Berlin, Springer-Verlag, 1928

Coote JH: Somatic sources of afferent input as factors in aberrant autonomic, sensory and motor function. In Korr IM (ed): Neurobiologic Mechanisms in Manipulative Therapy. New York, Plenum, 1978

Coote JH: The integrative role of the sympathetic preganglionic neuron. In Koepchen HP, Trzebski A, Hilton SM (eds): Central Interactions between Respiratory and Cardiovascular Systems. Berlin, Springer-Verlag, 1979

Coote JH, Downman CBB: Central pathways of some autonomic reflex discharges. J Physiol 183:714, 1966

Coote JH, Downman CBB, Weber WV: Reflex discharges into thoracic white rami elicited by somatic and visceral afferent excitation. J Physiol (Lond) 202:147, 1969

Coote JH, Macleod VH: The influence of bulbospinal monoaminergic pathways on sympathetic nerve activity. J Physiol (Lond) 241:453, 1974

Coote JH, Macleod VH: The effect of intraspinal microinjections of 6 Hydroxydopamine on the inhibitory influence exerted on spinal sympathetic activity by the baroreceptors. Pfluegers Arch 371:271, 1977

Coote JH, Sato A: Supraspinal regulation of spinal reflex discharge into cardiac sympathetic nerves. Brain Res 142:425, 1978

Coote JH, Westbury DR: Intracellular potentials from sympathetic preganglionic neurons. Neurosci Lett, December 1979

Dahlstrom A, Fuxe K: Evidence for the existence of monoamine neurons in the central nervous system. II. Experimentally induced changes in intraneuronal amine levels of bulbospinal neuron systems. Acta Physiol Scand [Suppl] 62:5, 1965

Fernandez de Molena A, Kuno M, Perl ER: Antidromically evoked responses from sympathetic preganglionic neurons. J Physiol (Lond) 180:321, 1965

Gebber GL, Barman SM: Inhibitory interaction between preganglionic sympathetic neurons. In Meyer P, Schmitt H (eds): Nervous System and Hypertension. Paris, Wiley-Flammarion, 1979

Horeyseck G, Janig W: Reflexes in postganglionic fibers within skin and muscle nerves after noxious stimulation of skin. Exp Brain Res 20:125, 1974

Illert M, Gabriel M: Descending pathways in the cervical cord of cats affecting blood pressure and sympathetic activity. Pfluegers Arch 335:109, 1972

Janig W: Central organization of somato sympathetic reflexes in vasoconstrictor neurons. Brain Res 87:305, 1975

Koizumi K, Brooks CM: The integration of autonomic system reactions: A discussion of autonomic reflexes, their control and their association with somatic reactions. Ergeb der Physiol 67:1, 1972

Konishi M: Fluorescence microscopy of the spinal cord of the dog with special reference to the autonomic lateral horn cells. Arch Histol Jpn 30:33, 1968

Korr IM: Sustained sympathicotonia as a factor in disease. In Korr IM (ed): The Neurobiologic Mechanisms in Manipulative Therapy. New York, Plenum, 1978

Lebedev VP, Petrov VI, Skobolev VA: Recurrent inhibition of sympathetic preganglionic neurons of the lateral horns of the spinal cord. Neurophysiology 9:294, 1978

Lipski J, Coote JH, Trzebski A: Temporal patterns of antidromic invasion latencies of sympathetic preganglionic neurons related to central inspiratory activity and pulmonary stretch receptor reflex. Brain Res 135:162, 1977

Loewy AD, Burton H: Nuclei of the solitary tract: Efferent projections to the lower brain stem and spinal cord of the cat. J Comp Neurol 181:421, 1978

Petras JM, Cummings JF: Autonomic neurons in the spinal cord of the rhesus monkey: A correlation of the findings of cytoarchitectonics and sympathectomy with fiber degeneration following dorsal rhizotomy. J Comp Neurol 146:189, 1972

Poljack S: Die Struktureigentümlichkeiten des Ruckermarkes beiden Chiropteren. Zugleich ein Beitrag zu der Frage uber die spinalen Zentren des Sympatheticus. Z Anat Entwicklungsgesch 74:509, 1924

Polosa C: Spontaneous activity of sympathetic preganglionic neurons. Can J Physiol Pharmacol 46:887, 1968

Rethelyi M: Cell and neuropil architecture of the intermedio-lateral (sympathetic) nucleus of cat spinal cord. Brain Res 46:203, 1972

Saper CB, Loewy AD, Swanson LW, Cowman WM: Direct hypothalamic-autonomic connections. Brain Res 117:305, 1976

Sato A: The spinal and supraspinal somato sympathetic reflexes. In Kao FF, Koizumi K, Vasalle M (eds): Research in Physiology. Bologna, Auto Gaggi, 1971

Sato A: Spinal and supraspinal inhibition of somatosympathetic reflexes by conditioning afferent volleys. Pfluegers Arch 336:121, 1972

Sato A, Schmidt RF: Somato sympathetic reflexes: afferent fibers, central pathways, Discharge characteristics. Physiol Rev 53:916, 1973

Sato Y, Terui N: Changes in duodenal motility produced by noxious mechanical stimulation of the skin in rats. Neurosci Lett 2:189, 1976

Sato A, Sato Y, Shimada F, Torigata Y: Changes in gastric motility produced by nociceptive stimulation of the skin in rats. Brain Res 87:151, 1975

Schramm LP, Stribling JM, Adair JR: Developmental reorientation of sympathetic preganglionic neurons in the rat. Brain Res 106:166, 1976

Sears TA: The slow potentials of thoracic respiratory motoneurones and their relation to breathing. J Physiol (London) 175:404, 1964

Seller H: The discharge pattern of single units in thoracic and lumbar white rami in relation to cardiovascular events. Pfluegers Arch 343:317, 1973

Smith OA: Anatomy of central neural pathways mediating cardiovascular functions. In Randall WC (ed): Control of the Heart. Baltimore, Williams & Wilkins, 1965

Uchizono K: Excitation and Inhibition. Synaptic Morphology. Tokyo, Igaku Shoin, 1975

Wurster RD: Spinal sympathetic control of the heart. In Randall WD (ed): Neural Regulation of the Heart. New York, Oxford University Press, 1977

CHAPTER SEVEN
The Neurophysiology of Spinal Pain Syndromes

SCOTT HALDEMAN

Pain of spinal origin is one of the most common and costly problems with which health care practitioners are faced. Nagi et al. (1973) conducted a survey in Columbus, Ohio which led to the conclusion that 18 percent of the general population between the ages of 18 and 64 suffered from persistent back pain. Other workers have estimated that as high as 50 percent of the general population and 65 percent of industrial workers suffer from back pain (McBeath 1970). Benn and Wood (1975) estimated that 13.2 million workdays were lost in Britain in 1970 due to back pain. Pheasant (1977) extrapolated the California survey he conducted to the population of the United States to conclude that the cost of hospital treated patients with back pain was about $1.38 billion or 1.4 percent of all dollars expended for health care in the United States in 1974. These figures do not include the cost of nonhospitalized treatment of back pain, the treatment costs of pain originating from the cervical and dorsal spine, lost workdays, or inflation.

Patients with spinal pain syndromes make up by far the major portion of the average chiropractor's workload. Breen (1977) found that 53 percent of patients seeking chiropractic help in Britain did so for low back pain and 90 percent for conditions affecting the musculoskeletal system. Vear (1972) came to similar conclusions following a survey of patients who sought chiropractic care in Ontario. This area of pathophysiology is therefore one of the most important topics for a practicing chiropractor to understand.

Spinal Pain Syndromes

The noxious stimulation of spinal and paraspinal structures can result in a wide variety of pain syndromes. The variation in pain occurs in such factors as age of onset, nature of injury, location in the spine, intensity, duration, aggravating factors, relieving factors, areas of radiation, and response to treatment.

The literature on the spinal pain syndromes is so confusing that any systematic classification is impossible. There are, however, a large number of named pain syndrome or diagnoses which have been considered to originate from the irritation of spinal or paraspinal tissues. These diagnoses can be divided into syndromes in which the pain is primarily felt close to the spine and those in which the pain radiates some distance from the spine.

SPINAL PAIN SYNDROMES
Suboccipital headache
Anteflexion headache
Cervical syndrome
Acute neck pain
Chronic neck pain
Myofascial pain
Fibrositis
Trigger point tenderness
Acute disc syndrome
Lumbago
Lumbo-sacral strain
Lumbar hyperextension syndrome
Quadratus lumborum syndrome
Psoas syndrome

RADIATING PAIN SYNDROMES

Occipital-frontal tension headache
Brachial neuralgia
Cervical or pseudo-angina
Intercostal neuralgia
Pseudo-appendicitis
Pseudo-cholecystitis
Sciatica
Neurogenic claudication
Notalgia paresthetica

Certain of the syndromes, such as suboccipital headaches, brachial neuralgia, and lumbago, simply describe the area where pain is felt. Anteflexion headache and lumbar hyperextension syndrome describe syndromes that are aggravated by a particular movement. Sacroiliac sprain, postural low back pain, and cervical tension headaches refer to the supposed etiology of the syndromes, whereas myofacial pain and acute disc syndrome suggest that the pathogenesis of the pain is understood. This type of terminology reflects the confusion which now exists in our understanding of spinal pain and the difficulty clinicians are having in communicating their impression of the ailment from which a particular patient is suffering.

The problem, in part, is due to a general lack of understanding of the pathogenesis of spinal pain. If one reviews the literature in search of a single etiologic factor which could explain all spinal pain, one can become frustrated very easily. There are clinicians and scientists of considerable repute who have implicated each of the various spinal and paraspinal tissues in the etiology of spinal pain, and for most of the tissues there are at least two or three pathological processes which are considered possible causes of the noxious stimulus. Table 1 gives a breakdown of the more commonly quoted etiologic factors which are thought to be responsible for spinal pain.

In order for a clinician to make sense of the growing scientific and clinical literature on spinal pain and to utilize the available knowledge on the subject in the practical management of patients, it is necessary that he or she develop a working model of spinal pain. A logical place to start is with the neurophysiological processes

TABLE 1. Factors Implicated in the Pathogenesis of Spinal Pain Syndromes

Tissue	Pathological Process
Intervertebral disc	Degeneration
	Herniation
	Discitis
Posterior joints	Congenital asymmetry
	Subluxation
	Fixation or locking
	Sacrolization or lumbarization
	Rheumatoid or osteoarthritis
Vertebral body	Spondylosis
	Osteoporosis
	Intraosseous hypertension
Ligaments	Acute strain
	Chronic strain
	Laxity
Muscles	Poor muscle tone
	Muscle spasm
	Myofascial pain
Nerve root	Compression
	Stretch
	Inflammation
Sacroiliac joint	Subluxation
	Trauma
	Fixation
	Inflammation
Psychological status	Depression
	Anxiety

which are involved in the genesis of pain from spinal and paraspinal tissues.

Stimulus for Spinal Pain

The adequate stimulus for pain as defined by Sherrington (1906) is any event which threatens or causes tissue damage. The noxious stimulus may be mechanical, chemical, or thermal. An adequate stimulus for spinal pain could, therefore, conceivably include:

1. Stretching, tearing, compression, or crushing of tissue;

2. The release intrinsically or injection extrinsically of chemical agents such as acids, alkali, hypertonic solutions, or a variety of pain producing agents such as kinins, acetylcholine, or histamine;
3. The burning or freezing of tissues;
4. Ischemia, especially of muscle.

Most body tissues have the ability to react to noxious stimuli by releasing chemical compounds such as histamine, substance P, kinins, acetylcholine, serotonin, or acids. These agents have been demonstrated to cause pain when applied to free nerve endings (Lim 1970; Keele and Armstrong 1964, 1968). These agents are also considered important in the mediation of the inflammatory reaction which usually accompanies pain. Mediators of inflammation and pain have been shown to be released from degenerating intervertebral discs (Nachemson 1969), traumatic injury or inflammation of diarthrodial joints and ligaments (Melmon et al. 1967; Zvaifler 1973), and muscle hypoxia (Lim 1970).

These mediators, in turn, are thought to diffuse from the injured tissue to the vicinity of free nerve terminals where they bring about partial depolarization resulting in a lowering of membrane electrical threshold for the initiation of action potentials. The sequence of events leading to the initiation of nerve impulses in second-order nociceptor neurons in the spinal cord is illustrated in Figure 1.

The demonstration that serotonin (Sicuteri 1967) and prostaglandins (Flower 1973) can cause a decrease in pain threshold to the kinins, has led to the suggestion that it may be a combination of pain-producing substances which activate the nonciceptive chemoreceptors. It has been further suggested that prostaglandins released from the site of a lesion could sensitize afferent pain fibers to other mechanical or chemical stimuli (Flower 1973).

A number of high-threshold sensory receptors have been described in animals and man which, when stimulated, give rise to pain sensation. These receptors include:

1. Sharp point receptors which respond to

Stimulus
(threatened or actual tissue damage)
↓
Tissue reaction
(release of inflammatory agents)
↓
Transduction
(depolarization of nerve terminals)
↓
Initiation of impulses
in A Δ and C nerve fibers
↓
Conduction of nerve
impulses to spinal cord
↓
Release of synaptic
transmitter agent
↓
Depolarization of
second-order neuron

FIG. 1. **Hypothesized chain of events following application of noxious stimulus to tissue.**

pin-prick but not to a blunt probe (Burgess and Perl 1967; Iggo 1960);
2. High-threshold mechanoreceptors which respond to firm pressure or squeezing (Burgess and Perl 1967; Iggo 1961);
3. Polymodal receptors which respond to a variety of stimuli including changes in temperature and squeezing (Iggo 1959);
4. Low-temperature receptors which respond to cold (Iggo 1959);
5. Chemosensitive receptors which respond to a variety of chemical agents such as acetylcholine, 5-hydroxytryptamine, angiotensin, histamine, blood serum, etc. (Keele and Armstrong 1964, 1968; Lim 1970);
6. pH receptors which can be activated by either excessively acid or alkaline tissue changes; Lindahl (1961) demonstrated that pain is felt when tissue pH falls to 6.2;
7. Muscle ischemia receptors; it appears that muscle ischemia alone will not cause pain

until the muscle is exercised (Lewis et al. 1931; Iggo 1960). Lim 1970 has postulated that ischemia causes local hypoxia and acidosis which sensitize the chemoreceptors for pain in the muscle.

Pain-Sensitive Structures in Spinal and Paraspinal Tissues

The nerve terminal which is considered to act as the pain receptor is the free nerve ending. These free nerve endings appear as complex arborizations of fine, unmyelinated axons under the light microscope (Weddell et al. 1954; Wyke 1970; Fig. 2). The ending, which is thought to undergo continuous fragmentation and regeneration, is separated from the intercellular matrix by a basement membrane (Cauna 1968). Lim (1970) suggests that the anionic receptor sites in pain terminals may be located in the basement membrane which surrounds each Schwann cell and its contained axon.

Free nerve endings that have the capacity to react to noxious stimuli have been found in a number of spinal and paraspinal tissues. These structures with their nerve supply make up a spinal nociceptor system which, according to Wyke (1976), includes the following:

1. The skin and subcutaneous tissues of the back which contain a dense subepithelial meshwork of thin unmyelinated fibers with fine nerve terminals ramifying between epithelial cells of the skin surface;
2. The paraspinal ligaments, including longitudinal, flaval, interspinous, and sacroiliac ligaments, contain fine nerve endings which have been shown to weave between bundles of ligamentous fibers (Jackson et al. 1966; Wyke, 1970). These fibers are most dense in the posterior longitudinal ligament and least dense in the flaval and interspinous ligaments;
3. The fibrous capsules of the posterior zygapophyseal and sacroiliac joints are innerved through a plexus of fine unmyeli-

nated fibers (Pederson et al. 1956; Wyke 1970);
4. The periosteal covering of the vertebral bodies and arches has a dense plexus of unmyelinated nerve fibers that is continuous with the plexus innervating the articular capsule, fasciae, aponeuroses, and tendons (Jackson et al. 1966; Hirsch et al. 1963; Wyke 1970);
5. The dura mater and epidural adipose tissue contain a plexus of unmyelinated fibers that is more dense in the anterior dural fibers than in the posterior fibers and more dense in the dura itself than in the epidural adipose tissue (Edgar and Nundy 1966; Wyke 1970);
6. The walls of arteries and arterioles supplying spinal and paraspinal tissues contain nerves that are carried into the cancellous bone of the vertebral bodies, sacrum, and ilium by blood vessels which supply the bone and can therefore be irritated by pathological changes occurring within the bone (Jackson et al. 1968; Hirsch et al. 1963);
7. The adventitial sheaths of the epidural and paravertebral veins have a nerve supply which extends the nociceptor system throughout the epidural and extravertebral connective tissue (Pederson et al. 1956; Wyke 1970);
8. The paraspinal muscles obtain their nociceptive innervation primarily through the perivascular plexus of nerves which lies within the adventitial sheaths of arteries, arterioles, and veins (Lim et al. 1962; Iggo 1962).

The only spinal structures which do not have direct nociceptive innervation are the nucleus pulposis and inner layers of the annulus fibrosis of the intervertebral discs and the superficial layers of the articular cartilage of the posterior facet joints. A number of researchers have found a fine plexus of nerve fibers in the outer loose connective tissue fibers of the annulus fibrosis which is continuous with the periosteum of the vertebral bodies (Stilwell 1956; Hirsch et al. 1963).

These observations should not be interpreted as suggesting that degeneration or trauma of

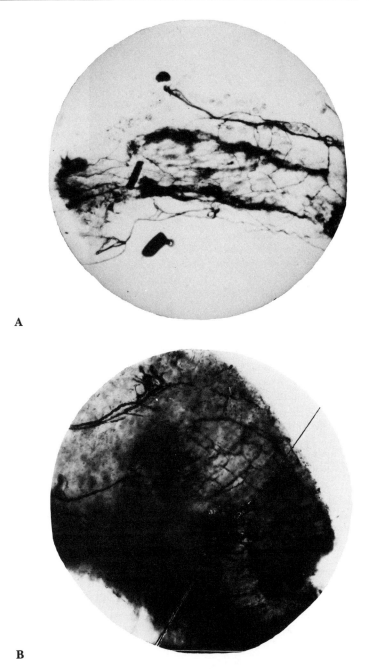

A

B

FIG. 2. (A). A small blood vessel, showing the plexus of unmyelinated nerve fibers that ramifies through its adventitial sheath (gold chloride method, ×210) (B). The plexus system of nerve fibers that ramifies with the blood vessels through the fibrous capsules of joints and through periosteum and dura mater (gold chloride method, ×210). (From Wyke B: Rheumatol Phys Med 10:365, 1970)

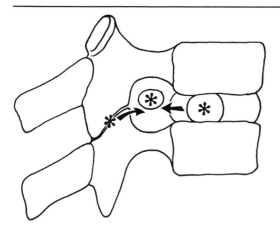

FIG. 3. **The posterior joints, nerve root, and intervertebral disc are in close proximity to each other. Inflammatory agents released from trauma to these structures may stimulate the same nociceptive receptors. (From Haldeman S. In Buerger and Tobis 1978)**

the disc and posterior joints are unable to cause pain. Nachemson (1969) has shown that degenerated intervertebral discs released acidic substances which may diffuse through the annulus fibrosis and activate nerve endings in the posterior longitudinal ligament, dura mater, and epidural tissues. It has also been demonstrated that degenerating articular cartilage can release inflammatory agents which may irritate nerve endings in the joint capsule (Melmon et al. 1967; Zvaifler 1973). The close approximation of the posterior facets, nerve root, and disc and the possibility that inflammatory agents released by irritation of any of these structures could stimulate the same plexus of nerve fibers might be one reason why it is so difficult to differentiate clinically the pain originating from these structures (Haldeman 1978; Fig. 3).

The possibility that spinal pain may, in certain patients, be due to the subthreshold stimulation of more than one spinal structure has been presented (Haldeman 1978). This multifactorial theory of back pain is based in part on the observation by Smith and Wright (1944) that pressure on a nerve root was more likely to cause sciatica if the nerve root was sensitized by disc herniation. The fact that disc herniation by itself need not be painful (Friberg and Hirsch

1949) also suggests that more than one factor may be responsible for spinal pain. This possibility is further supported by the work of Perl (1971) and Sicuteri (1967) who have demonstrated that in skin and muscle the threshold for pain may be lowered by previous tissue damage, repeated nerve stimulation, or muscle ischemia. This lowering of threshold may be so great that previously innocuous stimuli could become painful.

Afferent Pathways From Spinal and Paraspinal Tissues

The plexus of unmyelinated nerve fibers which make up the spinal nociceptor system sends impulses to the spinal cord via unmyelinated (less than 2 μ in diameter) C or group IV nerve fibers and to a lesser extent via small myelinated (2–5 μ in diameter) A delta or group III nerve fibers. These slow-conducting nerve fibers reach the spinal cord through three main peripheral pathways (Wyke 1970, 1976; Brodal 1969; Fig. 4):

1. *Posterior primary division of the spinal nerves:* The afferent nerve fibers which segmentally innervate the skin of the back in a dermatomal fashion, join with muscular branches from the dorsal paraspinal muscles to form the lateral branches of the posterior primary rami of the spinal nerves. The medial branch of the posterior primary rami of the spinal nerves is made up of afferent fibers from sensory receptors in the posterior apophyseal joints, the sacroiliac joints, the interspinous ligaments, the walls of blood vessels supplying the paraspinal muscles, the vertebral bodies and their arches, as well as the periosteum, fascia, tendons, and aponeurosis of the spine and paraspinal tissues. The apophyseal joints and posterior structures commonly receive an overlapping innervation from the nerve root above and below the structure making exact segmental localization of pain very difficult. A further complication to the problem of segmental pain localization is the observation that cer-

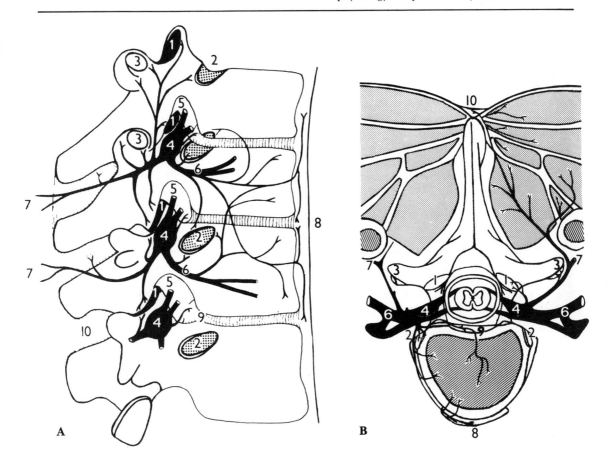

FIG. 4. **Nerve supply of the joints, ligaments, and periosteum of the thoracic spine, as seen in transverse (A) and vertical (B) section. 1, Apophyseal joints; 2, costovertebral joints; 3, costotransverse joints; 4, spinal nerve ganglia; 5, intervertebral foramina, containing dorsal and ventral nerve roots; 6, anterior primary rami of spinal nerves; 7, posterior primary rami of spinal nerves; 8, anterior longitudinal ligament; 9, posterior longitudinal ligament; 10, interspinous ligament. (From Wyke B: Rheumatol Phys Med 10:356, 1970)**

vical and lumbosacral nerve roots commonly have intersegmental connections (Pallie 1959; Pederson et al. 1956; Mulligan 1957). The fact that these connections do not exist in the dorsal spine might explain the apparent ability of patients to localize dorsal spine pain more accurately (Wyke 1970);

2. *Recurrent meningeal (sinuvertebral) nerves:* These nerves arise from each spinal nerve just distal to the dorsal root ganglion and turn back through the intervertebral fora-

men to supply the posterior longitudinal ligament, the ligamentum flavum, the anterior dura mater, epidural fat tissue and veins, and the walls of blood vessels which supply the vertebral bodies. Wiberg (1949) describes three patterns of distribution of the sinuvertebral nerve in the lumbar spine and notes that in certain people an afferent branch may descend up to two vertebral segments to innervate the posterior longitudinal ligament at that level. This anatomical observation is used as one explanation for poor localization of lumbar pain which may thus be felt to arise one or two segments removed from the irritable lesion (Wyke 1970);

3. *Centripedal branches of the paravertebral plexus of nerve fibers:* These small nerves extend the length of the vertebral column and innervate the paravertebral venous plexus, the longitudinal ligaments, dura mater, epidural fat, vertebral periosteum, and related connective tissue structures (Wyke 1970).

Spinal Cord Connections

The dorsal nerve root splits into two divisions as it enters the spinal cord. Most of the small-diameter nerve fibers which subserve pain assume a lateral or anterior position in the nerve root whereas the large-diameter nerve fibers tend to separate from them more medially (Ranson 1914; Brodal 1969). Evidence that pain sensation enters the spinal cord in the lateral aspect of the dorsal root comes from Ranson and Billingsley (1916) who found that vasomotor and respiratory reactions typical of pain responses were dependent upon the integrity of the lateral but not the medial division of the dorsal root.

The nociceptive afferent fibers penetrate the spinal cord and give off fine collateral branches which ascend or descend in the dorsolateral tract of Lissauer no further than one segment before sending filaments into the dorsal grey matter (Szentagothai 1964). In this way, the primary sensory fibers may influence up to two or three spinal cord segments.

The synaptic connections of primary nociceptive afferent fibers have not been clearly defined as yet. There is a direct excitatory connection with the posteromarginal cells in lamina I (Christenson and Perl 1970) which in turn have been found to contribute to the crossed anterolateral spinal thalamic tracts in the spinal cord (Foerster and Gagel 1932; Kumazawa et al. 1971). This monosynaptic pathway between pain receptors and the thalamus appears to be

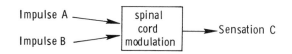

FIG. 5. **Implications of central convergence. Poor two-point discrimination; A and B cause an equal response in C. Referred pain: C interprets A as coming from B. Summation: A or B alone gives no response in C, while A + B gives a response. Inhibition (gate control): A alone gives a response in C, while A + B gives no response.**

the most direct method of transferring pain sensations to higher center.

In addition to the marginal cells, connections between afferent nociceptive fibers and neurons in lamina II, III, IV, and V have been found by means of degeneration studies (Ralston 1968; Scheibel and Scheibel 1968). There is a complex interaction between cells in these lamina which serves to modify the incoming neural information from nociceptors by interaction with impulses from nonnociceptive afferents and with descending excitatory and inhibitory impulses from higher brain centers. The convergence of impulses from multiple receptors onto the same spinal neurons and their interaction and modulation at this level has a number of important clinical implications (Fig. 5).

Poor Spinal Two-Point Discrimination. The observations that there are considerably more incoming afferent fibers than there are ascending spinal cord fibers (Ruch 1947) suggest that there is considerable convergence of afferent input in the spinal cord. The degree of convergence is considered one of the factors in two-point discrimination. The spine and paraspinal regions of the body have the poorest ability to two-point discriminate (Weinstein 1968) which further explains why patients have difficulty localizing spinal pain.

Referred Pain From Spinal Structures. The convergence of afferent fibers from skin, viscera, and muscles onto the same cells of the spinal cord (Pomeranz et al. 1968; Selzer and Spencer 1967) has served as an explanation for

FIG. 6. **Neuronal circuitry used by small and large primary afferent neurons in the dorsal horn of the spinal cord. In circuit A, small afferents (s) activate marginal cells (M) at the level of their distal dendrites. They also excite gelatinosa neurons (g), which probably provide modest inhibitory feedback to soma and proximal dendrites of marginal neurons. Circuit B is activated by large afferents (l) that excite dendrites of P cells as well as great numbers of gelatinosa neurons. The latter provide powerful inhibitory feedback to marginal neurons. Marginal neurons are thus excited by small afferents, many of which are nociceptive, and modulated by the combination of small-fiber and especially large-fiber excitation of inhibitory gelatinosa neurons. (From Kerr FWL: Mayo Clin Proc 50:685, 1975)**

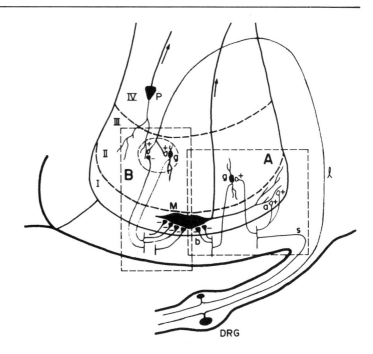

the clinical phenomenon of referred pain. The classic experiments of Kellgren and Lewis (1939) recently confirmed by Feinstein (1978) that irritation of spinal and paraspinal tissues by the injection of hypertonic saline can mimic a variety of visceral pain syndromes is one example of referred pain from the spine. The ability of a spinal lesion to mimic the pain of such disorders as angina pectoris, appendicitis, cholecystitis (Kellgren and Lewis 1939) may, in part, explain the anecdotal reporting of successful treatment of such disorders by practitioners of spinal manipulative therapy.

Summation of Pain From Spinal Lesions. The clinical observation that patients with back pain may have multiple factors which appear to influence their pain and may respond partially to the treatment of one of these factors can be explained, in part, by the phenomenon of summation. This physiological process is one of the characteristics of convergence, whereby input from two separate sensory stimuli may be inadequate to excite a response by themselves, but when stimulated together may summate to

bring about a central excitatory response (Haldeman 1978).

Interaction Between Nociceptive and Non-nociceptive Afferents. The activity of second-order neurons carrying sensory information to the brain can be influenced by the stimulation of other somatic afferent nerves (Pomeranz et al. 1968; Price and Wagman 1973). This observation, together with a number of hitherto unexplained clinical phenomena, led Melzack and Wall (1965) to propose the so-called "gate-control" theory for pain modulation in the dorsal horn. Since much of the original model for this theory has not withstood the close scrutiny of further research (Nathan 1976; Burgess 1978) it would not serve any purpose to present it in detail. The primary observation that pain sensation can be inhibited by other sensory input and input from higher brain centers, however, has been confirmed (Burgess 1978; Kerr 1975). Kerr has proposed a circuit diagram of the interaction between small and large nerve fibers in the dorsal horn of the spinal cord (Fig. 6). This model conforms more closely to current anatomical and physiological research than the model first proposed by Melzack and Wall in 1965. The interaction of peripheral sensory input has a number of important clinical applications when one considers the spinal pain syndromes.

Counterirritation and Acupuncture. These traditional methods of relieving pain have as their primary goal the stimulation of a large number of sensory receptors, often in the vicinity of the primary painful lesion (Kerr 1975). There are a number of reports in the literature which have demonstrated that these procedures can relieve pain (Gammon and Staff 1941; Stewart et al. 1977). The utilization of trigger point manipulation for the relief of spinal problems may well work through this neural mechanism. The fact that the trigger and acupuncture points have a very similar distribution (Melzack et al. 1977) further suggests a similar mode of action.

Partial Nerve Injury Causing or Potentiating Pain. There are a number of disorders which selectively destroy large-diameter nerve fibers. These disorders include postherpetic neuralgia (Noordenbos 1959), tabes dorsalis (Brodal 1969), rheumatoid vasculitis (Weller et al. 1970), and diabetes (Greenbaum et al. 1964). These disorders are often associated with a severe, painful peripheral neuropathy which at times can mimic radicular pain (Child and Yates 1978). Nerve compression similarly affects large nerve fibers before small nerve fibers (Haldeman and Meyer 1970). The question arises as to whether chronic neuropathies of this type might potentiate the pain which results from minor spinal injuries. Wyke (1976) quotes the observation by Ochoa and Mair (1969) that there is a selective degeneration of large-diameter nerve fibers with increasing age in adult life to explain the diminishing pain tolerance that characterizes older patients. There is, however, some disagreement with this point of view. Dyck et al. (1976) was unable to find any correlation between the amount of pain in peripheral neuropathies and the ratio of small to large nerve fiber degeneration. They also pointed out that certain diseases, such as Friedrich's ataxia, which are characterized by a highly selective large-diameter nerve fiber loss are not inevitably accompanied by pain. It is likely that many other factors play an important role in the modification of pain.

Spinal Nociceptive Reflexes

Stimulation of spinal pain receptors results in both segmental contraction of paravertebral muscles and discharges in sympathetic nerves (Wyke 1968). The somatosomatic reflexes occur through polysynaptic connections with alpha motor neurons in the anterior horn of the spinal cord (Lloyd 1960). The association of muscle spasm with spinal pain is a well-known clinical observation. The question often arises whether the muscle spasm is the cause of, or the response to spinal pain. It is possible that muscle spasm which occurs as a reflex may itself become painful causing a type of positive feedback circuit.

The visceral sympathetic response in the cardiovascular, respiratory, genitourinary and gastrointestinal tracts are being reviewed in this volume by Sato (Chapter 5). The clinical significance of these reflexes is still debated. Nonetheless, it is of interest that clinicians have reported a high incidence of spinal dysfunction in patients with such visceral disorders as chronic obstructive pulmonary disease (Miller 1975), ischemic heart disease (Rychlikova 1975), and peptic ulcer disease (Lewit and Rychlikova 1975). Again the question of cause and effect arises.

Descending Inhibitory System

The observation that severely wounded soldiers could block out pain completely was, in part, responsible for the proposal by Melzack and Wall (1965) of the existence of a central mechanism for inhibiting pain sensation. Since then, a number of researchers (Reynolds 1969; Mayer and Liebeskind 1974; Adams 1976) have found that direct stimulation of medial brainstem structures in animals and man can produce almost complete analgesia. The most consistent results occur on electrical stimulation of the central periaqueductal grey matter of the brainstem reticular formation. The effects are not considered causally related to the reward properties of certain brain centers since it often occurs at electrode sites which do not support self-stimulation (Mayer and Liebeskind 1974). The inhibition of spinal cord neurons on stimulation of the central grey matter can persist for up to 5 minutes beyond the actual period of brain stimulation (Liebeskind et al. 1973) and may develop gradually, achieving maximum effect after about 5 minutes of stimulation (Melzack and Melinkoff 1974). This latter observation has been considered to be due to recruitment of additional inhibitory neurons and has led to the suggestion that acupuncture analgesia, which shows a similar buildup of inhibition, may be due to activation of the reticular formation. Direct stimulation of dorsal column tracts can similarly cause significant inhibition of pain (Brown and Martin 1973) presumably by activating inhibitory descending pathways originating in the reticular formation.

The neurons in the periaqueductal grey matter that are responsible for the descending inhibition of spinal neurons have been shown to be the site of action of the opiate analgesics (Adams 1976; Fields and Anderson 1978; Kuhar et al. 1973). These sites have been found to be rich in peptides with morphinelike analgesic properties known as endorphins (Hughes et al. 1975; Simantov et al. 1976). The importance of these endorphins in the modulation of pain is becoming increasingly more obvious as research progresses. Recently, a relationship between pain tolerance and cerebrospinal fluid (CSF) levels of endorphins was noted (Knorring et al. 1978) which led to the suggestion that endorphins are one of the physiological factors that contribute to pain threshold and pain tolerance levels. Patients with psychological depressive disorders have been found to be relatively insensitive to pain (Knorring et al. 1974) and to possess increased CSF endorphin levels (Almay et al. 1978). Of similar interest is the observation that acupuncture analgesia can be blocked by

naloxone, an antagonist of the opiate analgesics (Sjölund and Eriksson 1976), and in certain patients increased endorphin levels in the CSF can be found after electroacupuncture (Sjölund et al. 1977). This suggests that in addition to a spinal gate-control inhibitory mechanism, acupuncture may have a central analgesic action mediated through a release of endorphins.

Another neurochemical agent which appears to be intimately involved in the central inhibitory mechanism is serotonin or 5-hydroxy-tryptamine. This agent is thought to be one of the primary neurotransmitters in both ascending and descending spinal pathways involved with the modulation of pain sensation. The evidence in favor of this role for serotonin has been reviewed by Messing and Lytle (1977). Brain serotonin, which is synthesized from the amino acid precursor tryptophan, has been found to decrease when animals have been fed tryptophan-free diets (Fernström and Wurtman 1971). These animals have, in turn, been found to be hyperalgesic to electroshock (Lytle et al. 1975) thus creating a potentially clinical relevance to the neurotransmitter. Moldofsky and Warsh (1978) have further suggested that there may be a measurable change in plasma-free tryptophan levels in patients with chronic pain such as "fibrobrositis." Attempts to treat these patients with dietary tryptophan, however, proved to be unsuccessful.

The primary pathways which are thought to be important in the descending inhibitory mechanism are shown in Figure 7. The periaqueductal grey matter can be activated through both ascending dorsal column system pathways (Brown and Martin 1973) or via descending pathways from higher centers. It, in turn, appears to inhibit the spinal cord nociceptor neurons directly through tryptaminergic inhibitory pathways and indirectly through pathways utilizing substance P as a transmitter which causes the release of endorphins in the spinal cord (Hughes 1978). The transmitter released at primary sensory terminals appears to be either glutamate (Haldeman and McLennan 1972) or substance P (Hökfelt et al. 1975; Krnjević and Morris 1974). This complex interaction of neural pathways and chemical

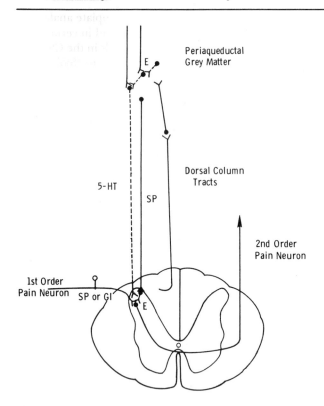

Periaqueductal
Grey Matter

E

5-HT

SP

Dorsal Column
Tracts

2nd Order
Pain Neuron

1st Order
Pain Neuron

SP or Gl

E

FIG. 7. **The major components of the descending inhibitory system for pain. Dotted lines, inhibitory neurons; solid lines, excitatory neurons. The chemical agents thought to be important in this system have been included. SP, Substance P; E, encephalin; 5-HT, 5-Hydroxytryptamine; Gl, glutamate. (Modified from Hughes J 1978)**

transmitters determines whether pain impulses will be permitted to pass from primary to second-order neurons in the spinal cord.

Ascending Pathways in the Spinal Cord and Brainstem

Nociceptive information is transmitted from the spinal cord dorsal horn cells to the nuclei of the brainstem and thalamus through a variety of ascending pain-signaling systems. In a detailed review of the literature Dennis and Melzack (1977) have listed six ascending pathways which appear to be capable of transmitting nociceptive information to the brainstem. From a purely anatomical point of view, these pathways can be divided according to their location in either the dorsal or ventral spinal cord. However, most authors find that a functional division is of greater value (Wyke 1976; Dennis and Melzack 1977). The so-called "discriminative system" is responsible for determining the location and quality of the painful stimulus, while the "motivational-affective system" is responsible for the emotional responses to pain.

Discriminative Ascending Pain Pathways

The Neospinothalamic Tract. The neospinothalamic tract has been known to be involved in the transmission of pain impulses since Spiller (1905) discovered that pain sensation in humans was diminished following lesions of the ventrolateral quadrant of the spinal cord. Mehler et al. (1960) states that this tract contains the phylogenetically more recent of the anterolateral tracts which are involved in pain transmission. This tract is considered to be the most direct pathway through which pain impulses from the spinal cord can reach the thalamus (Dennis and Melzack 1978). It is made up of large-diameter fibers with the ability to conduct impulses rapidly (Wyke 1976). This pathway is not exclusively for the passage of pain impulses. Pomeranz et al. (1968) found that 30 percent of the nerve units in this tract responded exclusively to noxious stimulation while the other 70 percent showed polymodal responses to a wide variety of tactile, temperature, and noxious stimuli. The nerve fibers in this tract cross the midline in the spinal cord and ascend in the ventrolateral spinal funiculus. They pass through the lower brainstem in close association with the medial lemniscus and end in the ventral posterolateral nucleus of the thalamus (Getz 1952; Lund and Webster 1967). These tracts have also been found to terminate on other thalamic nuclei and certain subthalamic nuclei.

The Dorsal Column System. This system has traditionally been viewed as carrying only innocuous tactile and proprioceptive impulses and this is still considered the major function of these large tracts.

Uddenberg (1968), however, found that over 25 percent of axons in the dorsal columns of the cat exhibited sustained, high frequency discharges to noxious stimuli. These observations have been confirmed by Anquat-Petit (1975) but, as yet, have only been observed in the cat. The nociceptive relays in the dorsal columns differ from the relays of other sensations carried in this funiculi. The proprioceptive relay is via the primary afferent neuron with its cell body in the dorsal root ganglia. The nociceptive relay, on the other hand, is via second-order neurons or postsynaptic dorsal column fibers whose cell bodies are in the dorsal horn of the spinal cord (Anquat-Petit 1972, 1975). The final destination of these neurons is as yet undetermined. Dennis and Melzack (1977), however, feel that they very likely follow the same course as the other dorsal column fibers to the thalamus, especially the ventroposterolateral nucleus.

The Spinocervicothalamic Tract. This pathway ascends in the dorsolateral funiculus to the lateral cervical nucleus. The efferents from the lateral cervical nucleus cross the midline to ascend in the medial lemniscus to the ventroposterolateral nucleus of the thalamus (Dennis and Melzack 1977). This tract, which was originally thought to be present only in lower animals, has now been demonstrated in humans (Kircher and Ha 1968). The fact that the lateral cervical nucleus can only be demonstrated in 50 to 60 percent of human cadavers (Truet et al. 1970) has led to the suggestion·that it may be "vestigial" in humans. This pathway is intimately involved with the transmission of pain impulses in cats, and Dennis and Melzack (1977) feel that it probably serves a similar function in humans.

In reviewing the literature and comparing the properties of these three pathways, Dennis and Melzack (1977) feel that the modalities they represent are qualitatively similar and include touch, pain, and temperature. However, there do appear to be minor differences in the type of sensation carried by each pathway—the neospinothalamic tract having a greater pain representation than the other pathways. These tracts all originate from the dorsal horn of the spinal grey matter, conduct at similar velocities, and project predominantly to the nuclei of the lateral thalamus as illustrated (Fig. 8). The tracts differ somewhat in the anatomical pathways they follow and the specific thalamic nuclei to which they project. There are also, apparently, some differences in the type of central inhibitory control which can be exerted on these three systems.

Dennis and Melzack have utilized these data to speculate on the rationale of having three systems for discriminative pain transmission. They feel that this arrangement may allow the response to pain to vary depending on what the person is doing at the time. Conceivably this could occur through inhibition or facilitation of these three nociceptive systems depending on the behavioral state of the body. This may be one explanation of why patients with spinal pain show such tremendous variation in their response to the pain at different times of the day and under differing circumstances.

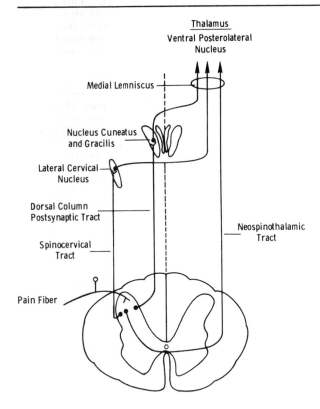

FIG. 8. **Diagram illustrating the oligosynaptic discriminative ascending pain pathways between the primary afferent fibers and the thalamus. (Modified from Dennis and Melzack 1977)**

The Motivational-Affective Ascending Pain Pathways

The Paleospinothalamic Tract. The paleospinothalamic tract projects to the midline and intralaminar thalamic nuclei rather than to the ventroposterolateral thalamus which is the terminal nucleus of the discriminative system. The cells of this tract are located primarily in the deeper lamina (VI–IX) of the dorsal horn of the spinal cord (Albe-Fessard et al. 1974). The fibers for the most part cross the midline in the spinal cord. However, some fibers may ascend ipsilaterally. They ascend in the ventrolateral fasciculus together with the neospinothalamic nuclei separating medially from the latter tract in the diencephalon to terminate in the medial thalamic nuclei (Dennis and Melzack 1977).

The Spinoreticular Tract. The spinoreticular tract originates from similar spinal cord cells as does the paleospinothalamic tract and ascends in close approximation to this tract. It differs from the paleospinothalamic tract in that a high percentage of these fibers ascend ipsilaterally (Kerr and Lippman 1973). The fibers separate from the spinothalamic tracts in the brainstem at various levels to terminate in a number of reticular formation nuclei (Pompeiano 1973). Reticular formation neurons in turn project to the periaqueductal grey matter where they interact with the descending inhibitory system. There are projections to the mesencephalic nuclei, the dorsal and posterior hypothalamus, and the midline and intralaminar nuclei of the thalamus (Casey and Jones 1978). The nociceptive input to the reticular formation has been found to be diffuse, poorly somatotopic and highly convergent with other sensory modalities (Dennis and Melzack 1977). The paleospinothalamic and spinoreticular fibers have also been shown to conduct at a slower rate than either the dorsal column or neospinothalamic fibers (Feltz et al. 1967).

The Multisynaptic Ascending and Descending Propriospinal System. This system exists in the spinal cord and connects different levels of the cord. The various components of the fasiculi proprii have been reviewed by Nathan and Smith (1959) who include the ground bundles, Lissauer's tract, and the cornicommissural, coma, and septomarginal tracts under this heading. These fibers mediate all those functions that continue after the spinal cord has been transected. Hannington-Kiff (1974) feels

that these fibers also ascend to the brainstem reticular formation and are partly responsible for the diffuse, nonspecific, persistent responses to painful stimuli.

The three pathways of the nonspecific motivational-affective system are illustrated in Figure 9. They make up a system rather than individual tracts with specific functions. This system appears to be less important in the perception and localization of pain. Instead, it is responsible for the less conscious spinal, brainstem, and affective responses to pain. It is through this system that an individual automatically withdraws from pain, changes blood pressure, respiratory and heart rate, and passes information to the hypothalamus and limbic system to bring about emotional responses to noxious stimuli.

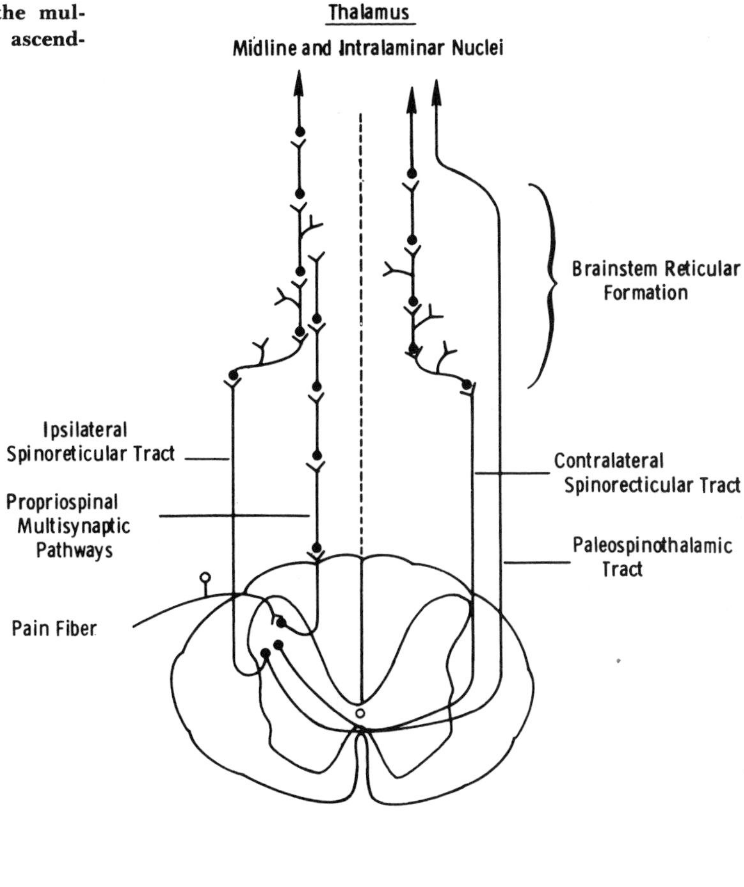

FIG. 9. **Diagram illustrating the multisynaptic motivational-affective ascending pain pathways.**

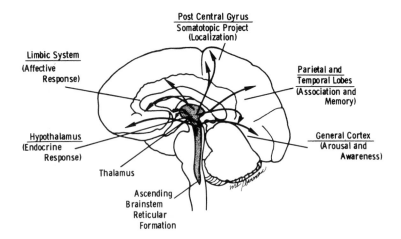

FIG. 10. **Diagram illustrating the major areas of the brain to which pain impulses project.**

Central Responses to Pain

The response of the brain to painful stimuli is an extremely complex one. There are very few higher functions which are not influenced to a greater or lesser extent by this extremely powerful sensory stimulus. Figure 10 illustrates those central functions which have been demonstrated to be influenced specifically by painful stimuli.

Perception and Localization

The major projection of the rapid oligosynaptic ascending pathway from the ventral posterolateral thalamus is to the postcentral region of the parietal cerebral cortex. This primary somatosensory cortex has a strict somatotopic spatial distribution of neurons which has been named the homunculus (Penfield and Rasmussen 1950). The back and neck have a relatively small homuncular area of representation in the lateral parasagittal region of the postcentral gyrus. This may account, in part, for the poor ability to accurately localize spinal pain.

Stimulation of the nociceptive pathways to the primary sensory cortex results in the specific anatomic localization of the stimulus and the recognition of the nature of the stimulus; i.e., whether it is throbbing, pricking,

pressing, bursting, or burning (Wyke, 1968; Nashold et al. 1972).

Much of the localization and perception of pain is felt to be secondary to concomitant stimulation of mechanoreceptors. This conclusion comes from the observation that exclusive stimulation of nociceptors results in little or no activation of postcentral cortical neurons (Mountcastle and Powell 1959). At the same time, direct stimulation of the primary and secondary cortex in unanesthetized patients does not result in the sensation of pain although it does evoke a variety of nonpainful somatic sensations (Penfield and Rasmussen 1950).

The Motivational-Affective Response

The distinctly unpleasant emotional sensation which is the hallmark of pain appears to arise from the phylogenetically older part of the brain known as the limbic system. This complex system of centers and pathways provides the mechanism whereby a pain stimulus is perceived as uncomfortable, aching, or hurting. Destruction of pathways or nuclei within the limbic circuit such as the orbitofrontothalamic projection system, the medial thalamus or cingulate gyrus results in a loss of this affective component to pain (White and Sweet 1969; Wyke 1968; Cassinari and Pagni 1969). When these pathways or nuclei have been surgically destroyed in man through procedures such as orbitofrontal leukotomies or stereotactic surgery in attempts to reduce pain, patients have noted that they are still aware of the fact that something is wrong with the body and can localize the sensation (through an intact somatosensory cortex). These patients, however, no longer complain of discomfort or pain (White and Sweet 1969; Nemiah 1962).

Activation of the limbic system by painful stimuli is primarily via neural connections between the intralaminar and medial thalamic nuclei and the cingulate gyrus and orbitofrontal cortex (Brodal 1969; Purpura and Yahr 1966).

General Arousal and the Focusing of Attention

In order for the cerebral cortex to receive and interpret a sensory stimulus and bring this sensation into conscious thought, it is necessary that the individual be awake and alert. The mechanism for achieving the state of general awareness or wakefulness and for focusing attention on a particular stimulus appears to lie in the brainstem reticular formation.

The reticular activating system extends from the medulla to the thalamus and has both ascending and descending components (Bowsher 1976). Activation of the ascending reticulothalamic pathways by stimulating specific reticular formation nuclei causes generalized cerebral arousal which can be determined both clinically and through electroencephalography (Pompeiano 1973). Similar arousal responses can be obtained by stimulating peripheral sensory receptors which connect directly with neurons in the reticular formation. Destruction of the medial reticular formation while sparing the long sensory tracts to the cortex results in permanent coma despite the fact that sensory input can still reach the cortex (French 1960).

The reticular formation is also, in part, responsible for the focusing of attention on specific sensations. The exact manner in which this takes place is still unknown. One possible mechanism is by modulating the input via the descending inhibitory pathways from the periaqueductal nuclei involved in the endorphin system. This mechanism could, conceivably, close the "gate" to all sensations other than that on which attention was being focused (Melzack and Wall 1965; Mayer and Liebeskind 1974).

The Establishment of Memory Engrams

The exact electrochemical process through which memory engrams are established in the brain is unknown. The storage and retrieval of memory, however, is of major importance in the interpretation of sensory input and allows an individual to correlate the nature, intensity, and associated sensations of the immediate stimulus with previous sensory experiences. This, in turn, allows for an appropriate response to the sensation.

The major storage site for memory engrams appears to be in the temporal lobes which receive thalamocortical projections from the medial thalamic nuclei (Brodal 1969; Purpura and Yahr 1966). The establishment of memory engrams for painful experiences has been noted to be a function of the intensity of the stimulus, the length of time the stimulus lasts and the frequency with which it is repeated (Wyke 1976).

The Visceral-Hormonal Response

The hypothalamus is considered to be one of the major centers for the control of sympathetic and parasympathetic activity as well as hormonal function (Haymaker et al. 1969). Input to the hypothalamus is via medial thalamic nuclei, the reticular formation and the limbic system (Martini et al. 1971). It is via these inputs that the viscerohormonal responses to pain are mediated. These responses include cardiovascular, gastrointestinal and hormonal changes (Engel 1959; Black 1970). Many of the cardiovascular and gastrointestinal responses are mediated through spinal or lower brainstem reflexes (Chapters 5 and 6, this volume). These responses are, in turn, modified and coordinated by higher centers in the cortex and hypo-

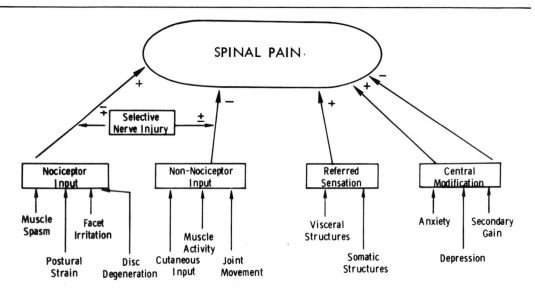

FIG. 11. **A diagramatic model for evaluating the various factors which might produce or influence spinal pain.**

thalamus. The discovery of a direct effect of the enkephalins and opiate antagonists on the secretion of pituitary hormones (Stubbs et al. 1978; von Graffenreid et al. 1978; Rivier et al. 1977) together with the growing number of metabolic and neuronal functions which are being found to be influenced by these natural peptides, has led to the suggestion that there may be an enkephalinergic system which has a physiological role in providing a link between perception, behavior, neuroendocrine regulation, endocrine secretion, and metabolism (Stubbs et al. 1978).

A Conceptual Approach to Spinal Pain Syndromes

When reviewing the neurophysiology of pain in the above manner, it is very easy to disassociate physiology from a specific clinical situation. However, an understanding of the physiological mechanisms of pain and the specific anatomical, physiological, and psychological characteristics of the spinal pain syndromes is essential

if one is to approach patients with these problems in a logical manner.

Figure 11 presents a conceptual model that provides one method of evaluating a patient with spinal pain. In this model, spinal pain is not equated with any one pathological disturbance, such as disc disease or myofascial pain. Instead, it is viewed as the sum of all the anatomical, physiological, pathological, psychological, and environmental processes which are known to influence pain. These processes may be present to a greater or lesser extent in any one patient, but it is unlikely that any patient with pain can be considered to have only a single localized pathological lesion uninfluenced by psychological factors or sensory input from other receptors.

Figure 11 has been simplified to include only five major components to pain, ignoring for simplicity's sake environmental, metabolic, and other factors which may be of importance. Similarly, the input to each of these major components to spinal pain has been reduced to a few examples rather than an extensive list of all possibilities. The component marked "nociceptor input" could include any one or combination of pathological processes which were listed in Table 1. These processes will result in tissue destruction and are potential causes of primary back pain (Wyke 1976). The nonnociceptor input comes from rubbing, heating, or cooling the skin, muscle activity, joint movement, or any therapeutic (mustard plaster, electrocutaneous stimulators, etc.) means of stimulating peripheral receptors. This input may have the effect of closing the "gating mechanism" in the central nervous system thereby inhibiting pain. Selective nerve injury caused by systemic diseases such as diabetes and rheumatoid arthritis, or by nerve compression, may influence the manner in which the painful and nonpainful sensations interact. The possibility that the pain is being felt some distance from a pathological process must be taken into account. This referred pain may be from visceral or somatic structures and may be the primary cause of pain or simply contribute to the discomfort from which the patient is complaining. Finally, the psychological factors for anxiety, depression, or secondary gain are important components in the central modification of the pain signal and play a large part in determining just how the patient will respond to his or her pain.

If a complaint of spinal pain is viewed as a composite of all these factors, then it should be possible to determine, with thorough examination procedures, the relative importance of these factors in any particular patient.

References

Adams JE: Naloxone reversal of analgesia produced by brain stimulation in the human. Pain 2:161, 1976

Albe-Fessard D, Levante A, Lamour Y: Origin of spinothalamic and spinoreticular pathways in cats and monkeys. In Bonica JJ (ed): Pain. Advances in Neurology, vol 4. NY, Raven Press, 1974

Almay BGL, Johansson F, von Knorring L, Terenius L, Wahlstrom A: Endorphins in chronic pain. Differences in CSF endorphin levels between organic and psychogenic pain syndromes. Pain 5:153, 1978

Angaut-Petit D: Post-synaptic fibers in the dorsal columns and their relay in the nucleus gracilis. Brain Res 48:380, 1972

Angaut-Petit D: The dorsal column system. I. Existence of long ascending post-synaptic fibers in the cat's fasciculus gracilis. Exp Brain Res 22:457, 1975

Benn RT, Wood PHN: Pain in the back: An attempt to estimate the size of the problem. Rheumatol Rehabil 14:121, 1975

Black P: The Physiological Correlates of Emotion. New York, Academic Press, 1970

Bowsher D: Role of the reticular formation in responses to noxious stimulation. Pain 2:361, 1976

Breen AC: Chiropractors and the treatment of back pain. Rheumatol Rehabil 16:46, 1977

Brodal A: Neurological Anatomy in Relation to Clinical Medicine, 2d ed. London, Oxford University Press, 1969

Brown AG, Martin HF: Activation of descending control of the spinocervical tract by impulses ascending the dorsal columns and relaying through the dorsal column nuclei. J Physiol (Lond) 235:535, 1973

Burgess PR: Peripheral Modulation: Neurophysiological observations. Neurosci Res Program Bull 16:160, 1978

Burgess PR, Perl ER: Myelinated afferent fibers responding specifically to noxious stimulation of the skin. J Physiol (Lond) 190:541, 1967

Casey KL, Jones EG: VI Suprasegmental mechanisms. An overview of ascending pathways: Brainstem and thalamus. Neurosci Res Program Bull 16:103, 1978

Cassinari V, Pagni CA: Central Pain. A neurosurgical survey. Cambridge, MA, Harvard University Press, 1969

Cauna N: Light and electron-microscopical structure of sensory end organs in human skin. In Kenshalo DR (ed): The Skin Senses. Springfield IL, Thomas, 1968

Child DL, Yates DAH: Radicular pain in diabetes. Rheumatol Rehabil 17:195, 1978

Christensen BN, Perl ER: Spinal neurons specifically excited by noxious or thermal stimuli. Marginal zone of the dorsal horn. J Neurophysiol 33:293, 1970

Dennis SG, Melzack R: Pain-signalling systems in the dorsal and ventral spinal cord. Pain 4:97, 1977

Dyck PJ, Lambert EH, O'Brien PL: Pain in peripheral neuropathy related to rate and kind of fiber degeneration. Neurology 26:466, 1976

Edgar MA, Nundy S: Innervation of the spinal dura mater. J Neurol Neurosurg Psychiatr 29:530, 1966

Engel BT: Some physiological correlates of hunger and pain. J Exp Psychol 57:389, 1959

Feinstein B: Referred pain from paravertebral structures. In Buerger AA, Tobis JS (eds): Approaches to the Validation of Manipulative Therapy. Springfield, IL, Thomas, 1978

Feltz P, Krauthamer G, Albe-Fessard D: Neurons of the medial diencephalon. I. Somatosensory responses and caudate inhibition. J Neurophysiol 30:55, 1967

Fernström JD, Wurtman RJ: Effect of chronic corn consumption on serotonin content of rat brain. Nature (New Biol) 234-62, 1971

Fields LH, Anderson SD: Evidence that raphespinal neurons mediate opiate and midbrain stimulation produced analgesias. Pain 5:333, 1978

Flower RJ: Asprin-like drugs and prostaglandins. Am Heart J 86:844, 1973

Foerster O, Gagel O: Die Vorderseitenstrangdurchschaeidung beim menchen. Eine klinisch-pathophysiologisch-anatomische studie. Z Ges Neurol Psychiatr 138:1, 1932

French JD: The reticular formation. In Field J, Magoun HW, Hall VE (eds): Handbook of Physiology. Section 1. Neurophysiology. Washington, American Physiological Society, 1960

Friberg S, Hirsch C: Anatomical and clinical studies on lumbar disc degeneration. Acta Orthop Scand 19:222, 1949

Gammon GD, Starr J: Studies on the relief of pain by counterirritation. J Clin Invest 20:13, 1941

Getz B: The termination of spinothalamic fibers in the cat as studied by the method of terminal degeneration. Acta Anat (Basel) 16:271, 1952

Graffenried B von, del Pozo E, Roubiech J, Krebs E, Poldinger W, Burmeister P, Kerp L: Effects of the synthetic enkephalin analogue. FK 33-824 in man. Nature 272:729, 1978

Greenbaum D, Richardson PC, Salmon MV, Urich H: Pathological observations on six cases of diabetic neuropathy. Brain 87:201, 1964

Haldeman S, Meyer BJ: The effect of constriction on the conduction of the action potential in the sciatic nerve. South African Med J 44:903, 1970

Haldeman S, McLennan H: The antagonistic action of glutamic acid diethylester towards amino acid-induced and synaptic excitations of central neurons. Brain Res 45:393, 1972

Haldeman S: Why one cause of back pain? In Buerger AA, Tobis JS (Eds: Approaches to the Validation of Manipulative Therapy. Springfield IL, Thomas, 1978

Hannington-Kiff JG: Pain Relief. London, Heinemann, 1974

Haymaker W, Anderson E, Nauta WJH (eds): The Hypothalamus. Springfield IL, Thomas, 1969

Hirsch C, Inglemark BE, Miller M: The anatomical basis for low back pain: studies on the presence of sensory nerve endings in ligamentous, capsular, and intervertebral disc structures in the human lumbar spine. Acta Orthoped Scand 33:1, 1963

Hökfelt T, Kellerth JO, Nilsson G, Pernow B: Experimental immunohistochemical studies on the localization and distribution of substance P in cat primary sensory neurons. Brain Res 100:235, 1975

Hughes J: Intrinsic factors and the opiate receptor system. Neurosci Res Program Bull 16:141, 1978

Hughes J, Smith TW, Kosterlitz HW, Fothergill LA, Morgan BA, Morris HR: Identification of two related pentapeptides from the brain with potent opiate antagonist activity. Nature (London) 258:577, 1975

Iggo A: Cutaneous heat and cold receptors with slowly conducting afferent fibers. Q J Exp Physiol (London) 44:362, 1959

Iggo A: Cutaneous mechanoreceptors with afferent C fibers. J Physiol (London) 152:337, 1960

Iggo A: Non-myelinated afferent fibers from mammalian skeletal muscle. J Physiol (London) 155:52P, 1961

Jackson, HC, Winkelmann RK, Bickel WH: Nerve endings in the human lumbar spinal column and related structures. J Bone Joint Surg 48A:1272, 1966

Keele CA, Armstrong D: Substances producing pain and itch. London, Arnold, 1964

Keele CA, Armstrong D: Mediators of Pain. In Lim RKS (ed): Pharmacology of Pain. Oxford, Pergamon Press, 1968

Kellgren JH, Lewis T: Observations related to referred pain, visceromotor reflexes and other associated phenomena. Clin Sci 4:47, 1939

Kerr FWL: Pain, a central inhibitory balance theory. Mayo Clin Proc 50:685, 1975

Kerr FWL, Lippman HH: Ascending degeneration following anterolateral cordotomy and midline myelotomy in the primate. Anat Rec 175:356, 1973

Kircher C, Ha H: The nucleus cervicalis lateralis in primates including man. Anat Rec 160:376, 1968

Knorring L von, Almay BGL, Johansson F, Terenius L: Pain perception and endorphin levels in cerebrospinal fluid. Pain 5:359, 1978

Knorring L von, Espvall M, Perris C: Averaged evoked responses, pain measures and personality variables in patients with depressive disorders. Acta Psychol Scand Suppl 255:99, 1974

Krnjevic K, Morris ME: An excitatory action of substance P on cuneate neurons. Can J Physiol Pharmacol 52:736, 1974

Kuhar MJ, Pert CB, Snyder SM: Regional distribution of opiate receptor binding in monkey and human brain. Nature (London) 245:447, 1973

Kumazawa T, Perl ER, Burgess PR, Whitehorn D: Excitation of posteromarginal cells (Lamina 1) in monkey and their projection in lateral spinal tracts. XXVth Int Congr Physiol Sci 9:328, 1971

Lewis T, Pickering GW, Rothchild O: Observations upon muscular pain in intermittent claudication. Heart 15:359, 1931

Lewit E, Rychlikova E: Reflex and vertebrogenic disturbances in peptic ulcer. Rehablitacia VIII Suppl 10–11:116, 1975

Liebeskind JC, Guilbaud G, Besson JM, Oliveras JL: Analgesia from electrical stimulation of the periaqueductal grey matter in the cat: behavioral observations and inhibitory effects on spinal cord interneurons. Brain Res 50:441, 1973

Lim RKS: Pain. Ann Rev Physiol 32:269, 1970

Lim RKS, Guzman F, Rodgers DW: Note on the muscle receptors concerned with pain. In Barker D (ed): Symposium on Muscle Receptors. Hong Kong, Hong Kong University Press, 1961

Lindahl O: Experimental skin pain induced by injection of water soluble substances in humans. Acta Physiol Scand [Suppl] 51:75, 1961

Lloyd DPC: Spinal mechanisms involved in somatic activities. In Field J, Magoun HW, Hall VE (eds): Handbook of Physiology. Section I. Neurophysiology. Washington, American Physiological Society, 1960

Lund RD, Webster KW: Thalamic afferents from the spinal cord and trigeminal nuclei: an experimental anatomical study in the rat. J Comp Neurol 130:313, 1967

Lytle LD, Messing RB, Fisher L, Phebus L: Effects of chronic corn consumption on brain serotonin and the response to electric shock. Science 190:692, 1975

Martini L, Molla M, Fraschini F. (eds): The Hypothalamus, New York, Academic Press,1971

Mayer DJ, Liebeskind JC: Pain reduction by focal electrical stimulation of the brain: an anatomical and behavioural analysis. Brain Res 68: 73, 1974

McBeath A: The problem of low back pain, A Review. Wisc. Med. J. 69:208–210, 1970

Mehler WR, Feferman ME, Nauta WJH: Ascending axon degeneration following anterolateral cordotomy. An experimental study in the monkey. Brain 83:718, 1960

Melmon KL, Webster ME, Goldfinger SE, Seegmiller JE: The presence of a kinin in inflammatory synovial effusion from arthritides of varying etiologies. Arthritis Rheumat 10: 13, 1967

Melzack R, Melinkoff DF: Analgesia produced by brain stimulation: evidence of a prolonged onset period. Expt Neurol 43:369, 1974

Melzack R, Stillwell DM, Fox EJ: Trigger points and acupuncture points for pain: correlations and implications. Pain 3:3, 1977

Melzack R, Wall PD: Pain Mechanisms: A new theory. Science 150:971, 1965

Messing RB, Lytle LD: Serotonin-containing neurons: Their possible role in pain and analgesia. Pain 4:1, 1977

Miller WD: Treatment of visceral disorders by manipulative therapy. In Goldstein M (ed): The Research Status of Spinal Manipulative Therapy. NINCDS Monograph no. 15. Bethesda, MD, DHEW, 1975

Moldofsky H, Warsh JJ: Plasma tryptophan and musculoskeletal pain in non-articular rheumatism ("fibrositis syndrome"). Pain 5:65, 1978

Mountcastle VB, Powell TPS: Central nervous mechanisms subserving position sense and kinesthesis. Bull Johns Hopkins Hosp 105:173, 1959

Mulligan JH: The innervation of the ligaments attached to the bodies of the vertebrae. J Anat (London) 91:455, 1957

Nachemson A: Interdiscal measurements of pH in patients with rhizopathies. Acta Orthop Scand 40:23, 1969

Nagi SZ, Riley LE, Newby LG: A social epidemiology of back pain in a general population. J Chron Dis 26:769, 1973

Nashold BS, Somjen G, Friedman H: Paresthesias and EEG potentials evoked by stimulation of dorsal funiculi in man. Exp Neurol 36:273, 1972

Nathan PW: The Gate-Control Theory of Pain. A critical review. Brain 99:123, 1976

Nathan PW, Smith MC: Fasciculi proprii of the spinal cord in man. Brain 82:610, 1959

Nemiah JC: The effect of leukotomy on pain. Psychosomat Med 24:75, 1962

Noordenbos W: Pain. Problems pertaining to the transmission of nerve impulses which give rise to pain. Amsterdam, Elsevier, 1959

Ochoa J, Mair WGP: The normal sural nerve in man. II. Changes in the axons and Schwann cells due to aging. Acta Neuropathol (Berlin) 13:217, 1969

Pallie W: The intersegmental anastomoses of posterior spinal rootlets and their significance. J Neurosurg 16:188, 1959

Pederson HS, Blanch CFJ, Gardner ED: The anatomy of the lumbosacral posterior rami and meningeal branches of spinal nerves (sinuvertebral nerves) with an experimental study of their functions. J Bone Joint Surg 38A:337, 1956

Penfield W, Rasmussen T: The cerebral cortex of man: a clinical study of localization of function. New York, Macmillan, 1950

Perl EP: Is pain a specific sensation? J Psychiatr Res 8:273, 1971

Pheasant HC: Backache—Its nature, incidence and cost. West J Med 126:330, 1977

Pomeranz B, Wall PD, Weber WV: Cord cells responding to fine myelinated afferents from viscera, muscle and skin. J Physiol 99:511, 1968

Pompeiano O: Reticular formation. In Iggo A (ed): Handbook of sensory physiology. Vol. 2. Somatosensory System. Berlin, Springer-Verlag, 1973

Price DD, Wagman IH: Relationships between pre and postsynaptic effects of A and C fiber inputs to dorsal horn of M. Mulatta. Exp Neurol 40:90, 1973

Purpura DP, Yahr MD (eds): The Thalamus. New York, Columbia University Press, 1966

Ralston HJ: Dorsal root projections to dorsal horn neurons in the cat spinal cord. J Comp Neurol 132:303, 1968

Ranson SW: The tract of Lissauer and the substantia gelatinosa Rolandi. Am J Anat 16:97, 1914

Ranson SW, Billingsley PR: The conduction of painful afferent impulses in the spinal nerves. Am J Physiol 40:571, 1916

Reynolds DV: Surgery in the rat during electrical analgesia induced by focal brain stimulation. Science 164:444, 1969

Rivier C, Vale W, Ling N, Brown M, Guillemin R: Stimulation in vivo of the secretion of prolactin and growth hormone by B-endorphin. Endocrinology 100:238, 1977

Ruch TC: Visceral sensation and referred pain. pp. 385–404. In Fulton JF (ed): Howell's Textbook of Physiology. 15th ed, Philadelphia, Saunders, 1947

Rychlikova E: Reflex changes and vertebrogenic disorders in ischemic heart disease. Rehabilitácia [Suppl] 8:109, 1975

Scheibel ME, Scheibel AB: Terminal axonal patterns in cat spinal cord. II The Dorsal Horn. Brain Res 9:32, 1968

Selzer ME, Spencer WA: Convergence and reciprocal inhibition of visceral and cutaneous afferents in the spinal cord. Fed Proc 26:433, 1967

Sherrington CS: The integrative action of the nervous system. New Haven, Yale University Press, 1906

Sicuteri F: Vaso-neuroactive substances and their implication in vascular pain. Research and Clinical Studies in Headache. Basel, Karger, 1967

Simantov R, Keehar MJ, Pasternak GW, Synder SH: The regional distribution of a morphine-like factor enkephalin in monkey brain. Brain Res 106:189, 1976

Sjolund R, Eriksson M: Electro-acupuncture and endogenous morphines. Lancet 2:1085, 1976

Sjolund B, Terenius L, Eriksson M: Increased cerebrospinal fluid levels of endorphins after electroacupuncture. Acta Physiol Scand 100:382, 1977

Smith M, Wright V: Sciatica and the intervertebral disc. J Bone Joint Surg 40A:1401, 1944

Spiller WG: The occasional clinical resemblance between caries of the vertebrae and lumbothoracic syringomyelia, and the location within the spinal cord of the fibers for the sensations of pain and temperature. Univ P Med Bull 18:147, 1905

Stewart D, Thomson J, Oswald I: Acupuncture analgesia: An experimental investigation. Brit Med J 1:67, 1977

Stilwell DL: The nerve supply of the vertebral column and its associated structures in the monkey. Anat Rec 125:139, 1956

Stubbs WA, Jones A, Edwards CRW, Delitala G, Jeffcoate WJ, Ratter SJ: Hormonal and metabolic responses to an enkephalin analogue in normal man. Lancet 2:1225, 1978

Szentagothai J: Neuronal and synaptic arrangement in the substantia gelatinosa. J Comp Neurol 122:219, 1964

Truex RC, Taylor MS, Smythe MQ, Gildenberg PL: The lateral cervical nucleus of cat, dog and man. J Comp Neurol 139:93, 1970

Uddenberg N: Differential localization in dorsal funiculus of fibers originating from different receptors. Exp Brain Res 4:367, 1968

Vear HJ: A study into the complaints of patients seeking chiropractic care. J Can Chiropr Assn 16(3):9, 1972

Weddell G, Pallie W, Palmer E: The morphology of peripheral nerve terminations in the skin. Quart J Microscop Sci 95:483, 1954

Weinstein S: Intensive and extensive aspects of tactile sensitivity as a function of body part, sex and laterality. In Kenshalo DR (ed): The Skin Senses. Springfield, IL, Thomas, 1968

Weller RO, Bruchner FE, Chamberlain MA:

Rheumatoid neuropathy: a histological and electrophysiological study. J Neurol Neurosurg
Psychiatr 33:592, 1970

White JC, Sweet WH: Pain and the neurosurgeon: a
forty years' experience. Springfield, Thomas,
1969

Wiberg G: Back pain in relation to the nerve supply
of the intervertebral disc. Acta Orthopaed Scand
19:211, 1949

Wyke BD: The neurology of facial pain. Brit J Hosp
Med 1:46, 1968

Wyke B: Neurological basis of thoracic spinal pain.
Rheumatology and Physical Medicine. 10:356,
1970

Wyke B: Neurological aspects of low back pain. In
Jayson M (ed): The Lumbar Spine and Back
Pain. New York, Grune & Stratton, 1976

Zvaifler NJ: The immunopathology of joint inflammation in rheumatoid arthritis. Adv Immunol
16:265, 1973

CHAPTER EIGHT
Computer-Aided Spinal Biomechanics

C. H. SUH

Biomechanics can simply be defined as a study of the mechanics of the biological system. Doctors of chiropractic use their hands for manipulation and/or adjustment of the spine and other joints. This means that chiropractors are using a system of force to achieve a clinical end. Chiropractors, like many other clinicians, face patients with pain and discomfort; thus, neurophysiological, psychological, and neurochemical considerations are essential to the chiropractor. Nonetheless, in order to analyze the spine and deliver an adjustment chiropractors must become specialists in spinal biomechanics.

The term *subluxation,* or *spinal subluxation,* is among the most important and most frequently used words in chiropractic literature. Some discussion on this term is therefore in order. The definition of *subluxation* varies. For example, *Stedman's Medical Dictionary* (1972) simply defines it as: "Semiluxation; an incomplete luxation or dislocation; though a relationship is altered, contact between joint surfaces remains." Chiropractors, on the other hand, often include neurophysiological disturbances in the definition of subluxation. This implies that subluxation has a living character which includes both biomechanical and neurophysiological abnormalities. For this reason, any conclusion regarding subluxation that is based solely on the study of cadavers is unacceptable.

This chapter will concentrate on computer-aided biomechanics focusing on the following three major areas:

1. A computer-aided precision x-ray method for the measurement of spinal displacement;
2. A computer model of the spine for simulated study of spinal subluxation (elastostatic model);
3. A computer model of the spine for simulated study of spinal adjustments (viscoelastic dynamic model).

A Computer-Aided Precision X-ray Method for the Measurement of Spinal Displacements

A Review of X-ray Methods in Biomechanics

The x-ray has become one of the most valuable clinical examination tools available. The graphical output of anatomical structures of the human body produced by x-rays generally serves as a "true picture" of the x-ray object. However, due to the large amount of distortion in the routine x-ray image generated by its inherent central projection characteristic together with other geometrical errors associated with x-ray equipment, an accurate measurement of fundamental biomechanical data (i.e., distance, angle, and relative position) from the x-ray image is impossible unless more accurate techniques are developed and applied.

Techniques known categorically as *photo-*

grammetry, which have been developed mainly for geographical surveys and map production, have recently been extended to x-ray photography. Numerous contributions in this area have appeared in the literature (Hallert 1970; Dodge et al. 1960; Nelson and Lipchik 1966; Wictorin 1964, 1966). However, these techniques are generally not sufficiently well formulated to be of use to clinicians. Recent radiological literature has mentioned the use of three-dimensional correction techniques (Lusted and Keats 1967). Dawson and his co-workers (1970) in Lancashire, England published an outline of a new method which uses the computer to study the relative positions of the brain and the axes of operating instruments in stereotactic surgery. The spine, because of its close relationship to the nervous system, has been of particular concern in the development of accurate methods of positional x-ray analysis. Special processes and apparatus for spinal positional analysis have been developed and patented by Vladeff (1942), Fox (1956), and Kuhn (1960). The latter was known as a *protractorscope.*

This chapter presents a rigorous fundamental analytical method of precision analysis of spinal x-rays. It is based on the reconstruction of three-dimensional geometry from x-ray films. The analytical method is being developed in such a way as to utilize the efficiency and accuracy of digital computers. When developed it should be possible to utilize a typical x-ray machine in common clinical use in its application.

Reconstruction of X-ray Geometry

For practical reasons, it was found to be necessary to reconstruct the geometry from information appearing on the x-rays themselves without recording the relative positions of the focus points, the object and the image planes. To solve this problem, a reference frame was x-rayed along with the object. In cervical x-ray analysis a helmet-type reference frame was used (Fig. 1). It is made of plastic plates with lead wires embedded in them. When a cervical x-ray is taken with this helmet in place, the lead wires of the helmet are clearly projected and appear around the cervical vertebrae on the x-ray film. Each of these lines on the x-ray film will, in general, appear to be longer than the premeasured true lengths of the lead wires in the helmet.

For three-dimensional analysis, at least two different views are required. In general, orthogonal projections are preferred because of the clear identification of the images and better intersections of x-ray projection lines in the reconstructed geometry. This results in higher accuracy.

Figure 2 illustrates the reconstruction and notations used in the computation. The rectangular reference frame has dimensions A, B, C, A_1, B_1, B_2, C_1, ΔX, ΔY_1, ΔY_2, and ΔZ, which are constant, known lengths measured with extreme accuracy. Two of the opposite side frames are identical. For the sake of simplicity in illustrating the basic method involved in the reconstruction, assume that P and Q image planes are orthogonal and parallel to the corresponding faces BC and AB of the reference frame.

Fixed coordinate axes (X,Y,Z) are established as reference axes in the geometrical system. The right-hand rule axes (X,Y,Z) are attached to the reference frame in such a way that any point in the reference frame is measured in the positive direction of X, Y, and Z as shown in Figure 2. The reconstruction then requires the location of the two focus points P and Q and the image P_1 and Q_1 with respect to the fixed coordinate axes (X,Y,Z).

Since most biomechanical measurements, such as distance, angle, and relative position, can be calculated by using the coordinates of a series of points in one fixed coordinate system, the process of using only coordinates of points (rather than attempting to measure angles or other geometric features) is sufficient.

To illustrate the procedure, the problem may be stated as follows:

PROBLEM: Let it be required to locate the point (x_1, y_1, z_1) with respect to the localized fixed (X,Y,Z) coordinate axes using the two

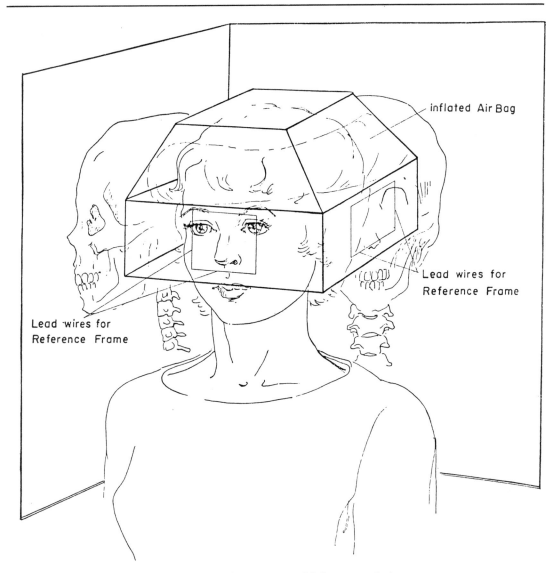

FIG. 1. **Helmet for computer aided x-ray analysis.**

x-rays; P image and Q image. Besides the two x-ray films, the only known parameters are the reference lengths A, B, C, A_1, B_1, B_2, C_1, ΔX, ΔY_1, ΔY_2, and ΔZ.

Solution of this problem has been presented in detail elsewhere with all the formula deriva-

tions and a numerical example (Suh 1972, 1974a). It consists of eight steps in a sequential method developed with analytical spatial geometry and algebraic manipulations. It gives four different sets of three linear equations which will give four different sets of solutions to x_1, y_1, and z_1 instead of one set.

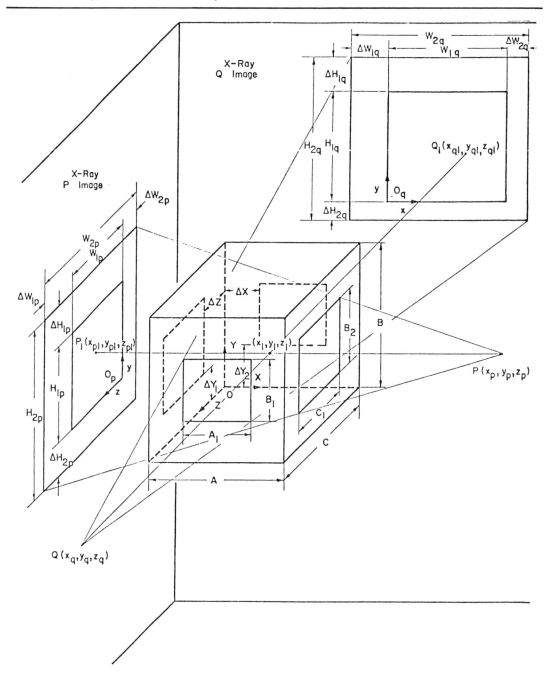

FIG. 2. **Geometry and notations for localized computer-aided x-ray analysis.**

Computer Implementation

The procedure, including error detection and discriminative measure, is a stepwise sequence and thereby renders itself to formulation with a simple computer program. Various computer programs written in BASIC and FORTRAN IV for conversational time-sharing terminals and conventional batch processing, respectively, are available together with appropriate user manuals. The simplicity of the program, as well as the recently improved time-sharing computing network, should make this system practical for any clinician or researcher with the mere addition of a single remote console and common telephone.

Discussion and Further Research

In securing the highest accuracy from computer aided x-ray analysis, the following three points should be kept in mind:

1. *Grid size of the reference frame.* A reduction in the lead wire grid in the frame has the advantage of being able to use a smaller x-ray and the production of better x-ray images of the lead wires themselves due to the wires being closer to the focal plane. However, a clear disadvantage must be noted which will limit the amount of grid reduction which is possible. The shortening of the reference lead wire lengths will make shorter images of these wires on the x-ray. This, in turn, will reduce the accuracy involved in the entire numerical procedure. Thus, an optimum size of the wire grid exists.
2. *Point identification.* Since an x-ray is actually a shadow of the object, there exists considerable inherent human error in locating the same geometrical points on the bones from different x-rays. This could be largely overcome by the following efforts:
   a. Through years of experience, clinicians and radiologists have acquired a great deal of anatomical insight which should increase the accuracy of locating corresponding points on the x-rays.
   b. Coordinate digitizers are commercially available which can more accurately determine point coordinates on the x-ray film. They also store the data automatically, eliminating the need for hand recording.
   c. Most of the x-ray analysis will involve positions and displacements. The rigid body condition of each bone should be used in the kinematic analysis to correct and/or improve the data points measured and stored.
3. *Structural errors.* The proposed method of x-ray analysis is based on correcting the distortion of central projection. However, the x-ray focus is not truly a geometrical point. Furthermore, the negative x-ray image planes are not true geometrical planes due to shrinkage and lack of flatness. Another source of structural error results from the opposite sides of the reference frame not being parallel.

In a series of experiments carried out with the prototype reference frames for cervical spinal analysis (Fig. 3), it was found that effects due to structural errors are much less serious than the two previously discussed factors. The total of these errors can be estimated by a calibration procedure using a precisely known object and placing it in the reference frame.

Our experience in using this x-ray method in a realistic environment has revealed a problem concerning point identification which requires further research in order to obtain higher accuracy with this method of x-ray analysis. Since a spinal subluxation is associated with the displacement of a vertebra with respect to other vertebrae, kinematic theories on rigid body displacement have been used (Suh 1973, 1974b). The x-ray data of spatial coordinates are required for the displacement analysis but unlike the other biomechanical analyses, such as distances between two points, angle between two lines, etc., displacement calculations require more accurate data. Therefore, it was necessary to correct the x-ray data before displacement analysis could be considered.

By definition, any displacement of a rigid body in three-dimensional space should not change its shape. In other words, the distance between any two points in a rigid body should

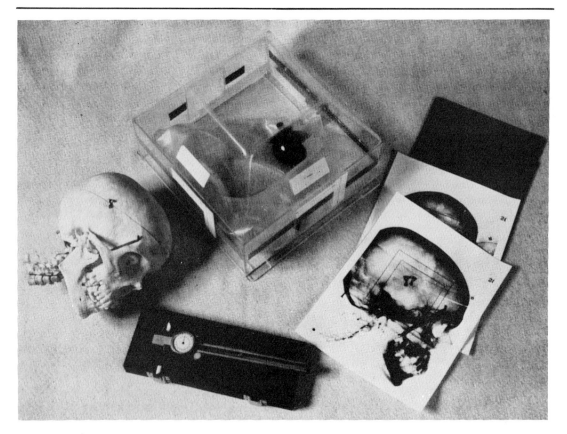

FIG. 3. **Experimental helmet of reference frame for cervical x-ray analysis.**

remain constant. Therefore, when the coordinates of the same points on a rigid body are measured in different positions and the distances between these points are calculated, they must be the same in any position. Since there is usually inherent measurement error, it is not necessarily true that the measured data will give the same lengths with accuracy. Two methods to correct the data which use the properties of a rigid body have been presented and discussed in an earlier report (Suh 1974b). Unfortunately, most of the facts discussed and developed in that report are difficult to prove by analytical geometry. Instead, numerical checks by computer outputs for the most possible cases are given.

The most essential part of the optimization problem is the construction of an objective function which can be minimized. It is known that the establishment of an objective function in analytical form is a difficult matter and often there is no universal systematic way to approach it.

The data correction problem can be formulated as follows: Assume that three points on a rigid body are measured at the two positions with some degree of measurement error. The reason why the three-point problem is important will become clear from the kinematics. Figure 4 shows the symbols and coordinates for each point; these symbols are used throughout this chapter.

Assuming there is some measurement error in A_1, B_1, C_1, A_2, B_2, and C_2, the calculated distances with these data (between these points) may not be equal:

$$\overline{A_1 \; B_1} \neq \overline{A_2 \; B_2}$$

$$\overline{A_1 \; C_1} \neq \overline{A_2 \; C_2} \qquad (1)$$

$$\overline{B_1 \; C_1} \neq \overline{B_2 \; C_2}$$

The problem is to change the coordinates such that these constant-length equations hold; that is fulfill rigid body conditions. Let the corrected points be A_1', B_1', C_1', A_2', B_2', and C_2', then

$$\overline{A_1' \; B_1'} = \overline{A_2' \; B_2'}$$

$$\overline{A_1' \; C_1'} = \overline{A_2' \; C_2'} \qquad (1')$$

$$\overline{B_1' \; C_1'} = \overline{B_2' \; C_2'}$$

For a solution to this problem, which obviously has innumerable solutions, we know that the corrected points depend on the selection of the objective function. Let us intuitively define the objective function as the sum of the corresponding distances between the original data points (A_1, B_1, C_1, A_2, B_2, and C_2) and the corrected data points (A_1', B_1', C_1', A_2', B_2', C_2');

$$
\begin{aligned}
f(&x_{a1}', y_{a1}', z_{a1}', x_{b1}', y_{b1}', z_{b1}', x_{c1}', y_{c1}', z_{c1}', \\
&x_{a2}', y_{a2}', z_{a2}', x_{b2}', y_{b2}', z_{b2}', x_{c2}', y_{c2}', z_{c2}') \\
&= \overline{A_1 A_1'} + \overline{B_1 B_1'} + \overline{C_1 C_1'} \\
&\quad + \overline{A_2 A_2'} + \overline{B_2 B_2'} + \overline{C_2 C_2'} \\
&= \sqrt{(\Delta x_{a1})^2 + (\Delta y_{a1})^2 + (\Delta z_{a1})^2} \\
&\quad + \sqrt{(\Delta x_{b1})^2 + (\Delta y_{b1})^2 + (\Delta z_{b1})^2} \\
&\quad + \sqrt{(\Delta x_{c1})^2 + (\Delta y_{c1})^2 + (\Delta z_{c1})^2} \\
&\quad + \sqrt{(\Delta x_{a2})^2 + (\Delta y_{a2})^2 + (\Delta z_{a2})^2} \\
&\quad + \sqrt{(\Delta x_{b2})^2 + (\Delta y_{b2})^2 + (\Delta z_{b2})^2} \\
&\quad + \sqrt{(\Delta x_{c2})^2 + (\Delta y_{c2})^2 + (\Delta z_{c2})^2}
\end{aligned} \qquad (2)
$$

where $\Delta x_{a1} = x_{a1} - x_{a1}'$, $\Delta y_{a1} = y_{a1} - y_{a1}'$, $\Delta z_{a1} = z_{a1} - z_{a1}'$, etc.

Now the data correction problem can be stated as an optimization problem as follows: Minimize the objective function f of Equation 2 subject to the constant-length equations of Equation 1.

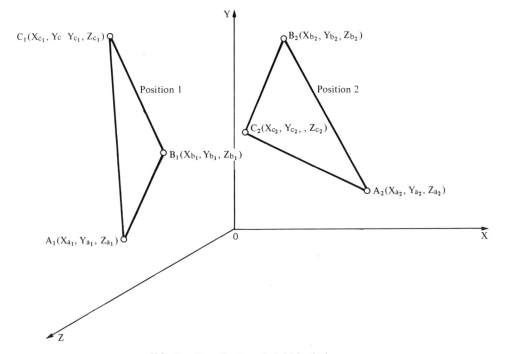

FIG. 4. **Coordinates of rigid body in space.**

Computer Model of the Spine for Simulated Study of Spinal Subluxation (Elastostatic Model)

A Review of Spinal Models

Creating a model of the complicated biomechanics of the spinal column presents a difficult challenge. The osteoid processes of the spinal column exhibit awesome complexity and multiple irregularities in structure. Supportive tissues of the spine express characteristically nonlinear behavior. Even static and dynamic tolerances of the spinal column seem erratic under various measurement attempts. Nevertheless, a model of the spinal column is obligatory for the eventual comprehension of relationships between imposed mechanical force and resulting spinal displacements.

Existing biomechanical data for the spinal column are not very appropriate for modeling attempts. While existing studies may represent creative simulations of automotive or aeronautical eventualities, they do not lend themselves to realistic approaches to most disorders seen by chiropractors. What one requires is a study on small, quasi-statis displacements of the spinal column. Unfortunately such studies are quite rare. It follows that the necessary biomechanical data for a comprehensive model of the spinal column are also rare or nonexistent. Precisely what measurements are required remains uncertain because only a comprehensive model will reveal the gaps in existing biomechanical information on the spine.

A model of the spinal column must accurately conform to mechanical constraints of geometry and force. In addition, such a model must provide some degree of anatomical reality. Recent advances in computer graphics make it possible to satisfy these requirements. By comparing the model with the results of a modified cineradiographic procedure used in continuous displacement analysis, it is possible to achieve a very accurate, realistic model applicable to clinical as well as research situations.

The spine as a major structure and the supporting column of the body has been a subject of biomechanics research for many years. In order to study mechanical and structural behavior of the spinal column numerous attempts to construct a model of the spine have been made. Most notable of these is the model by Illi (1951). He constructed a hardware model by placing an axis in the vertebral canal and by assembling wedged discs connected by wire. He used this model to demonstrate among other things that the spinal cord constituted the axis of the torsional movements of the spine itself.

In 1957 Werne described a conceptual biomechanical model of the odontoid ligaments in an attempt to illustrate the role of the delicate alar ligaments in spinal displacement. In 1969 Kopell described a spinal model and used this model to explain an acute back derangement by illustrating faulty stabilizing systems and muscle spasms. In 1972 Markolf, a research engineer at the University of California, Berkeley, constructed another hardware model of the spine. This model, made by bending and twisting metal, was developed as an aid in the design of braces and other supports developed to immobilize the spine.

These physical and mechanical hardware models are useful for the demonstration of basic spinal mechanics to laymen and researchers, especially if they are built with enough mobility. However, such modeling is seriously limited in its ability to represent the complex movements of the spine accurately. This is due mainly to the practically impossible task of finding or manufacturing artificial materials which duplicate the mechanical properties of the tissues involved, such as intervertebral discs, ligaments, and muscles. At the same time this type of modeling does not utilize many of the recent scientific and engineering developments made in modeling techniques.

A contribution, perhaps the most important and relevant work to our particular approach, has been made by Schultz (1974) at the University of Illinois. Since 1970 he has utilized digital computers and engineering mechanics to investigate spinal problems. Most of his work was closely associated with scoliosis and his attempt at solving spinal movement problems with highly nonlinear relations is still in its initial stages of development. The difficulty becomes obvious once one has to face a large number of highly nonlinear equations which must be solved simultaneously and repeatedly for continuous motion simulations. At the University of Colorado a highly efficient computer program has been developed to attack and overcome this difficulty. At the same time an investigation into relevant chiropractic spinal analysis procedures has been initiated with the development of the nonlinear-equation solver.

Mathematical Modeling of the Spine

Beginning in 1970, a research team was developed at the University of Colorado to initiate spinal modeling to meet the needs of biomechanic analysis. Since its inception, this model has utilized digital computers for numerical computations and computer graphics output. The development of this model can be followed by reading reports from the annual biomechanics conferences on the spine which have been held between 1970 and 1974 (Palsania 1972, Suh and Palsania 1973, Suh et al. 1973, Suh and Hong 1973, Suh and Kwak 1974).

In developing a three-dimensional computer model of the spine the following characteristics and capabilities are required:

1. The model should be basically elastostatic in nature to be useful at any particular position of equilibrium of the spine or spinal segment, whether the position is within the normal or abnormal range.
2. The model at the same time must possess the capability of performing voluntary spinal movements for the study of motion patterns and to investigate various kinematic parameters involved in the displacements.
3. The digital computer model should have the capability of storing the linear and nonlinear characteristics of discs, ligaments, muscles, and other tissues involved. All these characteristics of experimental biomechanics should continuously interact with the geometry involved in simulated spinal motion.

4. This model should also be developed simultaneously with computer graphic techniques so that the performing simulations are clearly, accurately, and continuously displayed graphically. Presently, at the University of Colorado most of the essential nonlinear computations involved are programmed and executed with the use of the University's dual CDC 6400 system with a CDC Computer Graphic system. New equipment, such as the Evans and Sutherland picture system are being proposed for future use to display the outputs in graphical forms, taking advantage of the increased line-drawing capacity.

Computer Graphics of Spinal Biomechanics

Computer graphics, which couples intuitive graphical presentations with high-speed computing, is being utilized in various health care systems and analyses. These are now major areas of research. The accelerating use of computer graphics has resulted in sophisticated diagnostic techniques. Clinicians are, however, often laymen in understanding computer techniques. Many times only computer-generated graphics can provide the "picture" necessary for a decision in intricate health care problems.

From a structural point of view the spine is the main column of the human body. Physiologically, it is the container of the spinal cord which, together with the brain, forms the central nervous system. A spinal subluxation is defined as abnormal displacement of one or more vertebrae with respect to others which may encroach upon or stimulate components of the nervous system or cause pain. Evaluation of the neurophysiological concomitants of mechanical displacements of the spinal segments demands accurate analysis of relative position and displacement of the various components of the spinal column in vivo.

Until recently the only technique available for continuous displacement analysis was cineradiography (Fielding 1957; Howe 1972). The development of a computer simulation model for the biomechanical study of the spine has added a new dimension to the study of spinal segmental displacement.

The development of spinal computer graphics at the University of Colorado, Boulder has been in two major areas: 1) three-dimensional computer graphics of the vertebra and 2) computer graphics of spinal displacement.

Three-Dimensional Computer Graphics of Individual Vertebrae. The investigation of three-dimensional computer graphics was initiated to obtain accurate perspective views of the complex, irregular, and anomalously shaped human vertebra (see Tsukutani 1972). Three examples of three-dimensional perspective plots of the atlas (the first cervical vertebra) generated by a Tektronix 4010-1 interactive graphics terminal (with Hard Copy Unit Tektronix 4610) are shown (Fig 5). These views reflect use of the program PPLOT package based on program PICPER developed by L. D. Matheson of the National Oceanic and Atmospheric Administration of the U.S. Department of Commerce, Boulder Laboratories, and H. Akima's smooth-curve fitting procedures (Akima 1970). The data of three-dimensional points are taken from a human atlas with a mechanical XYZ measuring device designed and developed at the biomechanics laboratory.

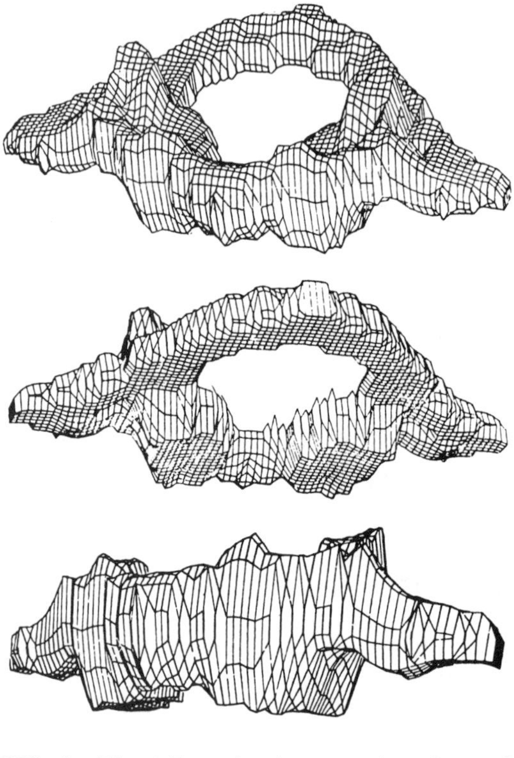

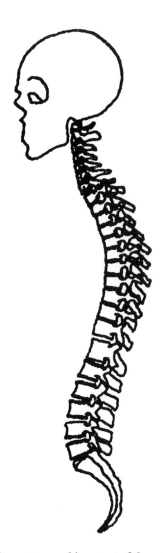

FIG. 5. **Three-dimensional perspective views of the atlas (1st cervical vertebra).**

FIG. 6. **Computer graphic output of the spine from skull to sacrum.**

Computer Graphics of the Spine. The major objective in developing computer graphics routines (Suh and Hong 1973) is to compare the displacement predicted from the mathematical and biomechanical model of the spine with those of a living human spine determined from cineradiographs.

In order to digitize the spine in the sagittal plane, a series of lateral spine x-rays are taken from skull to sacrum. Using these x-ray films and an overlay method, approximately 7000 data points are digitized by the cursor on the screen of the Tektronix 4610-1. These points are used to generate any segment of the spine in real scale or the full spine with skull in reduced scale as shown in Figure 6.

In order to simulate displacement the spinal discs are mathematically modeled (Suh and Dalsania 1973) using data obtained from the measurement of the mechanical properties of discs obtained from a fresh human cadaver (Markolf 1972). At the same time representations of various spinal ligaments and muscles are included in the model. In order to study the individual effects of some of these ligaments and muscles during spinal displacement, the names of these structures are given three letter codes (Fig. 7), which are displayed on the computer screen. The modeling of these ligaments and muscles has been derived from anatomical

```
LGA=CERVICAL LIGAMENT AND LIGAMENT NUCHAE
DSK=CERVICAL DISK
SCM=STERNOCLEIDOMASTOIDEUS
SCP=SCALENUS POSTERIOR
LOC=LONGUS CAPITIS
RCA=RECTUS CAPITIS ANTERIOR
RCL=RECTUS CAPITIS LATERAL
SCA=SCALENUS ANTERIOR
SME=SCALENUS MEDIUS
LCS=LONGUS COLLI SUPERIOR
LCI=LONGUS COLLI INFERIOR
LCU=LONGUS COLLI VERTICAL

LLG=LUMBAR LIGAMENT
LDS=LUMBAR DISK
PSO=PSOAS
EOB=EXTERNAL OBLIQUE
IOB=INTERNAL OBLIQUE
RAB=RECTUS ABDOMINIS
```

FIG. 7. **Coded muscle names and ligaments.**

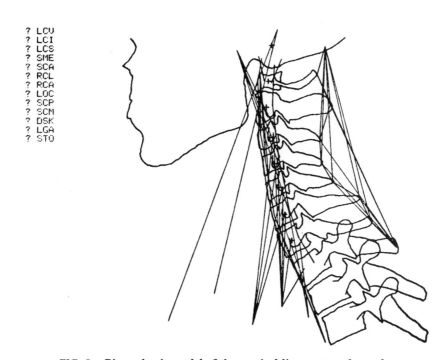

FIG. 8. **Biomechanic model of the cervical ligaments and muscles.**

studies to determine the geometric shapes of these structures connecting end points of the ligaments, as well as the origins and insertions of the muscles. Ligament and muscle models for the cervical and lumbar spine, respectively, are displayed in Figures 8 and 9.

Spinal Curvature Study. The spine is partitioned into primary and secondary curvatures. Physiologically, the thoracic curve is known to be present during fetal life and is called a primary curve, while the cervical and lumbar curves are due to development after birth under gravitational force and are called compensatory or secondary curvatures.

Applying different sets of muscular forces which act on the spine and are statically bal-

anced with the gravitational force, the changes of curvatures are observed on the screen and studies along with the change of the center of the curvatures. The computer is programmed to draw three circles for each of the major spinal curvatures and to print out the radius and center of each of the curvatures on the screen (Fig. 10).

Spinal Displacement Study. Cineradiographic studies of normal and abnormal spinal motion (Fielding 1957; Howe 1972) suggest that certain spinal disorders are closely related to patterns of voluntary movement of the spine.

The spinal model developed here has the ability to calculate each vertebral position under the influence of applied muscular forces. The elastostatic equilibrium positions are computed using displacement matrices by either a nonlinear simultaneous equation solver or a nonlinear optimization program, depending on whether the equations are based on a free body force and moment summation or the principle of minimum potential energy of the spinal system. Figure 11 shows the computer graphics output generated by this system for three different superimposed positions of the cervical spine including the skull. Inclusion of the skull enables us to study the motion pattern of the altantooccipital joint.

The superimposition technique allows one to study the path of each vertebra during flexion of the cervical spine. A similar study has been completed on the lumbar spine utilizing the same computer model (Fig. 12).

Three-dimensional simulation of the cervical spine was first developed in 1975 utilizing elastostatic systems analysis (Hong and Suh 1975). The cervical spine was chosen for the initial study because of the larger range of motion it provides thus making it easier to evaluate gross motion. Figures 13 through 16 illustrate the computer graphic presentation of the intervertebral discs, ligaments, articulating facets, and muscles. Each of the intervertebral discs in Figure 13 are modeled directly from the experimental data of cadaver spine discs by expressing the mechanical properties in nonlinear algebraic functions and then programming these functions as computer subroutines. All

```
? RAB
? IOB
? EOB
? PSO
? LDS
? LLG
? STO
```

FIG. 9. **Biomechanic model of the lumbar ligaments and muscles.**

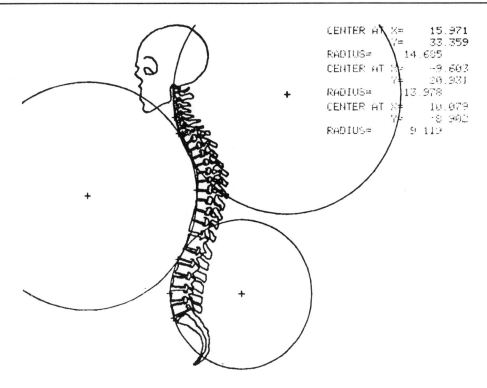

CENTER AT X=   15.971
         Y=   33.359
RADIUS=   14.685
CENTER AT X=   -9.603
         Y=   20.931
RADIUS=   13.978
CENTER AT X=   10.079
         Y=   -8.302
RADIUS=   9.113

FIG. 10. **Computer graphic display of primary and secondary spinal curvatures.**

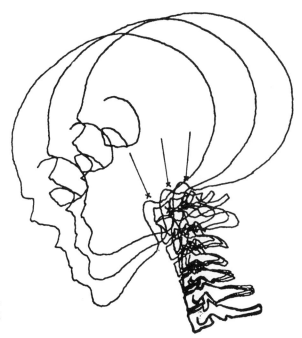

FIG. 11. **Three superimposed displacement positions of the cervical spine.**

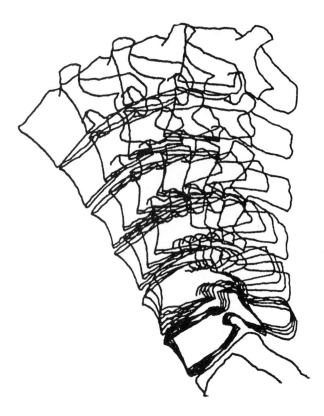

FIG. 12. **Four superimposed displacements of the lumbar spine.**

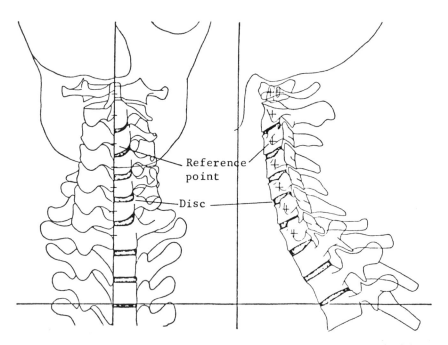

Reference point

Disc

FIG. 13. **Computer graphic presentation of the location of the cervical intervertebral discs and reference points.**

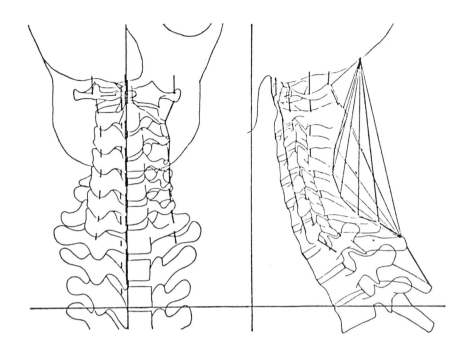

FIG. 14. **Computer graphic presentation of the cervical paraspinal ligaments.**

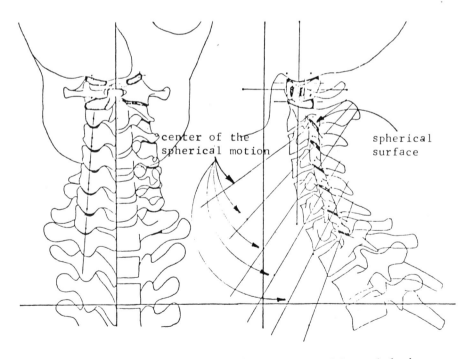

FIG. 15. **Geometric data for the articulating joints of the cervical spine.**

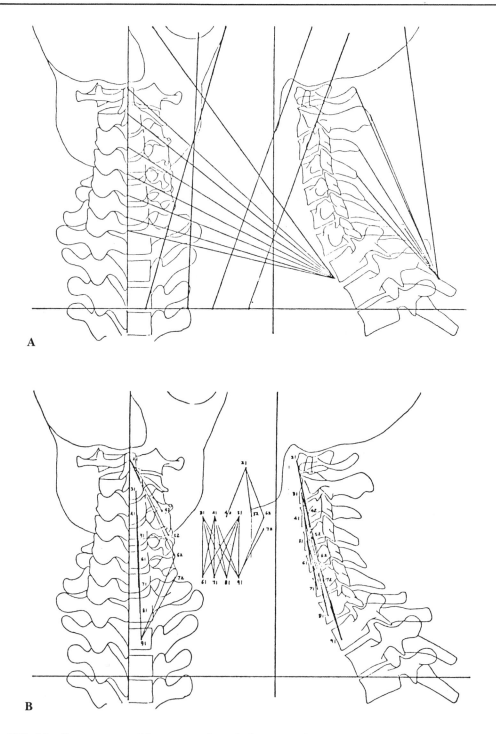

FIG. 16. **Computer graphic presentation of the cervical paraspinal muscles. (A) Sterno-cleidomastoideus and trapezius. (B) Longus colli.**

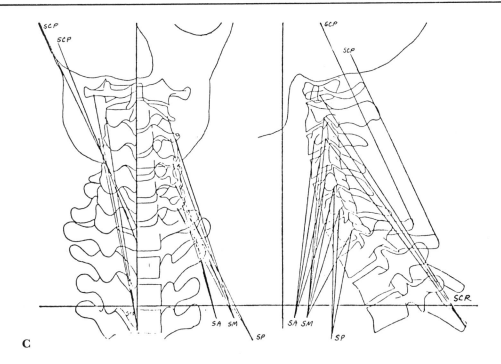

C

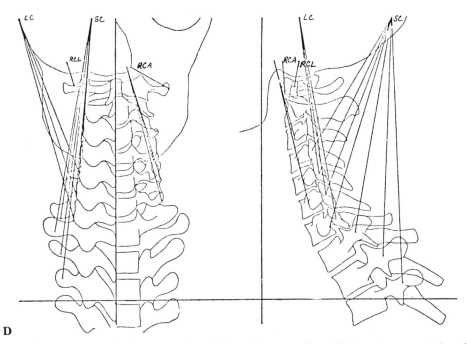

D

FIG. 16. (*cont.*). **(C) Scalenus anterior (SA), scalenus medius (SM), scalenus posterior (SP), splenius capitis (SCP), splenius cervicis (SCR). (D) Longus capitis (LC), rectus capitis anterior (RCA), rectus capitis lateralis (RCL), longissimus capitis (LCP), semispinal capitis (SC).**

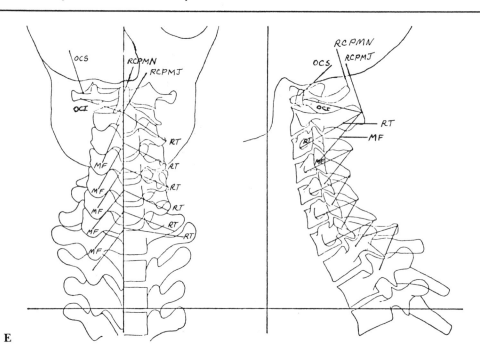

E

FIG. 16 *(cont.).* **(E) Rectus capitis posterior major (RCPMJ) minor (RCPMN), obliquus capitis superior (OCS) and inferior (OCI), rotatores (RT), and multifidus (MF).**

the ligaments shown in Figure 14 and the muscles shown in Figure 16 are geometrically modeled by straight lines. The surfaces of posterior facets that constrain movement of the cervical spine are geometrically modeled by spherical surfaces as shown in Figure 15. Figure 17 shows a typical result of this simulation study. In this case the muscle of Scalenus anterior is evaluated with three-dimensional computer graphics output.

Computer Model of the Spine for Simulated Study of Spinal Adjustments (Viscoelastic Dynamic Model)

Dynamics of Spinal Motion in Clinical Research

A spinal adjustment involves the introduction of a dynamic force directed at the spine in an attempt to correct a subluxation. It is possible to study the dynamics of spinal motion of a patient during and after adjustment by means of distortion-free x-ray analysis. In order to observe the actual mechanical history of vertebral displacements by this method one must compare two positions of the vertebra seen in pre- and postadjustment x-rays.

Another method which could be of value in studying the effect of the adjustment is mathematical modeling of the spine using a digital computer. Computer simulation has several advantages over cadaver studies and mechanical models. Once the program has been developed, it is simple to use and obtain reproducible data, and the parameters in the simulation can be changed quite easily, enabling many different cases to be analyzed. In addition, the mathematical model could be more accurate than a physical model, since no transducers are required for quantification. An efficient computer model of the cervical spine is, in the author's opinion, the best way to approach the problem of dynamic analysis of the spine.

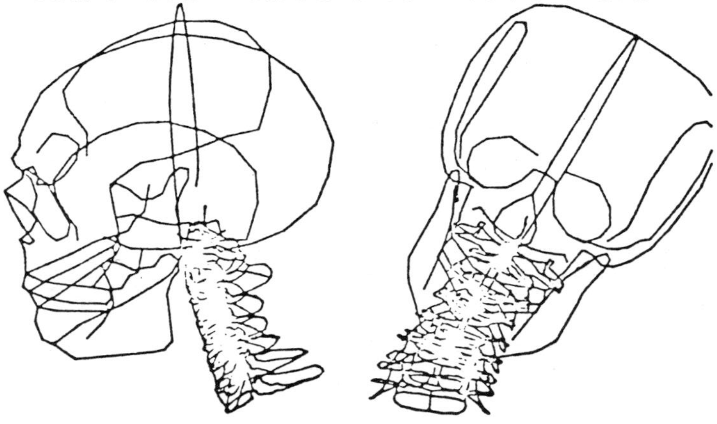

FIG. 17. Evaluation of the action of the scalenus anticus muscle by means of three-dimensional computer graphics. (Left) Both-side action. (Right) Single-side action.

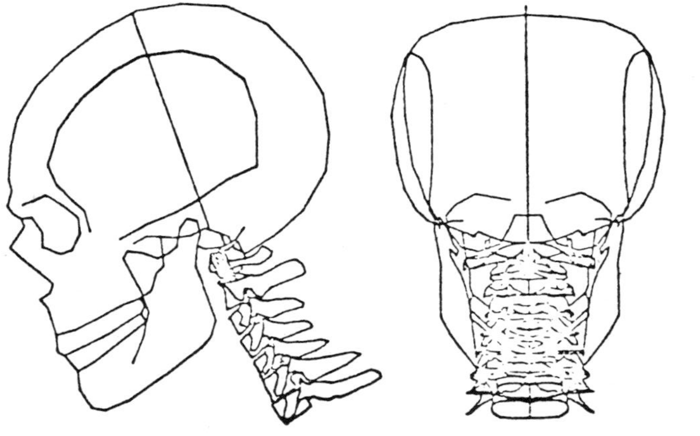

Modeling the Anatomical Features of the Spine

The first step in the development of a discrete element model for the spine is to determine how the actual anatomical features can best be represented in the computer model. The body parts that need to be modeled are the skull, the seven cervical vertebrae, the intervertebral discs, the connecting ligaments, the muscles attached to the skull and vertebrae, and the joints and articulating facets between the bony tissue. Once model elements are established for these parts, a method for writing and solving the equilibrium equations can be developed.

Ligaments

Ligaments are composed mainly of bundles of collagenous fibers placed parallel or closely interlaced with one another; they have a white, shining, silvery appearance. They are flexible, but strong, tough, and inextensible. Certain ligaments consist entirely of yellow elastic tissue; i.e., the ligamenta flava. The elasticity of these ligaments serve as a substitute for muscle power. In this model, the following assumptions are made about the ligaments:

1. A bundle of ligament fibers is modeled by one or more massless nonlinear spring-damper parts.
2. A ligament is connected at a point.
3. No moments are generated at the connecting points as the ligaments are assumed to be perfectly flexible.

Intervertebral Discs

Intervertebral discs are complex to model. Ligaments are basically tension devices and can easily be modeled by an element like a spring. The discs, however, attach over a large area and carry loads in all possible ways, and thus cannot be replaced by a few simple elements. Instead, the discs are modeled using experimental data directly. Data are collected by first establishing a reference frame on each of two adjacent vertebrae at their geometric centers. One vertebra

is fixed while the other is displaced in the desired way and force readings are taken. The positive and negative directions of the six degrees of freedom of the moving vertebra provide 12 different movements that must be tested. However, the lateral symmetry of the vertebrae eliminates three of these movements, as the positive and negative directions of those three should be the same. This symmetry leaves nine movements to be tested, namely: flexion, extension, rotation, lateral flexion, a transversal plane motion along the coronal direction, a positive and negative transversal plane motion along the midsagittal direction, elongation, and compression.

The data for each motion in each vertebral pair are then put into equation form through a curve fitting technique where

$$Y = f(X)$$

such that

$$Y = aX + bX^2$$

where Y is the moment or force, X is the displacement (rotation or translation), and a and b are determined by the curve filling. This testing of actual vertebral pairs must also include the dynamic properties of the intervertebral disc to establish the damping properties of the disc. This information about the curves is then written into a subroutine which will calculate the forces and moments exerted by the disc, given the relative displacement and velocity of the two adjacent vertebrae. It is assumed that the discs are massless. Since the relative displacements between adjacent vertebrae will be small, every displacement is assumed to be independent and the overall effect of a complex displacement is the sum of each independent displacement.

Muscles

Muscles work in two modes. They can exert force by contraction, or they can be passive and function similar to an elastic ligament. They are connected by flexible tendons. In the passive mode, the muscle is modeled exactly like a ligament with the same assumptions. In the active mode the muscle is considered to be a source of force, attached with a flexible joint that generates no moments at the connecting points.

Joints and Articulating Facets

Biomechanical joints are very difficult to model exactly. The function of a joint is to allow specific movement and restrict other types of movement. Biomechanical joints, however, usually are somewhat compliant to other types of movement. These joints could be modeled as complex mechanical joints, but the equations describing such a joint are complex and time consuming. This model assumes that the biomechanical joints can be modeled with a system of nonlinear spring-damper pairs, compliant in tension while stiff in compression, fashioned in such a way as to allow for easy movement of the desired type while restricting other types of motion. The compliance in tension allows for the fact that the bone joints are not connective. Forces may be transmitted only in compression.

It should be noted that the formulation of this model is based on qualitative information, not quantitative data. The anatomical features of the spine determine the configuration of the model. Unfortunately, accurate values for spring constants and damping coefficients are not as yet known. The geometrical information used in this model (location of muscle attachments, joints, masses, etc.) are more easily measured. Hong and Suh (1975) tested these data in a static model of the cervical spine and felt that the data used were valid. Values for the spring constants and damping coefficients used in this model are based on estimates and should not be taken as accurate.

Formulation of Equilibrium Equations

In a previous section, the anatomical features of the spine were modeled as a system of massless, nonlinear spring-damper pairs, rigid bodies, and applied forces. The single exception is the intervertebral discs, which were modeled using experimental data directly in an equation form obtained by curve fitting techniques. The discs can be viewed as a system of springs and dampers whose configuration is not known. However, the overall effect of the system is known. Therefore, dynamic analysis of the human spine now becomes the analysis of a system of nonlinear spring-damper pairs connected to a set of rigid bodies which may be acted upon by applied forces.

The analysis of this elastodynamic system requires the formulation of the equilibrium equations for each rigid body. Since a rigid body in three-dimensional space has six degrees of freedom, six equations for each rigid body are required. These six equations are defined by the simple relationships $F = ma$ and $T = I\alpha$, where F = force, m = mass, a = acceleration, T = torque, I = moment of inertia, and α = angular acceleration. The forces and torques in the x, y, and z directions are summed and equated to the accelerations multiplied by the inertial components in those directions. Since acceleration is the second derivative of position, the six equations will be second-order differential equations. Once these differential equations are formed, they must be solved at many points in time to establish the time relationship of the positions and velocities of the rigid bodies.

Formulation of Differential Equations Using Displacement and Differential Displacement Matrices

In order to calculate the forces and moments acting on the rigid bodies, the forces and positions of the spring-damper pairs, as well as the positions at which the applied forces act, must be determined. The positions of the geometric centers of each vertebra must also be known in order to find the forces and moments imposed by the intervertebral discs. It is possible to include the x, y, and z coordinates of each of these points as unknowns. However, there are only six equations for each rigid body necessary to determine its dynamic behavior. Additional constraint equations would have to be imposed to guarantee the rigid behavior of the rigid bodies. Obviously, if there are eight rigid bodies and 100 spring-damper pairs, several hundred equations and unknowns would have to be solved simultaneously.

By utilizing the characteristics of the displacement matrix (Suh 1968, 1975; Suh and Radcliffe 1978) and the differential displacement matrix (Suh and Radcliffe 1978; Suh 1971; Suh and Seo 1976) these several hundred equations may be reduced back to the original six equilibrium equations for each rigid body. A displacement matrix describes the displaced position of a rigid body in terms of its original position and a set of input quantities. Any point on that rigid body can be determined in the new position by multiplying the displacement matrix on the vector describing the original position of that point. The differential displacement matrix, or velocity matrix, similarly describes the velocity of a point in terms of the position of that point and another set of input quantities. The input quantities for the displacement matrix are the linear and angular displacements of the rigid body, and the inputs for the velocity matrix are the linear and angular velocities of the rigid body. Since these input quantities are the variables in the six second-order equilibrium equations, no more constraining equations are needed (Suh and Seo 1976).

In the model of the cervical spine, for example, intervertebral discs are modeled directly from data taken from actual spinal measurements. Since the geometric centers are the reference points for these data and the vertebrae are not symmetric in every plane, the center of mass may not coincide with the geometric center. Therefore, the displacement matrix is used to find the new position of the geometric center. The new positions of the geometric centers are inputs to a subroutine that calculates the forces and moments exerted on adjacent vertebrae due to that displacement. These forces and moments are also summed with the forces and moments due to the spring-damper parts and applied forces in the equilibrium equations.

Each rigid body has six second-order equilibrium equations. In the cervical spine model, there is a total of 48 equations to be solved si-

multaneously. The differential equations are solved on the computer by a routine called DASCRU (Suh and Seo 1976). DASCRU has proven to be a fast and accurate differential-equation solving routine. However, it can solve only first-order equations. The equilibrium equations must be transformed into first-order equations in order to be solved in DASCRU. To illustrate how this is done, consider the following second-order equation:

$$\ddot{A} = B\dot{A} + CA$$

Let the two unknowns (V_1 and V_2) in the solution be: $V_1 = A$ and $V_2 = \dot{A}$. The second-order equation is then transformed into two first-order equations:

$$\dot{V}_2 = BV_2 + CV_1$$
$$\dot{V}_1 = V_2$$

In the cervical spine model, a set of 96 equations are produced in terms of 96 unknowns describing the position and velocity of each of the eight rigid bodies. These 96 equations are then solved in DASCRU, starting at time $t = 0$ and progressing in small increments up to some final time. This is actually an integration process as the velocities are found by integration of the accelerations and the displacements are integrations of the velocities. The accuracy of these integrations increases as the time increment size decreases. The DASCRU routine automatically decreases the time increment size until sufficient accuracy is obtained (four-place accuracy).

The input to the system can be an initial velocity or position, or some forcing function. An initial velocity input would likely be used in the simulation of an auto accident. An initial position input might simulate a spinal adjustment. A forcing function input would be used to simulate muscular activity. Whatever the input, a useful form of output must be developed in order to fully utilize the information produced by the model.

Form of Output and Computer Graphics

A great deal of information is produced during a dynamic simulation of the cervical spine, namely the linear and angular displacements and velocities of eight rigid bodies at many points in time. The accelerations of the rigid bodies are also calculated. The model might calculate well over a million pieces of data in only a few seconds of simulation time. Obviously, the interpretation of these numbers into useful information could be a tedious and expensive task. Therefore, the ultimate value of a cervical spine model depends not only on the accuracy of the model, but also on the form of the information produced.

The particular application of the cervical spine model will determine what form of output is the most useful. The best form could indeed be the numerical results. For example, a researcher studying injury to the brain might know that values of acceleration would cause brain damage. For him, the most valuable information would be the maximum values of velocity and acceleration of the skull. These may be all that he is interested in. On the other hand, an engineer designing the interior of an automobile may only be interested in the path traveled by the skull during a simulated accident. For him, a graphic display of this motion may be sufficient. He probably has worked with accident simulation using mechanical dummies and high-speed cameras, and could best work with an output that simulates a high-speed film recording. Other types of research may require other forms of output from the cervical spine simulation either to relate to their current knowledge, or to provide new methods of analysis not possible with conventional techniques.

Sketching Method

In this method, a line sketch is drawn to represent each bone in the cervical spine. Enough points on those lines are measured from the sketch so that when the measured points are connected with straight lines, an approximation of the original sketch is reproduced. Examples of the graphics produced by the sketching method are shown in Figures 18, 19, and 20.

The sketching method eliminates the biggest problem of the grid and x-ray methods—the need for large amounts of data to be collected and stored in order to define the bones. For example, the sketching method uses 233 points to sketch the skull, and much less for each vertebra. Although the sketching method simplifies the collection and storage of data, the hidden-line elimination process cannot be used as the sketching lines do not define the boundaries of the body. If depth is required to make the three-dimensional effect clear, a varying intensity method is the most efficient. In other words, the intensity of a line varies according to the distance from the observer.

While the sketching method is the simplest method of graphically displaying the cervical spine, it is also the most readable for most people. Motion pictures can be generated using the same technique described in the x-ray method. As the dynamic simulation is being computed, the solution for each point in time can be drawn by the computer, either electronically or mechanically, and recorded with a movie camera or videotape. Rather than record every calculated solution, however, each second of simulation time is divided into a specific number of segments. If there were 200 segments per second, then the solutions for each multiple of .005 seconds would be drawn and recorded. The specific number of segments for each second depends on the type of playback device available and whether a real time viewing of the motion simulation is required. If so, the playback equipment must be capable of matching the recording intervals (200 frames per second in this case).

Example of Graphic Output

Consider the case of a passenger in an automobile. The car is struck on the left rear corner while stopped at an intersection. The passenger is wearing both lap and shoulder

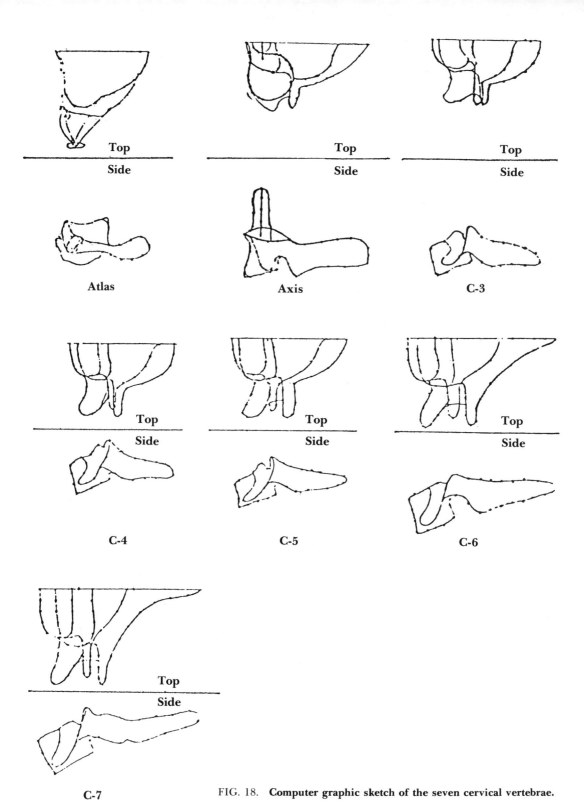

FIG. 18. **Computer graphic sketch of the seven cervical vertebrae.**

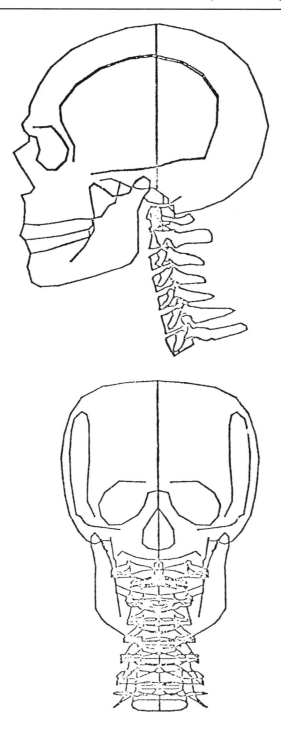

FIG. 19. **Completed front and side views of the skull and cervical vertebrae.**

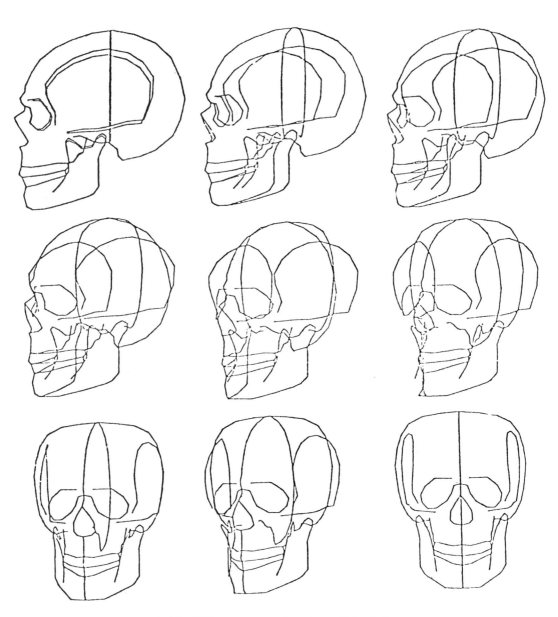

FIG. 20. **Different perspective views of the skull.**

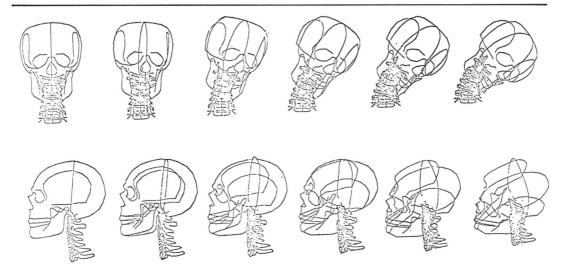

FIG. 21. **Simulated motion of "whiplash" reaction.**

belts and the car is not equipped with head restraints. This "whiplash" can be simulated using this cervical spine model. Assume that the first thoracic vertebra is given a velocity at time $t = 0+$. The velocities of the components of the cervical spine are of course still zero—the head will snap back and to the left. The muscles can be considered to be passive since the passenger will have no time to react to the accident.

A sample of the graphic output of this simulation at various points in time is shown in Figure 21. The solution has many points between these five pictures that would constitute a motion picture. The final motion picture records the total simulation in a form convenient for study later in time and not requiring the computer simulation to be repeated (Suh 1977).

REFERENCES

Akima H: A new method of interpolation and smooth curve fitting based on local procedures. J Assoc Comput Mach, 17:589, 1970

Dalsania V: A mathematical model for elasto-static systems and application to spinal analysis. In Biomechanics Lab Report, Boulder, University of Colorado, 1972

Dawson BH, Dervin E, Heywood OB: Geometrical problems in stereotactic surgery: a three dimensional analysis for use with computer techniques. J Biomech 3:175, 1970

Dodge HT, Sandler H, Ballew DH, Lord TD: The use of biplane angiocardiography for the measurement of left ventricular volume in man. Am Heart J 60:762, 1960

Fielding JW: Cineroentgenography of the normal cervical spine. J Bone Joint Surg 39A:1280, 1957

Hallert B: X-Ray Photogrammetry, Basic Geometry and Quality. Amsterdam, Elsevier, 1970

Hong SW, Suh CH: A mathematical model of the human spine and its application to the cervical spine. Proc 6th Ann Biomech Conf, Boulder, University of Colorado. December 1975

Howe JW: Cineradiographic evaluation of normal and abnormal cervical spinal function. J Clin Chiropr [Arch Ed] 2:76, 1972

Illi FW: The Vertebral Column. Chicago, National College of Chiropractic, 1951

Kopell HP: Help For Your Aching Back. New York, Grosset & Dunlap, 1969

Kuhn J: Protractorscopic and Stereoprotractorscopic Spinograph Analysis. Nashville, Parthenon Press, 1956

Lusted LB, Keats TE: Atlas of Roentgenographic Measurement. 2nd ed. Chicago, Chicago Yearbook, 1967

Markolf KL: Deformation of the thoracolumbar intervertebral joints in response to external loads. J Bone Joint Surg 54:511, 1972

Nelson CN, Lipchik EO: A computer method for calculation of left ventricular volume from biplane angiocardiograms. Invest Radiol 1:139, 1966

Schultz AB: Mechanics of the human spine. Appl Mech Rev, November 1974, p 1487

Stedman's Medical Dictionary, 22nd ed. Baltimore, Williams & Wilkins, 1972

Suh CH: Design of space mechanisms for rigid-body guidance. J Eng Ind Trans Am Soc Mech Eng (Ser B) 90:499, 1968

Suh, CH: Differential displacement matrix and generation of screw axes surfaces in kinematics. J Eng Ind Trans Am Soc Mech Eng (Ser B) 93:1, 1971

Suh CH: Computer-aided x-ray analysis of the spine (Parts I and II). Biomechanical Lab Report. Boulder, University of Colorado, November 1972

Suh CH: Displacement analysis of spinal system. Proc 4th Ann Biomech Conf, Boulder, University of Colorado, November 1973

Suh CH: The fundamentals of computer-aided x-ray analysis of the spine. J Biomech 7:161, 1974a

Suh CH: Researching the fundamentals of chiropractic. Proc 5th Ann Biomech Conf, Boulder, University of Colorado, December 1974b

Suh CH: Computer Aided Design of Mechanisms. Boulder, University of Colorado, 1975

Suh CH: Dynamic simulation of the cervical spine with use of the differential displacement matrix. Proc 3rd Int Conf Impact Trauma. Amsterdam, Free University of Amsterdan, 1977

Suh CH, Dalsania V: Computer implementation of spinal discs in biomechanical models. Proc 4th Ann Biomech Conf, Boulder, University of Colorado, November 1973

Suh CH, Dalsania V, Hong SW: Program "spine" for solution of elastostatic system. Proc 4th Ann Biomech Conf, Boulder, University of Colorado, November 1973

Suh CH, Hong SW: Computer aided x-ray data correction method with use of rigid body conditions. Proc 5th Ann Biomech Conf, Boulder, University of Colorado, December 1974

Suh CH, Hong SW: Computer graphics for spinal analysis. Proc 4th Ann Biomech Conf, Boulder, University of Colorado, November 1973

Suh CH, Kwak YK: Initial investigation for three-dimensional simulation of the spine as an elasto-static system. Proc 5th Ann Biomech Conf, Boulder, University of Colorado, December 1974

Suh CH, Radcliffe CW: Kinematics and Mechanisms Design. New York, Wiley, 1978

Suh CH, Seo YT: An elasto-dynamic model of the human spine by differential displacement matrix method. Proc 7th Ann Biomech Conf, Boulder, University of Colorado, December 4–5 1976, pp 143–212

Tsukatani T: Computer Graphics of Spine. Biomech Lab, Boulder, University of Colorado, November 1972

Werne S: Studies in spontaneous atlas dislocation. Acta Orthop Scand [Suppl] 23:1, 1957

Wictorin L: Bone resorption in cases with complete upper denture. A quantitative roentgenographic-photogrammetric study. Acta Radiol Suppl 228:97, 1964

Wictorin L: Measurements on roentgenographs, A comparison between two methods. Acta Odontol Scand 24(4):517, 1966

CHAPTER NINE

Symptomatology in Terms of the Pathomechanics of Low-Back Pain and Sciatica

H. F. FARFAN

To date there is no uniform or generally accepted interpretation of many of the terms commonly applied to the patient with low-back pain and sciatica. It is therefore justifiable to refer back to the terminology of Goldthwaite (1911) when referring to the patient suffering from low-back pain or sciatica. According to Goldthwaite, *sciatica* refers to the type of pain that often succeeds and occasionally precedes lower-back pain. In his terminology, there are two types of sciatica:

1. Neuropathic sciatica, along with other neuropathies, is usually accompanied by an impairment in nerve conduction resulting in diminished sensation, loss of muscle tone or strength, diminished tendon reflexes and occasional autonomic phenomena. The pain and tenderness follow the nerve trunks in the lower extremity, that is, the posterior midline thigh. As Goldthwaite stated, this syndrome occurred in 20 percent of patients. It was an unwelcome but not unexpected complication of ordinary sciatica.

2. The remaining 80 percent of patients with sciatica do not have these neuropathic signs. This common form of sciatica can be referred to as the *nonneuropathic syndrome*. The pain and tenderness is located over the gluteus medius, the greater trochanter, and the iliotibial band to the lateral calf. There are no neurological signs.

This definition of the neuropathic syndrome, or neuropathic sciatica, has the clear advantage of being in the same class as ulna, median, or other peripheral neuropathies; these syndromes are caused by compression or a combination of pressure and stretch and not by direct trauma or primary nerve inflammation.

The nonneuropathic type of pain appears to be pain stemming from any part of the somite. In this instance from any damaged structure, be it muscle, ligament, or joint in that segment. At the intervertebral joint this type of pain is most readily elicited from the facet joints, posterior longitudinal ligament, and posterior annulus. It can also be elicited from the healthy disc, interspinous and supraspinous ligaments, and muscle. This "mental" separation of the lower extremity pain types has helped considerably in the assessment of patients.

Degeneration or Trauma

The terms *degeneration* or *degenerative arthritis* should not be used when relating to the patient. These are misnomers and are seriously misleading to the patient. There is abundant evidence to suggest that degeneration is healing in the presence of repeated trauma. A simple comparison will make this clear.

Consider a sprained interphalangeal joint of

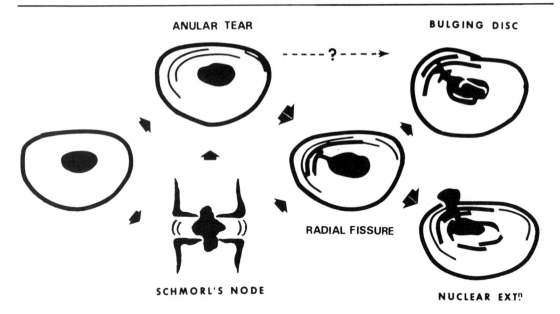

FIG. 1. Disc degeneration. Solid arrows, torsion trauma; open arrows, compression trauma. (Farfan HF: Mechanical Disorders of the Low Back. Philadelphia, Lea & Febiger, 1973. Modified from Farfan HF: J Bone Joint Surg 54A:492, 1972)

a finger. The injury is to the ligament that holds the joint surfaces together. When the ligament is ripped, the articular surfaces just slide off. They receive no injury. When the dislocation is reduced, the ligament heals by scar formation outside of the articular surfaces. The scar, like all scars, contracts thus returning the injured ligament to its original state.

But consider the disc. When the disc is sprained again it is the ligament which holds the end plates together that is torn. This ligament is, of course, the annulus and differs from the finger joint. This ligament is located between the end plates. Scarring of this ligament will cause the end plates to come closer together. Hence the radiographic finding of a narrowed disc. Would it not be better to tell the patient that there has been a cumulative injury to the disc which is healing rather than imply that his back is degenerating or falling apart? It is worse to compound the felony by telling him that it is going to spread to other joints (by telling him that he has degenerative arthritis); the usual connotation of the word *arthritis* is that of a

spreading disease. Truly, there is no place for the term *degeneration* in the diagnosis or treatment of the patient with low-back pain and sciatica.

The purpose of this chapter is to show that the etiology of disc degeneration is trauma. The basis of treatment is the understanding of the mechanism of injury. We propose to try to explain the major incidents of the degenerative process (Fig. 1). We can say that, like the finger, it is relatively difficult to injure the spine in the performance of its natural function which is flexion-extension. In flexion-extension motion, the main damaging force is overload in compression. On the other hand, like the finger, the spine is readily injured in performing an unnatural motion such as rotation. Similarly, it is relatively easy to injure the intervertebral joint by torsion.

In life, the spine is never subjected to pure compression or pure torsion. It is always subjected to a combination of loads. It is nevertheless reasonable to say that the spine suffers an injury mainly due to compression or one mainly due to torsion admitting a certain amount of arbitrariness and a certain degree of reservation because other modes of force application have not yet been studied.

Pathological Sequence of Fractured End Plate

The fractured end plate is the commonest pathological finding in the lumbar spine. Original descriptions of this lesion are to be found in the pathological studies reported by Andrae (1929) and Schmorl (1929). In studying these lesions at a later date, Key (1949) came to the conclusion that the Schmorl's nodes, as they came to be called, represented healing fractures of the end plates.

Four types—not necessarily four grades—of this injury exist in the laboratory (Fig. 2):

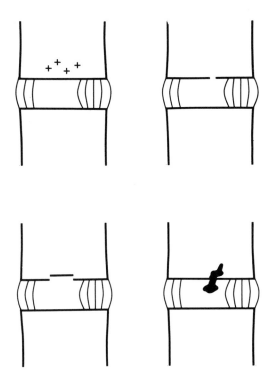

FIG. 2. **Various types of fractured end plate: (A) subchondral; (B) fissure fracture; (C) depressed fracture; (D) fracture with trapped disc material.**

1. Sub-end plate compression fractures of cancellous bone. The overlying end plate and cartilage is intact and so still maintains the normal fluid barriers between disc and vertebral body.
2. Fractures of the end plate and cartilage which open a communication between disc and vertebral body. These fractures are of three types: a) fissure fractures of the end plate; b) depressed fractures of the end plate; and c) fissures or depressed fractures with disc material forced into the vertebral body.

These fractures can all be created in the laboratory by compression of the vertebra-disc-vertebra unit. The application of axial load through the annulus causes bending stresses in the end plate. A linear fracture of the end plate can be produced in this manner even when the nucleus has been removed (Lamy 1978). Larger bending stresses can be induced in the end plate when the nucleus is present. This is not to say that the fracture occurs because the pressure in the disc is increased. Any bit of firm material in the center of the disc, such as degenerated disc material, will act like a punch and produce a punched-out fracture of the end plate.

A rise of pressure in the disc will not cause a fractured end plate, but by stretching the disc apart, the increased pressure ruptures the annulus. A fracture of the end plate can result if the end plates are restrained by a compressive force which is the normal state of affairs when intradiscal pressure is increased. The fractured end plate, though it heals, remains a weakness. Under normal conditions, the end plates can withstand high injection pressures in the disc. However, when Schmorl's nodes are present, very little injection pressure is required to re-open the communication between disc and vertebral body (Farfan 1973). The disc with a fractured end plate loses some of its stiffness. However, it does retain, in great measure, its capacity to support axial compression because the main resistance to axial compression is provided by the vertebral body cortex, the peripheral ring of the end plate, and the annulus.

The loss of the fluid seal between disc and

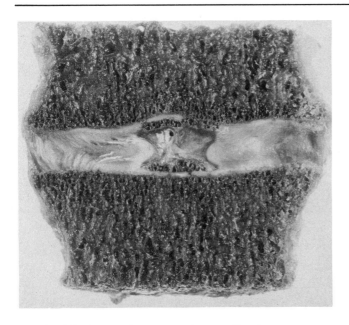

FIG. 3. **Natural fractured end plate. (Farfan HF: Mechanical Disorders of the Low Back. Philadelphia, Lea & Febiger, 1973. Modified from Farfan HF: J Bone Joint Surg 54A:492, 1972)**

vertebral body may have great import for the disc-vertebra unit as a whole when accelerated loadings are applied as in heavy lifting, rapid flexion-extension, or repeated motions. This is because of the hydraulic augmentation of the vertebral body's resistance to compression. As the vertebral body is compressed its fluid content is expelled through the resistance of its cancellous bone. The more rapidly the fluid has to be expelled, the greater will be the resistance offered by the porous cancellous bone. In other words, this mechanism ensures that with rapid loading, the vertebral body becomes strengthened by this mechanism. With fractures of the end plate, as with fractures of the peripheral cortex, this mechanism is impaired (Fig. 3).

Following a fractured end plate, the spine cannot be expected to handle loads which can only be manipulated at high speed. For people of great strength this limit would be in the neighborhood of 57 kg-m but for people of average strength this limit would be much less, probably half of this.

Schmorl's nodes tend to propagate from one end plate to the next in a sequence consistent with the hydraulic compartmentalization of the spine. Discs and vertebral bodies are initially separate compartments. Fractures of one end plate extend the compartment to include one disc and one vertebra, the second fracture will extend the compartment to include either the neighboring disc or else to the adjacent vertebral body and so on. The most common location of the Schmorl's node in the lumbar spine is in the upper two lumbar vertebrae where they seem to be of little clinical significance. They may, however, occur in the lower lumbar spine caused by the sudden impact of a fall on the buttocks or possibly by heavy lifting. There seems to be no reason to expect these injuries to be painless, but because they are undisplaced fractures in cancellous bone, one may expect rapid healing accompanied by rapid resolution of symptoms.

In those instances where disc material is trapped in the fracture it is not known whether the healing is delayed. In the laboratory, such displaced fragments may sometimes be extracted from the vertebral body by distracting the disc. Though this in vitro situation does not compare with that in life, it is possible that this phenomenon might well account for the success of a sudden manipulative elongation of the spine.

The axial compression overload does its principal damage to the disc and not to the facet joints. The facet joints of L1–2, L2–3, and L3–4 in all positions of the spine are in line with the axial overload. Those of the last two lumbar vertebrae come close to this alignment when the spine is in flexion, the position assumed for a heavy lift. This leaves them safe from the compressive overload.

The late sequelae of the end plate fracture have not been studied in any experimental model. We must extrapolate from what we know of the healing process to arrive at the probable sequence of events. At the onset, the disc loses its content and there is bleeding into the disc from the vertebral body. This is rapidly followed by the invasion of the disc cavity by granulation tissue which accounts for the digestion or gradual resolution of the avascular end plate cartilage and inner annulus. With the loss of disc material, the disc loses its thickness and the adjacent vertebrae come closer and closer together. The remaining viable outer annulus is pushed gradually over the end plate rim causing osteophyte formation.

Accompanying the loss of disc thickness, the facet joints subluxate becoming arthritic and painful, especially when subjected to weight bearing; i.e., long standing or sitting, particularly if the spine is forced in extension or flexion (Figs. 4 and 5). Furthermore, the subluxation of the facets may result in lateral entrapment of the nerve root, the superior facet coming quite close to the nerve as it passes outward around the pedicle of the vertebra above (Fig. 6). Such a joint does not have any increased mobility and it gets stiffer and stiffer with passing years. Its natural progression often leads to a natural ankylosis or fusion. It seems unlikely that mobilization of such a joint could do anything except produce an inflammatory response which, in turn, would only increase the stiffness or at worse initiate the lateral entrapment syndrome.

In the entire sequence outlined above, there is no mention of disc protrusion. This is simply because with compression axial overload the disc may bulge but never sufficiently enough to interfere with the neural canal content. The high axial loads in life are generated in the

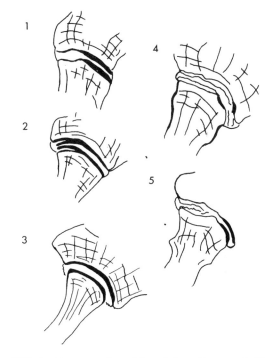

FIG. 4. **Degeneration of facet joints. (1) normal; (2) fragmentation of cartilage; (3) loss of cartilage, early osteoporosis; (4) crush fracture of base articular process, synovial invasion of widened joint and advancing osteoporosis; (5) almost total loss of cartilage, further synovial invasion of joint space, osteoporosis. (Farfan HF: Mechanical Disorders of the Low Back. Philadelphia, Lea & Febiger, 1973. Modified from Farfan HF: J Bone Joint Surg 54A:492, 1972.)**

flexed position and with forward flexion, the posterior disc annulus does not bulge backward into the canal. In fact, it becomes flattened or even slightly concave.

In a very special set of circumstances, high compression loads may result in disc protrusion into the neural canal. This particular situation may arise with a sudden fall on the buttocks which finds the intervertebral joint unconstrained by tight ligaments (spine not fully flexed) and the muscles inactive.

In the laboratory, the intervertebral joint is found to be very resistant to compression axial load withstanding nearly one ton of compres-

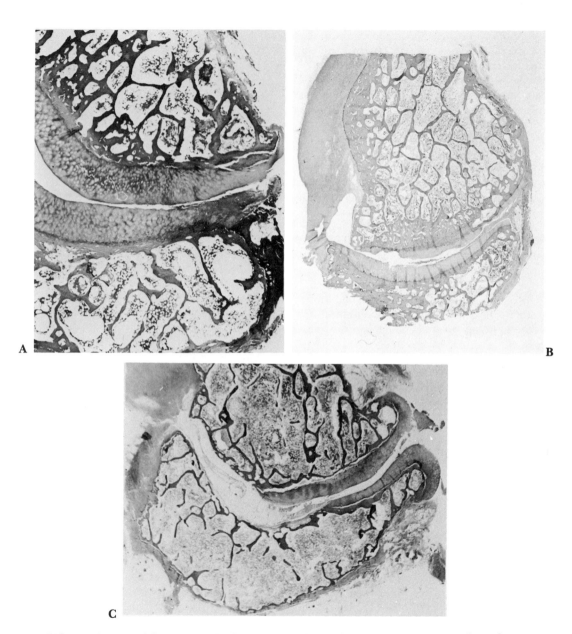

FIG. 5. (A) Normal facet. (B) Early degeneration of articular cartilage. Note mass of new bone formation at the inferior margin of the lamina closer to the facet. (C) Ulcerations are more advanced. Note tongue of synovial tissue growing into the joint from its ventral aspect.

D

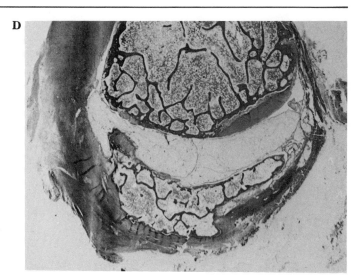

FIG. 5 (*cont.*). (D) Marked erosion of articular cartilage on both sides of joint with loss of subchondral bone and thinning of the bony trabeculae on both sides of the joint. Large fatty synovial mass separating the articular surfaces. (Farfan HF: Mechanical Disorders of the Low Back. Philadelphia, Lea & Febiger, 1973. Modified from Farfan HF: J Bone Joint Surg 54A:492, 1972)

sion before failure. It requires a lift of over 180 kg to produce compression loads of this order in young healthy individuals. By comparison, the intervertebral joint is very susceptible to torsion requiring a one-handed lift of less than 45 kg to generate the 9.4 kg-m of torque required to damage the joint (Farfan et al. 1970).

The Pathological Sequence of Torsional Overload

Lumbar joints are not all equally sensitive to torsion. The joint with a more rounded disc shape tends to be less sensitive to torsion than that with a more oval shape. The lower lumbar joints should, therefore, be expected to be the first to fail (Farfan et al. 1972). Furthermore, the L5 vertebra in 60 to 70 percent of individuals is either deeply seated in the pelvis or else articulated closely with the pelvis by means of short iliotransverse ligaments. In either case, the L5 vertebra and therefore the joint between it and the sacrum is protected from torsional stresses (MacGibbon and Farfan 1979). The L5–S1 joint is also protected from torsion by reason of the lumbar curve. Generally speaking, L5 joints with large lumbosacral angles

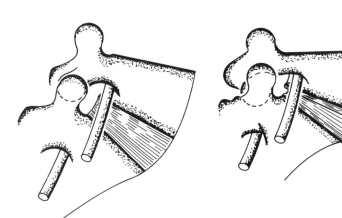

FIG. 6. Collapse of lumbosacral joint brings superior facet of L5 close to the exiting nerve root particularly when the spine is extended.

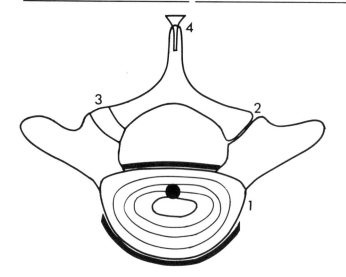

FIG. 7. **Parts of the intervertebral joint that resist torsion. These include: 1) disc and its anterior and posterior longitudinal ligaments which may be considered as integral components of the disc; 2) bony facet articulations; 3) capsules of the facet articulations; 4) the supraspinous and other intervertebral ligaments; as well as the musculature. (Farfan HF: Mechanical Disorders of the Low Back, Philadelphia, Lea & Febiger, 1973; modified from Farfan HF: J Bone Joint Surg 54A:492, 1972)**

would tend to feel less torsional strain than those with small lumbosacral angles (Kraus 1976). These combinations of antitorsional devices make the L4–5 disc, two to one, the commonest lumbar joint affected by torsion.

In the presence of such antitorsional devices, the L5–S1 disc can still be injured by axial compression loads and it is exactly in such "protected" joints that one can look for the probable sequences of "pure" axial compression overload.

When torsion is applied to an intervertebral joint, the center of motion is found to be within the disc (Fig. 7). Resistance to torsion is offered mainly by the facet joints and discs in almost equal proportion. When injuries occur, they occur simultaneously in the posterior elements and in the disc (Farfan et al. 1971).

Injuries in the facet joints are basically those of compression subchondral fractures on either side of the articulation. One can confidently expect the tissue response to be effusion, synovitis, and limitation of motion which are probably all pain producing responss. One can expect fibrillation of cartilage, loss of articular cartilage, possibly the presence of loose bodies in the joint, and chronic synovitis (see Fig. 5). In over 500 operations on facet joints all of these cardaveric pathologies have been confirmed. Of these, loose body formation is quite a rare finding, and in no case has a nipped synovial

fringe been recognized. By the same token, it can be said that isolated injuries to supraspinous or interspinous ligaments, ligamentum flavum, and facet capsules have not been recognized during operations. This is supported by laboratory studies which, while indicating that facet capsules and supra- and interspinous ligaments contribute to torque strength, have shown no gross injury at the point of failure of the whole joint.

As can be expected, the tissue reaction to intraarticular damage and chronic synovitis affects the juxtaarticular bone of the articular processes. Bone in this region becomes osteoporotic and subject to compression fracture. These compression fractures have been found in cadaver specimens, and also at surgery. Facet joint arthritis and fractures of the articular process, both in the same spinal segment, can be expected to give rise to referred pain. Putti (1927) was of the opinion that facet joint arthritis alone could explain most of the symptomatology in mechanical disorders of the back. There are many indications of the importance of these joints in symptomatology. However, it is not necessary to list the arguments pro and con.

However, one comment relative to the classical loss of lumbar lordosis accompanying intervertebral joint disease should be made. It is known that the loss of lordosis cannot be ascribed to "muscle spasm." Without exception the paravertebral muscles are behind the axis of flexion-extension motion which is in the disc. Contraction of these muscles, therefore, would produce extension or increased lordosis. On the other hand, axial rotation at the intervertebral joint is accompanied by flexion at the joint. This would emplain both the loss of lordosis and the rotoscoliosis. However, this cannot be the whole story because it does not offer an explanation for alternating scoliosis, a problem which shall be referred to later.

The effects of torsion on the disc are spectacular. At the point of maximal torsion, the disc "gives" suddenly with loud snapping sounds. In fact, it can be said to "slip" in almost exactly the same sense that a car clutch slips. The annulus becomes distorted all around its periphery but in greater degree at the posterolateral angles. Here the outer annular fibers subjacent to the longitudinal ligaments are ripped off the end plate on one side over a considerable distance. The inner annular layers and nucleus remain undistributed and there is no injury to the end plate.

The distortion of the outer annulus may be large enough to interfere with neural canal content and it may stretch the posterior longitudinal ligament. In the rabbit, this annular ligament injury calls forth a polymorphonuclear response followed by granulation tissue accompanied by an invasion of the outer annulus with new small vascular channels. There is some reason to believe that the same reaction occurs in humans (Sullivan et al. 1971).

Such soft-tissue distortion of annulus and posterior longitudinal ligament, both well supplied with nerve endings, is undoubtedly a source of pain whether or not the distortion interferes with the nerve roots. Theoretically, at this stage, the distorted annulus may be reduced, possibly by derotation in flexion. It is certain that at this stage, the circular cicatrization of the damaged annulus may return the annulus to its original shape and location.

When torsion is repeatedly applied to the disc in the laboratory over a given angle of arc, its resistance to torsion to this arc of motion is almost completely lost. Left to recover, much of its torque strength will return. If the test is performed after removing a small window of annulus for purposes of observation, it is seen that the inner annular layers begin to separate and gradually work themselves free, bulging up and out through the window. This separation of inner annular fibers is not uncommonly seen in degenerated discs where almost entire whorls of loose tissue can be found.

It is not evident that loose annular tissue found in degenerated discs is caused by repeated torsion. It is only important that they occur. Furthermore, there is some evidence that under certain conditions, these loose bits of material can be induced to move within the disc cavity. It is clear that disc protrusions could not occur unless disc material could be induced to move. When a disc cavity is injected with silastic glue and the glue is allowed to set, the glue sets with a firm rubbery consistency not unlike that of disc material removed at surgery. (The normal disc accepts only a small amount of material somewhat less than one milliliter.) To accept more, the disc must be already to some degree degenerated. When a disc prepared in this manner is subjected to repeated torsion, the little pellet of silastic is found to track through the disc material toward the posterolateral angle. When larger volumes of silastic have been used the material has, on occasion, been forced out through the annulus.

Thus, we have the phenomenon of material loose in the disc which, under certain circumstances, can be induced to move, even in the presence of discs with a still intact outer annulus. It is possible that such loose material may be forced up under the sensitive posterior outer annulus by a compressional or torsional force, much like a melon seed from between the finger and thumb. A manipulation might possibly dislodge this fragment from its pain-producing position to a more medial one, nearer the center of the disc. Also, this material might be moved from one side to the other, resulting in a sudden switch of clinical signs and symptoms. Needless to say, it can readily be imagined that manipulation could force loose material irretrievably through the annulus.

The Areas of Maximum Stress

As previously mentioned, torsion affects the disc, causing distortion and eventual avulsion of the annulus from one end plate. The site of maximum distortion and avulsion is at the location of maximum stress. This point of maximal stress is dictated by the shape of the disc in the following areas: 1) midpoint posteriorly in discs with rounded posterior outlines; 2) the posterolateral angle at the medial pedicular margins in discs with flat posterior outlines; and 3) laterally in discs with lozenge-shaped outlines (Fig. 8).

Were the disc shapes absolutely symmetrical, then highest stress concentrations would be bilaterally placed and similar. When the disc is asymmetrically formed, however, stress concentrations occur on only one side, usually on the more hypoplastic side. The hypoplastic side is indicated by axial tomography, or sometimes in simple radiographs when it is marked by a more oblique or smaller facet joint (Fig. 9). The hypoplastic side is, therefore, the weak side, the side on which disc problems arise and to which the rotoscoliosis occurs in the majority of instances. Repeated torsion will, therefore, repeatedly affect the weakest side, rupturing annular fibers in deeper and deeper layers until finally a communication between the outer annulus and the disc nucleus is created. This radial fissure, as it is known, indicates that the joint has reached the point of instability and abnormal motion that can often be demonstrated (Fig. 10).

Besides indicating the stage of instability attained, the radial fissure provides a channel through the outer annulus through which disc material can be extruded. Though relatively late in the process, the radial fissure may form early with a rapidly progressing clinical course. It remains, nevertheless, relatively uncommon to find a true extrusion of disc material.

In the vast majority of disc injuries, ingrowth of granulation tissue occurs with its concomitant vascularization from the end plate or from the outer layers of annulus. This tissue response digests or hydrolizes the disc content. Though not commonly thought of as scar formation, this reaction in the normally avascular

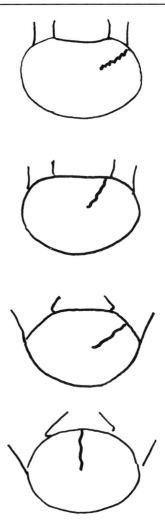

FIG. 8. **Radial fissures seem to occur at locations of torsional stress concentrations which in turn depend on the shape of the disc. The various lumbar disc outlines are shown. A. upper lumbar, fissures from lateral to the pedicle. B. commonest, L4. C. common, L5 (more commonly the L5 has a shape as in D). D. not uncommon at L4. (From Farfan HF: Orthop Clin N Am 8:13, 1977)**

disc removes loose fragments of tissue and tends to stabilize the remainder. The usual outcome is a loss of loose material for extrusion, a good reason for temporizing and allowing nature to do its bit.

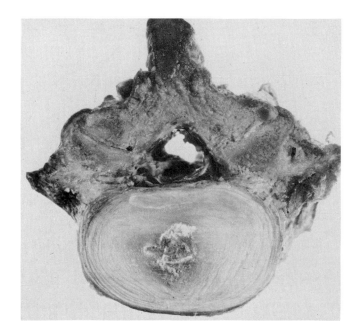

FIG. 9. **Grossly asymmetric intervetebral joint, obvious in both facet joint and disc. (Farfan HF: Mechanical Disorders of the Low Back. Philadelphia, Lea & Febiger, 1973. Modified from Farfan HF: J Bone Joint Surg 54A:492, 1972)**

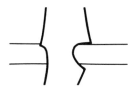

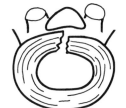

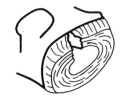

FIG. 10. **The nature of disc protrusion. Note separation of annulus only on one side. The lesion in life is covered partly by posterior longitudinal ligament and by inflammatory exudate. (From Farfan HF: Clin Neurosurg 25:284, 1979)**

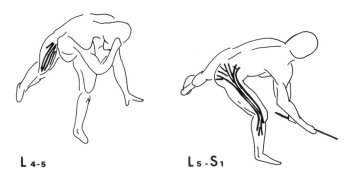

L 4-5 **L 5 - S 1** FIG. 11. **Facet syndromes. (See text.)**

The healing process in this instance is also imperfect, as it was in the case of the fractured end plate. In cadaveric material the disc, with even the earliest signs of degeneration, always shows less resistance to torsion than a normal disc. This ensures that when torsional overload is applied a second time, it will be the same joint that is injured, the other joints in the column being protected, as it were, by the presence of the one which is strained. The progression here, then, is always at the same joint, in contrast to the compressional overload which strikes successively neighboring discs.

Combined Posterior Facet and Disc Damage

It remains now to consider the combined effects of arthritic facets and damaged discs on the patient. Because of the arthritic facets, positions of extension or of flexion, if prolonged, will give backache and with further aggravation will cause referred pain in the buttocks and lateral thigh (Fig. 11).

Because of loss of annular tissue, resistance to both compression and torsional loads is impaired. Heavy lifting of any kind, especially when the load is carried asymmetrically, as in one-hand lifting, may cause the patient to experience difficulty. Such a condition is, of course, a serious threat to normal lifestyles.

Healing cannot be expected to progress any faster than that of a healing ligament which is the major component of the annulus. It takes at least six weeks for a damaged ligament to re-

gain 80 percent of its tensile strength. The acute inflammatory response of the facet joints may recover rapidly but the induced synovitis also takes a long time to settle.

Certain other conditions occur in a joint which has been damaged by torsion and these conditions are best understood if we keep clear the idea that the disc and posterior elements are injured simultaneously.

The deformation of the neural arch on one side may be so severe that it may never regain its original shape. When rotation is forced, the long superior articular process of the rotated vertebra is jammed against the short, sturdy, unyielding, superior facet of the vertebra below. The result is that the superior articular process is bent backwards and medially (Fig. 12).

In the meantime, the inferior process on the opposite side is not greatly distorted because the only resistance to its motion is the capsular ligament of the distracted facet. The pedicle on this side however is displaced medially taking its nerve root with it. In this way, with a rotation of 9°, the displacing pedicle may stretch the nerve root by 1 cm, which is probably enough to result in compromise of its function leading to a neuropathic syndrome without the necessity of having a disc protrusion or extrusion (Fig. 13).

This type of nerve root impairment may be of extreme clinical importance, both for the practitioner of spinal manipulation as well as for the surgeon. Relief of symptoms could be expected with restoration of normal alignment by rotation. For the surgeon, it explains a large group of patients explored without disc protrusion being found (the "hidden" disc of Dandy

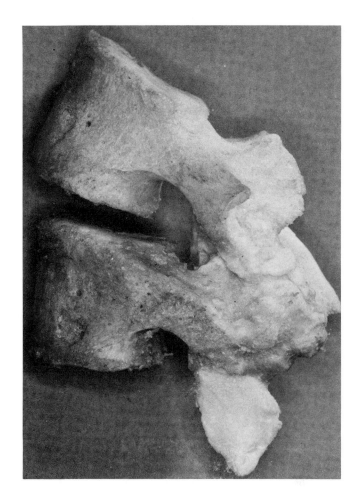

FIG. 12. The wide angle between the inferior articular process and pedicle is well demonstrated. This deformation allows the vertebra above to slip forward. (Farfan HF: Mechanical Disorders of the Low Back. Philadelphia, Lea & Febiger, 1973. Modified from Farfan HF: J Bone Joint Surg 54A:492, 1972)

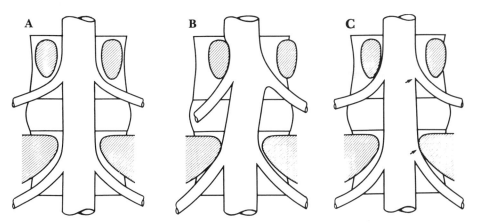

FIG. 13. The rotation effect on nerve roots. (A) Neutral. (B) L4 has been rotated to the patient's left stretching L4 and L5 roots on patient's left side. A temporary situation. (C) The spine has been derotated but because the vertebral body is now forward on the right side, it is the L5 nerve root that remains tight and may be stretched around the pedicle of L5 (arrow) or at the lamina of L4 (arrow).

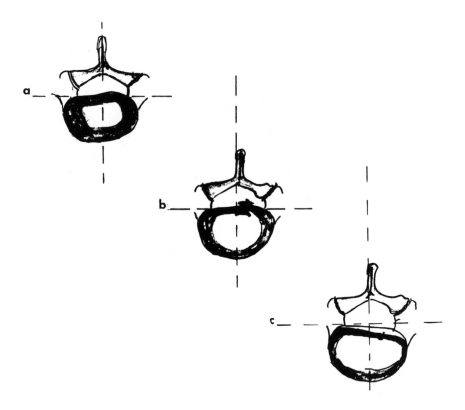

FIG. 14.   **Degenerative spondylolisthesis: the progression from original rotation injury. (A) Left facet joint is cracked and there is distortion of the annulus with subsequent degeneration. (B) The degeneration has progressed in both facet joints, making the arch weaker so that it is subject to crush fracture and deformation. (C) Deformation of arch allows listhesis to develop. (From Farfan HF: Orthop Clin N Am 8:15, 1977)**

[1942]). It could also explain certain false positive myelograms where the defect in the column of dye results from inability to fill the nerve sheath because the nerve root was tightly drawn against the pedicle.

When torsion is removed, the deformed arch may not recover and may remain with a skewed look. The disc, because it is damaged at the same time, permits the deformed neural arch to settle once more so that the gross relationship of lamina and facet joints are restored. The vertebral body, however, has now rotated forward on the deformed side. This has the effect of causing an abrupt change of direction of the neural canal causing the neural content to be drawn tight to the undisplaced side. This may

cause a restriction of the cauda equina. If, in addition, we consider that the facet joints may be swollen and arthritic and the disc distorted, we can see that the cauda equina as well as its circulation may be impeded thereby giving rise to the syndrome of spinal stenosis. When the displacement of the vertebral body becomes obvious, the condition is known as degenerative spondylolisthesis (Fig. 14).

In these late gross disturbances of the intervertebral joint, there seems little to gain by mobilization of the joint. As with the lateral entrapment syndrome due to collapse of disc thickness, the condition has passed beyond the scope of the practitioner of spinal manipulation.

REFERENCES

Andrae R: Uber Knorpelnoschiten am Hinter en-deder wirbelandechelben in berech des spinal-kanals. Beitr Pathol 82:464, 1929

Dandy WE: Recent advances in the diagnosis and treatment of ruptured intervertebral disks. Ann Surg 115:514, 1942

Farfan HF: Mechanical Disorders of the Low Back. Philadelphia, Lea & Febiger, 1973

Farfan HF, Cossette JW, Robertson GH, Wells RV, Kraus H: The effects of torsion on the lumbar intervertebral joints: the role of torsion in the production of disc degeneration. J Bone Joint Surg 52A:468, 1970

Farfan HF, Huberdeau RM, Dubow HI: Lumbar intervertebral disc degeneration: the influence of geometrical features on the pattern of disc degeneration. J Bone Joint Surg 54A:492, 1972

Farfan HF, Cossette JW, Robertson GH, Wells RV: The instantaneous center of rotation of the third lumbar intervertebral joint. J Biomech 4:149, 1971

Goldthwaite JE: The lumbosacral articulation. An explanation of many cases of "lumbago," "sciatica," and "paraplegia." Boston Med Surg 164:365, 1911

Key JA: The intervertebral disc: anatomy, physiology and pathology. Am Acad Orthop Surg 6:27, 1949

Kraus H: Effect of lordosis on the stress in the lumbar spine. Clin Orthop 117:56, 1976

Lamy C: Mechanism of failure of the vertebral body end plate. Unpublished.

MacGibbon B, Farfan HF: Are all lumbar spines the same—radiological survey. Spine 4:258, 1979

Putti V: New conceptions in the pathogenesis of sciatic pain. Lancet 2:53, 1927

Schmorl G: Die pathologische anatomie der wirbelsaule. Verh Dtsch, Ges Orthop 21:3, 1926

Sullivan JD, Farfan HF, Kahn DS: Pathological changes with intervertebral joint rotational instability in the rabbit. Can J Surg 14:71, 1971

SECTION THREE
Practice of Chiropractic

CHAPTER TEN
The Use of X-rays in Spinal Manipulative Therapy

REED B. PHILLIPS

The introduction and use of the roentgen ray has provided the clinician with a diagnostic tool of inestimable worth. No longer bound by the limitations of human capabilities, the clinician now utilizes this unseen energy to visualize structures encased within the integument. The objective of this chapter is to provide the reader with an understanding of how those who employ spinal manipulative therapy use x-rays to aid them in making a pathological and biomechanical evaluation of the patient.

Spinal manipulative therapy (SMT) involves the application of force to a specific localized area of the body. This force is applied in a manner that is as variable as the number employing the technique.

Many pathological processes may weaken bony architecture. Application of a manipulative force to such a weakened structure may incur further tissue damage or result in greater patient pain and discomfort. Such mishaps should and can be avoided through the discriminate use of x-rays.

The application of force in SMT is often applied in a specific direction in an attempt to cause a change in vertebral relationships. Though much information may be obtained through proper palpation of spinal and paraspinal tissues along with postural analysis and other methods of structural examination, the x-ray is a major factor in demonstrating vertebral relationships. A biomechanical evaluation of vetebral relationships is helpful in determining how to best apply the force associated with SMT.

The biomechanical evaluation of vertebral disrelationship includes the analysis of simple intersegmental disrelationships (subluxations) as well as multiple disrelationships extending over large areas (scolioses).

Pathological Screening

Patients seeking spinal manipulation usually do so because of the presence of spinal related pain or discomfort. X-ray evaluation aids the clinician in evaluating the source of the patient's complaint as well as determining the appropriateness of spinal manipulative care. There are conditions demonstrable through x-rays where spinal manipulation is contraindicated, or at least relegated to a role secondary to a more radical (manipulation being conservative) form of therapy.

Critical (Life-Threatening) Pathological Changes

Multiple myeloma is a disease that may affect the spine in the geriatric age group. The radiological manifestation of this disorder is that of diffuse osteoporosis and associated vertebral body collapse. The entire body is usually collapsed rather than the anterior portion of the vertebral body as is often seen in a compression fracture.

Other painful spinal diseases that are often recognized only with x-rays are the metastatic

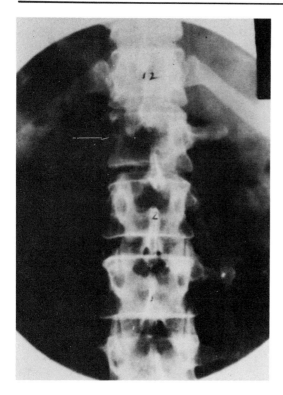

FIG. 1. **The absence of the pedicle on L-1 is evidence of lytic destruction of bone, most often due to metastatic disease, as in this case. Presenting symptom of the patient was "back pain."**

neoplasms. An early radiographic manifestation of these lesions is the lytic destrucion of the pedicle. Lytic destruction of a portion of a vertebra should be considered a contraindication to the application of a forceful manipulative thrust to the area of involvement (Fig. 1).

Patients presenting with spinal problems relating to trauma should undergo x-ray examination to determine the presence or absence of fractures and dislocation. Routine radiographic procedures may be sufficient for demonstrating obvious damage such as compression fractures of the vertebral body. More subtle and often more clinically significant posterior arch fractures may require the use of specialized procedures, such as tomography before visualization may be achieved.

Acute pyogenic arthritis of the disc or vertebral osteomyelitis may create severe spinal pain 2 to 4 weeks before radiologic changes may be made manifest. Such a disparity between symptoms of pain and radiologic signs of disease points out the importance of correlating clinical signs with patient symptoms and radiographic findings. Acute pyogenic infection of the spine may lead to destructive changes and spinal ankylosis in the absence of appropriate medical care.

Occasionally, radiographic manifestations of different spinal pathological changes are very similar, although their clinical significance differs considerably. For example, "ivory vertebrae" (vertebral bodies appearing more dense and sclerotic than adjacent structures) can be found in three different conditions. The clinical severity of these three conditions ranges from Paget's disease to Hodgkin's disease or malignant blastic metastatic disease. Subtle radiographic manifestations are helpful in differentiating which condition is producing the "ivory vertebrae." Enlargement of the vertebral contours and changes in the bony trabecular pattern would suggest the formation of Paget's disease. Erosion of the anterior vertebral body margin would suggest the presence of external pressure from an enlarged lymph node infiltrated with Hodgkin's sarcoma. Multiple sites of sclerotic change would cause one to consider metastatic disease.

Some relatively quiescent benign bone tumors may be overlooked if proper radiological evaluations are not done. Their presence may be insignificant. However, such conditions as neurofibromas (causing an enlargement of the intervertebral foramen) and aneurysmal bone cysts (causing expansile lesions of the vertebrae) may create considerable weakening of the osseous structure. Such weaknesses are a contraindiction to the application of forceful manipulation.

Noncritical (Non-Life-Threatening) Pathological Changes

Many pathological changes and anatomical variations which are not life threatening also require radiological evaluation. Although the clinical manifestations of a herniated intervertebral

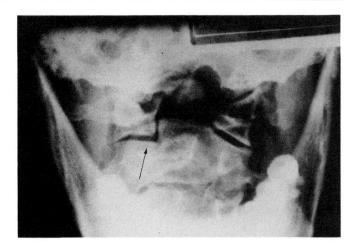

FIG. 2. **Structural asymmetry is common in spinal architecture. The facet surfaces between C1 and C2 are asymmetrical and will definitely influence the biomechanical motion of the involved segments.**

disc may be so classic as to leave little doubt regarding its presence, the radiographic evaluation helps to clarify the severity of the loss of disc space and the extent of any degenerative changes that may be associated with the disc pathology. Anatomical relationships of adjacent vertebral structures that may be affected by disc degeneration are also important to the clinician employing spinal manipulative therapy.

A knowledge of the presence of ankylosing spondylitis is essential before the application of spinal manipulation. Forceful manipulation to a partially fused joint may prove to be quite painful to the patient.

Developmental Variations

Scolioses are usually evident upon routine spinal examination. The etiology is often only appreciated on the radiograph. Hemivertebrae or congenital fusion may be the underlying cause. An understanding of such underlying conditions may affect the mode of therapy recommended.

Even when the mode of therapy is to be spinal manipulation, radiographic manifestations of congenital anomalies such as asymmetrical facet facings, spondylolysis with or without spondylolisthesis, shortened or elongated pedicles and incomplete posterior arch formation may play a significant role in determining how

spinal manipulative therapy should best be applied (Fig. 2).

Postural Evaluation From the Radiograph

When investigating the biomechanics of the spine that relate to the radiographic portrayal of the patient's posture, one must remember that the image portrayed on the x-ray film is actually a three-dimensional structure. As such, it is capable of movement in the following manner:

Flexion—anterior bending of the spine in the sagittal plane;
Extension—posterior bending of the spine in the sagittal plane;
Lateral flexion—lateral bending of the spine in the coronal plane;
Rotation—turning of the spine in a horizontal or transverse plane.

The portrayal of the above motions as visualized on a flat film is not easily described, and it is complicated by the fact that motion of the spine is often a combination of movement in two or more planes, e.g., lateral flexion and rotation are generally a combined movement (Illi 1951).

The following sections will attempt to correlate these general principles with more specific findings in the postural evaluation made from the radiograph. Terminology is usually describing patient position or movement relative to the plane of the film.

Gross Evaluations

Altered Curves and Body Unleveling. When observing the radiograph for postural evaluation, one should seek to determine if any abnormalities exist on a gross level. It should be determined if the head, trunk, and/or pelvis is rotated. If rotation is present, then it should be determined if the rotation is in the same or opposite direction and if the rotation is of near equivalent amounts for each area. Rotation of structures in the same direction and of near equivalent amounts would suggest faulty patient positioning at the time the x-ray was taken. Areas of opposing rotation may indicate the presence of significant structural problems.

After evaluating the presence or absence of rotation on a gross level, one should give consideration next to the effects of lateral flexion. By simple observation, one should be able to determine if one side of the head is higher than the opposite side, if one shoulder is higher than the other, or if one hip is higher than the opposite side.

The unlevel relationships of one side of the body to its opposing side may be the result of faulty patient positioning. On the other hand, significant structural problems may result in unleveling of body relationships.

Patient positioning can both increase and/or decrease spinal curvatures. A simple raising of the arms in a lateral lumbar view, may severely increase the lumbar lordosis. Pelvic rotation in an anteroposterior (A.P.) view may introduce a scoliosis in a normal lumbar spine and reduce a scoliosis in a crooked spine by presenting a lordotic curve to the x-ray beam at an oblique angle.

Arthritic Changes. Abnormal spinal relationships can be the result of arthritic changes such as thinning of the disc spaces; the presence of spur formation on the vertebral bodies or facets; breakdown of osseous structures; laxity of adjacent ligaments, and/or an imbalanced musculature.

Such changes may (but not necessarily) be pain producing or at least pain related. Pain producing arthritic changes often produce spasms, fixations, and antalgic posture and in this way alter the gross spinal relationships (it is assumed at this point that the radiograph has been previously screened for pathological entities).

Anomalous Changes. The presence of any altered posture should cause one to consider the possibility of the presence of an under- or overdeveloped structure. A structure may even be totally absent. If a vertebral segment is anomalous (such as a hemivertebra), normal spinal relationships may be distorted.

Specific Area Evaluations

Specific evaluation procedures are divided into biomechanically related regions (i.e., sacropelvic, lumbosacral, thoracolumbar, lower cervical, and upper cervical).

The procedures described in this section are a combination of the work of many authors (Janse 1954, 1963; Rich 1963; Santos 1965; American Chiropractic Association 1973; National College of Chiropractic 1960; Hildebrant 1974; Vladeff 1948; Winterstein 1970; Lind 1974; Dejarnette 1964; Gonstead 1968; Howe 1971). Authors will be recognized where the particular procedure described is unique. There is no attempt to suggest that one procedure is more ideal than the others. Most of the procedures are applicable to upright positioning of the patient.

Sacropelvic Region: Anteroposterior View

Short Lower Extremity. In order to establish the presence or absence of a short lower extremity a line is drawn that intersects the superior surface of each femoral head. A comparable line drawn parallel to the film base and near the line intersecting the femoral heads would indicate whether the femoral heads were equidistant

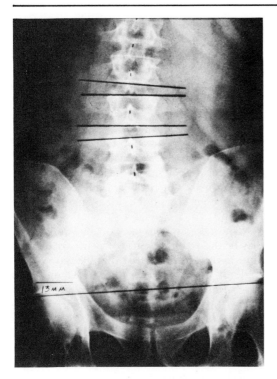

FIG. 3. The line connecting the two femoral heads is referred to as the femoral head line. A second line is drawn above the low femoral head. This second line is parallel with the level horizon and is drawn at the level of the high femoral head. The distance between the horizontal line and the femoral head line represent the amount of deficiency visualized on the radiograph between the height of the two femoral heads (13 mm). Vertebral end-plate lines are also present on L-2, L-3 and L-4.

from the film base. For this procedure to be valid, the film base within the cassette at the time of exposure must be parallel to the floor on which the patient is standing (Beilke 1936) (Fig. 3).

Pelvic Lateral Shifting. In order to establish whether or not the pelvis is in an acceptable weight-bearing position two vertical lines have been described. The first is a vertical line drawn in the center of the film running parallel with the side of the film and representing an ideal vertical. The second is a line extending

through the vertical center of the pelvis, passing through the second sacral tubercle and the center of the symphysis pubis (Fig. 4).

Deviation of the center line of the pelvis from the ideal vertical center line indicates that the pelvis was not centered to the x-ray beam and the film, when the radiograph was made. Lack of pelvic centering may simply be due to poor patient positioning. On the other hand, there may be a lateral shift of weight bearing because of a short lower extremity, or possibly an antalgic position. When there has been a lateral shift of the pelvis, it is often associated with an antero-inferior rotation of the pelvis on the side where the lateral shifting occurred. This rotation is usually on the side of a short lower extremity. If a true short lower extremity exists, then pelvic

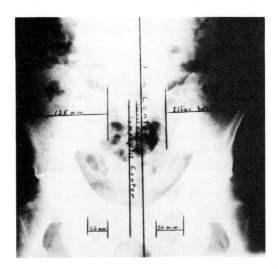

FIG. 4. The line extending the entire vertical length of the picture represents the film center. The adjacent short vertical line passes through the second sacral tubercle. The third vertical line (intermediate in length) passes through the symphysis pubis. Observing the film in a posteroanterior relationship, one suspects that the patient was positioned slightly left of center; both the second sacral tubercle and symphysis pubis are to the left of the film center. Also, the symphysis pubis is more to the left than the second sacral tubercle, indicating pelvic rotation where the right side of the pelvis has rotated anterior.

unleveling can be easily understood. Lateral shifting of the pelvis produces unequal weight bearing and unequal femoral alignment which causes the pelvis to shift inferior over a rotated femoral head. This pelvic shifting has been referred to as a "trochanter phenomenon" by Illi (1951).

A line drawn across the superior surface of the iliac crests, will usually indicate an unlevel pelvis when compared to the horizontal base of the film.

Pelvic Rotation. Rotation of the pelvis about a vertical axis may occur with or without a lateral shift. The presence of rotation would be indicated by the shifting of the second sacral tubercle (a structure on the posterior aspect of the pelvis) in a direction opposite to the shifting of the symphysis pubis (a structure on the anterior aspect of the pelvis) (see Fig. 4).

Pelvic rotation also produces other changes that can be visualized on the radiograph. These changes are subject to variability based on differing pelvic configurations.

The iliac bones normally are located somewhat oblique to the coronal plane of the film. Pelvic rotation about a vertical axis will cause the iliac bone on the side of anterior rotation to become more narrow in width compared to the opposite iliac wing that is rotated posterior.

The anteriorly rotated iliac wing is more parallel to the x-ray beam while the posteriorly rotated iliac wing is located more transverse to the x-ray beam. The minimal effects of magnification due to increased object-film distance do not offset the effects of rotation.

Changes occurring in the sacrum, a posterior pelvic structure, are similar to that occurring in the iliac wings although of a lesser magnitude. The posteriorly positioned sacrum will show a relatively greater width than the anteriorly rotated portion.

For consistency in measuring iliac and sacral widths, one should measure through the same horizontal level on each side.

Winterstein (1970) has proposed a hemipelvic measurement to indicate pelvic rotation. Measurements are made from the external iliac borders to a central pelvic line. The same rela-

tionship of narrowed anterior structures and widened posterior structures is maintained.

Another minor change indicating pelvic rotation includes an increased opening of the obturator foramen (an anterior pelvic structure) on the side of anterior rotation. This is once again due to the alignment of this foramen transversely across the x-ray beam. The posterior side shows the opposite changes, i.e., the obturator foramen appears decreased in size. The vertical opening of the pelvic basin (bordered primarily by the ileopectineal line) tends to decrease in size on the side of anterior pelvic rotation.

A short lower extremity on the radiograph may be the result or cause of pelvic rotation. It must also be remembered that, because of the angle of the x-ray beam (24° at 84 inches in target-film distance) (Leverone and Winterstein, 1974), a structure rotated anterior to the plane of the film will be projected inferiorly onto the film in the area of the pelvis. This phenomenon can produce an apparent short lower extremity which is nothing more than a projectional distortion (Fig. 5).

Most marking procedures have a mathematical formula regarding the correction of the femoral head height that has been projected low due to rotation (Winterstein 1970; Hildebrandt 1974; Gonstead 1968). The mathematical formulas are useful in that they make one aware of the effects of projectional distortion, but their reliability has not been properly validated.

Innominate Disrelationships. The innominate bone (ilium, ischium, and pubic bones combined) undergoes its own peculiar biomechanical changes within the pelvic unit. The extent of motion involved is minimal and results are usually described as one innominate position in relation to the other innominate.

Innominate motion occurs at the sacroiliac joints with a dispute as to whether the axis of motion in the coronal plane exists at the femoral heads or symphysis pubis (Kapandjii 1974; Hildebrandt 1974). The actual motion which occurs is generally analyzed on the film in two different ways.

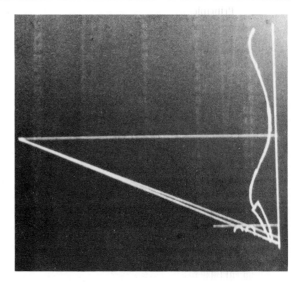

FIG. 5. **Projectional distortion. On a full spine film, rotation of the pelvis with one femoral head anterior to the other, the image of the anterior femoral head will appear on the film lower than will the femoral head closer to the film.**

Illi (1951) described innominate action as a rocking motion or anterior and posterior displacement in a sagittal plane. Hildebrandt (1974) is supportive of this concept, emphasizing that the pivotal point for this movement is at the symphysis pubis and not at the femoral heads. Hildebrandt contends that a shearing force would be present at the symphysis if the axis of the rocking motion were to occur at the hip joint.

Gonstead (1968) describes innominate motion both as a rocking motion similar to that described by Illi and also as a flaring motion where the iliac wings move in a medial to lateral direction (coronal plane) across the sacroiliac joints. The symphysis is described as having moved in an opposite direction to the iliac wings. The concept of innominate motion has many similarities to pelvic rotation.

The depiction of innominate disrelationship on the radiograph consists of an overall lengthening of the innominate that has rocked posterior. This can be measured from the superior surface of the iliacs to the superior surface of the pubic bone (Winterstein 1971) or to the inferior surface of the ischial tuberosity (Gonstead 1968). The anterior rocked innominate would show a decrease in its vertical dimension.

The vertical diameter of the obturator fora-

men would increase on the posterior rocked side, being aligned more transverse to the x-ray beam. The anterior rocked side would show a decreased vertical opening of the obturator foramen.

The pelvic inlet will decrease in vertical dimension on the posterior rocked side, and increase on the anterior rocked side.

The superior surface of the pubic body will be at a higher elevation on the side of the posterior rocked innominate at the symphysis pubis. The findings of pelvic flaring are similar to those of pelvic rotation.

Pelvic Rocking (Flexion and Extension). A description of pelvic rocking, flexion and extension, in the sagittal plane was purposely held until this point. The description of the radiographic changes given in the last section apply to the entire pelvis rocking as a unit. If the pelvis rocks posterior, both innominates would appear elongated, and if it rocks anterior, both innominates would appear to be shortened. Pelvic rocking is a motion occurring on the femoral heads (Kapandjii 1974).

Sacral Movement. The extent of sacral motion visualized on the radiograph will vary depending upon its angle of orientation with respect to the x-ray beam. If we consider the three planes of the body (sagittal, coronal, transverse) to be represented in the sacrum and use the sacral base as our plane of reference, then sacral motion can be described as a backward and forward rocking (flexion and extension) or nutation (Kapandjii 1974). The axis of this nutation motion has been suggested to be in three different areas. No doubt some variability exists, due to the variable nature of the sacroiliac joint iself. Visualization of forward rocking (flexion) of the sacrum on the A.P. film is demonstrated by a greater visualization of the sacral base as opposed to the body of the sacrum. Posterior rocking (extension) will show a decreased view of the sacral base and a larger proportion of the sacral body.

Hemisacral widening as viewed on the radiograph (on the side of posterior rotation) has already been mentioned. This is more definitive if the sacrum is positioned in a more vertical orientation. Lateral flexion of the sacrum is also visualized better in a more vertically oriented position. A line drawn across the sacral base or a line bisecting the sacral foramina from side to side will indicate lateral flexion when compared to the horizontal base of the film.

As a normal compensatory motion, such as dealing with a short leg, one usually finds the sacrum rotated anterior and laterally flexed, inferior on the side of the short leg. This also is the side where a posterior rocked innominate would be found (Illi 1951) (Fig. 6).

Fifth Lumbar Movement. Biomechanically, the fifth lumbar functions as part of the pelvis (Illi 1951; Kapandjii 1974). The fifth lumbar segment, resting on the sacral base, will tend to move with the sacral base. The fifth lumbar segment is also attached to the iliac wings via the iliolumbar ligaments. Therefore, movement of the innominates would influence L5 motion.

Radiographically, lateral flexion of any vertebral segment is usually accompanied by a wedging (narrowing) of the disc space towards the side of lateral flexion. This is graphically demonstrated by an intersecting of lines drawn through the adjacent end plates of each vertebra (see Fig. 3).

Forward flexion and backward extension are

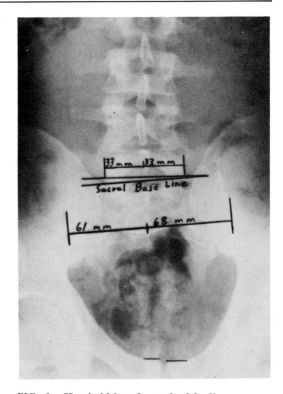

FIG. 6. **Hemiwidths of vertebral bodies, sacrum, iliacs, or the pelvis are indicators of the presence of rotation. In the structures noted, an increased hemi-width would indicate a rotation of that structure towards the film in a standard A.P. projection (posterior rotation). Narrowed hemiwidths would indicate anterior rotation. A line drawn across the sacral base will form an angle with a level horizontal line when lateral tilting of the sacrum occurs. Unleveling of the sacrum may be an individualized motion, or a part of the motion of the entire pelvis.**

best seen on lateral views. On the anteroposterior view, the way an endplate is visualized would give an indication of the position of a particular segment. One must be careful not to forget the angulation of the x-ray beam and how it would project a vertebral segment onto the film.

Rotation of a vertebral segment is determined radiographically in two ways. The more common method is to measure the distance between the lateral vertebral body margin and the

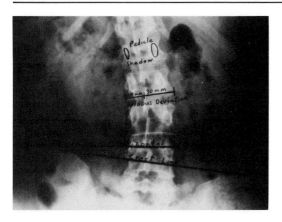

FIG. 7. **On the A.P. view, vertebral rotation is demonstrated two ways: 1) The spinous process moves away from the side of posterior body rotation. Measuring from spinous process to lateral vertebral body margin demonstrates a greater width on the side of posterior rotation. 2) Outlining of pedicle shadows will show a more oval structure of the side of posterior rotation. The pedicle shadow will also move towards the center (away from the lateral body margin) on the side of posterior rotation.**

spinous process. The spinous process is described as rotating away from the side of posterior vertebral body rotation. The pedicle shadow becomes more distinct on the side of posterior rotation (Nash and Mole 1969; Mehta 1973).

The fifth lumbar segment, working as a functional unit of the pelvis, will move with the sacral base, assuming the L5 disc is normal. If the innominate motion is counter to that of the sacrum, L5 becomes a unit where a translation of forces occur. Assuming the sacral base moves anterior and laterally flexes on the side of a short leg, L5 will move in a similar fashion. When the innominate rocks posterior on the same side, its ligamentous attachments will pull L5 posterior. Therefore, L5 will remain laterally flexed but rotated posteriorly on the side of the short leg (Fig. 7).

Sacropelvic Region: Lateral View.   A great deal of the mechanics in this region cannot be visualized due to the superimposition of pelvic structures.

The sacral-base angle is probably the most commonly used measurement. This measurement attempts to determine if the sacrum is rocked forward or backward relative to the base of the film. The angle is formed by intersecting lines drawn through the sacral base and a line drawn parallel to the horizontal base of the film. Kapandjii (1974) gives an average measurement of 30° for this angle. An increase of the angle suggests forward rocking of the sacral base and vice versa (Fig. 8).

The lumbosacral angle described by Hildebrandt (1974), is formed by intersecting lines drawn through the sacral base and the inferior

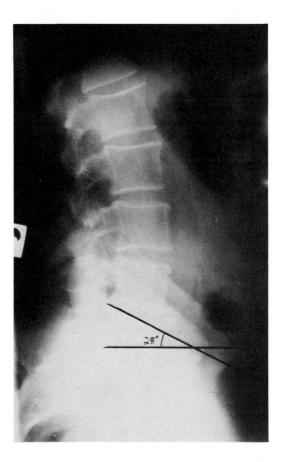

FIG. 8.   **Sacral base angle formed by intersection of horizontal base line and line drawn across the sacral base.**

Flexion and extension are not well visualized on the A.P. view.

Lateral flexion and rotation normally occur as a combined motion. Lateral flexion is depicted by an intersection of base lines across the vertebral endplates and rotation by deviation of the spinous process, or change in the pedicle shadows. In this region, rotation normally moves the vertebral body to the convex side of the curve that develops due to the lateral flexion that is taking place with the rotation. This motion is more demonstrable in the lumbar region because the axis of rotation is located posterior to the vertebral body. Thoracic segments have an axis of rotation anterior to the vertebral body and therefore move to a lesser extent than the lumbar vertebral bodies.

The appearance of scolioses is common in this region. Evaluation of scolioses can be done by drawing lines from the end plates of the segments at the beginning and the end of the curve into the concavity formed by the curve. An angle can be formed by intersecting perpendicular lines drawn from the end-plate

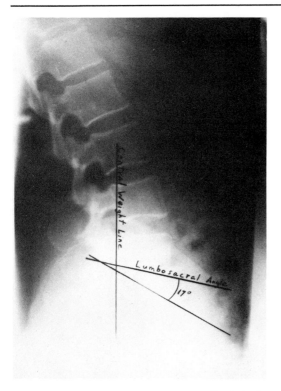

FIG. 9. **Lumbosacral angle after Hildebrandt (1974). Formed by the intersection of a line drawn through the sacral base and a line drawn through the inferior end plate of L5. Note also the central weight bearing line extending inferiorly from L3.**

end plate of L5. An average of 12° is given (Fig. 9).

Kapandjii (1974) designates the formation of the lumbosacral angle as being formed by the intersection of lines drawn through the vertical axis of L5 and the vertical axis of the sacrum. An average of 140° is given for this angle. An increase in Kapandjii's angle, or a decrease in Hildebrant's angle would suggest forward flexion of L5 relative to the sacral base (Fig. 10).

Thoracolumbar Spine (T4-L4): Anteroposterior View. Motion in this region again follows the pattern of flexion, extension, lateral flexion and rotation. The motion may be ascribed to an individual segment or any group of segments.

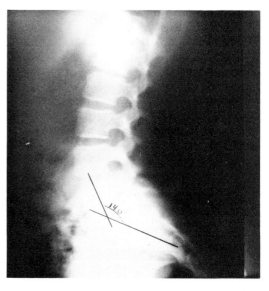

FIG. 10. **Lumbosacral angle after Kapanjii (1974). Formed by the intersection of lines drawn through the midportions of the sacrum and 5th lumbar vertebral body.**

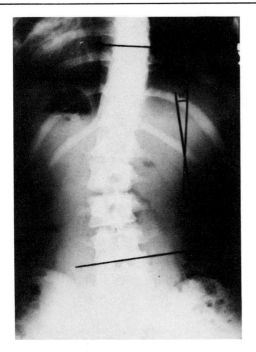

FIG. 11. Evaluation of scoliosis after Cobb (1948). A line is drawn through the end plate of the first and last segments that contribute to the formation of the curve. These two endplate lines are extended laterally from the spine to the concave side of the curve. The extension of perpendicular lines off the endplate lines form an angle at the point of intersection.

lines. This method was formulated by Cobb (1948) (Fig. 11; see also Hildebrant 1974).

The evaluation of scolioses is important to the clinician employing spinal manipulation. The radiograph provides a permanent record of the effects of treatment when posttreatment x-rays are taken.

Also, in the evaluation of scolioses, the use of stress or lateral-bending studies are often helpful to determine the amount of mobility that may be present within a scoliotic curve. Graphic evaluation can be done in a manner similar to that detailed by Cobb (see Hildebrant 1974).

It is interesting to note that the greatest mobility will be found in the direction that increases the curvature (Janse 1963) (Fig. 12).

Thoracolumbar Spine (T4-L4): Lateral View. An index of the depth of the lumbar lordosis can be measured by drawing a line from the posterior superior corner of L1 to the posterior inferior corner of L5. A perpendicular line drawn from the line joining the vertebral bodies is extended to the apex of the curve (usually L3 posterior body margin). The second line increases as the lordosis increases (Kapandjii 1974).

The normal lordotic curvature can be established by drawing a vertical line from the center of L3 to the sacral base. Ideally, this line should fall in the anterior one-third of the sacral base (Hildebrandt 1974). If the line passes through the posterior aspect of the sacral base the patient is usually in a swayback configuration (see Fig. 9).

Intersegmental flexion and extension is noted by disc space wedging. Flexion narrows the disc space anteriorly, and extension narrows the disc space posteriorly. Such changes can be demonstrated by drawing lines through adjacent vertebral end plates.

Cervicothoracic Spine (C3-T4): Anteroposterior View. This region is distinguished biomechanically primarily because the rotation of the individual segments is the reverse of what was found in the lumbar spine. The combined motion of lateral flexion and rotation results in the vertebral bodies rotating into the concavity of the curve formed. As one ascends from T4 upward, the amount of rotation that occurs increases considerably relative to the amount of lateral flexion that is present.

Radiographic depiction of these changes are the same as has already been described in other sections on the spine.

Cervicothoracic Spine (Occiput to T1): Lateral View. The cervical spine can be considered radiographically as a single unit.

Flexion and extension of individual segments is demonstrated with the use of end-plate lines. Ideally, the end-plate lines should converge to a point posterior to the cervical lordosis.

Flexion and extension views are often taken to demonstrate abnormal intersegmental mo-

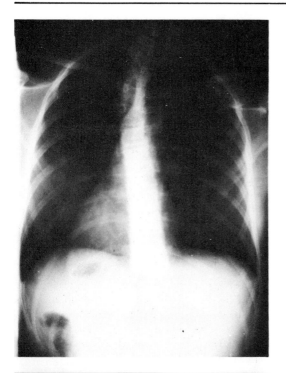

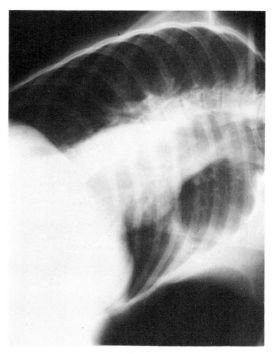

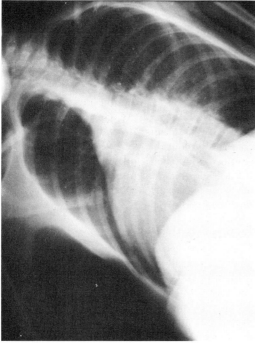

FIG. 12. (A) A.P. thoracic spine view with levoscoliosis present. (B) Right lateral bending of patient with levoscoliosis. Greatest mobility is present in the direction that increases the scoliotic deviation. (C) Left lateral bending of patient with levoscoliosis. The least amount of mobility is present when moving in the direction that decreases the scoliotic deviation.

tion as when an accident involving "whiplash" has occurred. Templating of three films (neutral lateral, flexion, and extension) by drawing lines up the posterior surfaces of each vertebral body may indicate levels of abnormal motion. The C7 level is used as a reference point on each film. Meschan (1975) describes a templating method using the occiput as a reference (Fig. 13).

An index for the depth of the cervical lordosis can be drawn in a manner similar to that of the lumbar lordosis.

Another evaluation of the lordosis is the intersection of a line drawn inferiorly off the

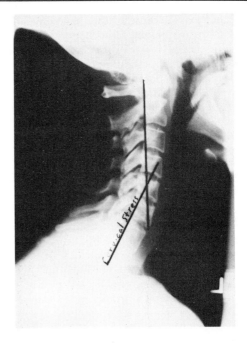

FIG. 14. **Cervical stress lines are formed by drawing a line inferiorly from the posterior margin of C2 and a line superiorly from the posterior margin of C7. They normally should intersect at the C4-5 interspace.**

posterior body of C2 and superiorly from the posterior body of C7. The two lines should intersect at the C4-5 disc space. Intersection above this level suggests a straightening of the lower portion of the lordosis. Intersection below C4-5 disc space suggests a straightening of the upper portion of the cervical lordosis (Fig. 14).

Upper Cervical Spine and Occiput (Open Mouth): Anteroposterior View. Lateral flexion in this region is minimal (8° in one direction is given by Kapandjii). This is predominantly a function of axis on C3 and occiput on atlas. Base lines extending through the individual segments or vertical bisecting lines compared to a vertical center line, will best demonstrate this motion.

Rotation is predominantly a motion between

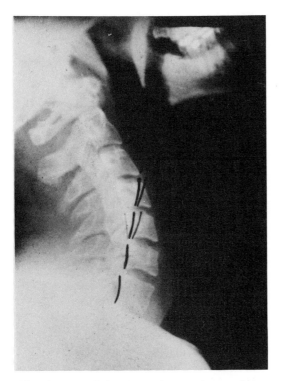

FIG. 13. **Templating is used to evaluate relative change in position through the use of a transparent overlay is demonstrated. The short vertical lines represent the position of the posterior aspect of the vertebral bodies in the positions of flexion, neutral, and extension. C6 shows a limitation of motivation because all three lines are superimposed.**

atlas and axis. Because of the dual convex nature of the articulating facets between axis and atlas, the act of rotation also produces an inferior inclination of that portion of the atlas that has rotated posterior. The occiput rotates with the atlas until maximum tension is achieved in the alar (check) ligaments which attach the occiput to the odontoid process.

From this point on (about 30°) (Kapandjii 1974), further atlas rotation results in lateral flexion of the occiput inferiorly on the side of anterior atlas rotation. Again, lateral flexion and rotation become combined movements of the spine.

Graphic representation of upper cervical rotation can be demonstrated by comparing differences in hemiwidths of various structures, i.e., spinous process to lateral body margin of C2, the lateral masses of C1, and the distance from internal occipital protuberance to the medial or lateral surface of the mastoid process. Occiput and C2 demonstrate posterior rotation on the side of increased width. The lateral mass of the atlas is an anteriorly located structure and therefore passes more transverse to the x-ray beam on the side of anterior rotation. Thus, on the atlas, the lateral mass of the greatest width is rotated anterior.

Lateral flexion of the atlas can occur when capsular ligaments are lax. This is evidenced by an overhang on the lateral mass of C1 relative to the lateral body margin of C2.

The space between the medial border of the atlas and the lateral border of the odontoid is also used as an indicator of movement. It will change when the atlas slips sideways leaving one side narrowed and the other widened. It will also change when the atlas rotates, narrowing on the side of anterior rotation and widening on the side of posterior rotation.

Factors Affecting Postural Evaluation

In view of the fact that spinal manipulative therapy is primarily directed toward structural relationships and their integrated function, the radiograph has become a prominent tool for determining technique. For a moment, the many facets that are involved in the clinician's evaluation of his patient's spinal x-rays will be considered.

Radiographic Magnification and Distortion

Classical physics will demonstrate that if we emit a light from a point source and project it a certain distance to a screen, any object placed in the beam between the source and the screen will cast a shadow greater than the actual object. The magnification of the projected object will be directly related to the relationship of the distances between the source, the object, and the screen. In x-ray projection, the light source is the x-ray tube, the screen is the x-ray film, and the object is the patient. Magnification is reduced by decreasing the object-film distance as much as possible. Distortion, which is most prevalent at the extreme ends of this projected object, can be reduced by increasing the target film distance (Fig. 15).

Therefore, a radiographic postural evaluation must include an understanding of the geometric effects of magnification and projectional distortion. The application of this understanding must precede the interpretation of the radiograph, and extend back to when the patient was positioned for the x-ray examination. Patient positioning is critical in radiographic postural evaluation.

Proper Patient Positioning for Spinal X-rays

Procedures used in patient positioning for spinal x-ray examination are not clearly defined. Several conflicting viewpoints have remained unresolved.

Conflict 1: Upright Versus Recumbent. The first conflict is upright versus recumbent positioning. The disagreement centers around film quality. Proponents for recumbent positioning contend that greater patient immobilization can be obtained during recumbency, thus reducing

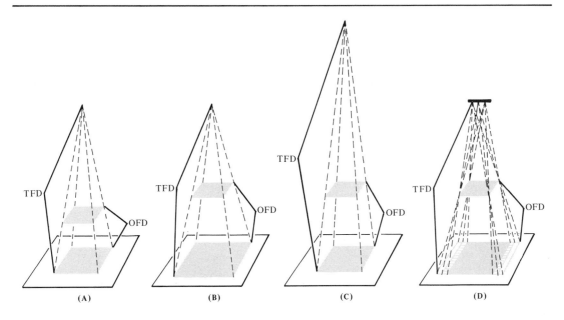

FIG. 15. **Radiographic magnification and distortion. (A,B) The effect of increasing the object-film distance (OFD), while the target-film distance (TFD) remains constant. (C, D) The effect of decreasing TFD while OFD remains constant.**

the loss of detail on the radiograph due to possible patient motion. (Traditional radiographic positioning texts illustrate spinal x-rays being obtained in the recumbent position [Greenfield and Cooper 1973]).

Those favoring upright spinal x-ray examination express a need for visualizing the patient's posture while being subjected to the effects of gravity. It is also the feeling of those favoring upright spinal x-ray examination that, with new powerful x-ray equipment (300 mamp, 125 kVp), adequate penetration of spinal areas can be achieved in a minimum amount of time, thus reducing the effects of motion. Film quality, it is felt, is not significantly sacrificed (Hildebrant 1974).

Conflict 2: Normal Posture. The second conflict is determining what represents normal posture. Abstracting the references from Solit's study in structural dynamics (1962), one finds recognized authorities supporting all of the following points of view:

1. In normal standing the feet should be (a) toes out at a 30° angle or (b) parallel.
2. A perpendicular line through the center of gravity should fall in the midline (a) between the ball and heel, (b) 1 cm anterior to the ankle joint, or (c) through the ankle joint.
3. Weight-bearing forces should be distributed predominantly (a) on the lateral aspect of the foot or (b) on the medial aspect of the foot.
4. The spinal curves should be (a) as shallow as possible, or one may accept as normal (b) a higher degree of lordosis of the lumbar spine so long as it is compensated by a commensurate kyphosis of the dorsal spine, so long as the line of gravity continues to intersect the spinal column at the conventional levels and so long as it still falls between hip and sacroiliac articulation (Solit 1962).

Several anatomical points have been designated as the most appropriate or most consistent for proper patient positioning. Denslow

(1955) used a midheel line that consisted of a point equidistant between the heels which, if projected vertically, would bisect the x-ray film and the central ray of the x-ray beam. The patient was positioned with each foot equidistant from the midheel line (6 inches between the medial border of each foot). The trunk above was allowed to assume its normal posture (Denslow 1955; Beilke 1936; Bailey and Beckwith 1937 [included a 20° angulation of each foot from the midheel line]; Beal 1950 [used a 45° angulation of each foot from the midheel line]).

Sausser (1947) felt the feet should be equidistant from a midline but was not rigid at 6 inches, and stated "feet [should] be permitted to assume a position characteristic to the individual."

Vladeff (1949) felt the sacrum was a more consistent landmark by which to center the patient to the x-ray beam, rather than the feet or the buttocks.

The importance of placing the feet directly beneath the hips to reduce pelvic sway was emphasized by Leverone and Winterstein (1974).

Pruitt (1953) positioned a single patient for three different x-rays using the sacrum for patient positioning first; the feet the second time; and the buttocks the third time. The fifth thoracic vertebra was found to be in a different position on each film.

In summary, it is important that the person interpreting the x-ray be aware of how the patient was positioned. A record of the position of the feet can be drawn onto the x-ray jacket simply by placing the jacket beneath the patient's feet when he is positioned. Positioning molds for the feet may also be used to secure foot placement. It is also important that the procedures followed in patient placement be consistent from patient to patient.

Conflict 3: Use of Positioning Devices. Because of the variability in "normal posture," some have advocated the use of various devices to predetermine patient positioning. Such devices have consisted of compression bands (Fox 1954), head clamps (Pettibon 1971), precision turntable (Vladeff 1948; Van Dusen 1968), and a spinal fixation and stabilization device (Rush and Steiner 1964). The use of such devices may

provide for a consistent procedure to be followed in patient positioning. The extent to which "normal posture" may be altered would vary with each device. Again, a knowledge of what procedures were used will aid in making a proper interpretation.

Conflict 4: Technical Conflicts. There is continual discussion as to whether a single x-ray should be taken of the entire spine, as opposed to localized views of smaller areas. Further debate continues on whether full-spine views should be done with split screens or filtration to the collimator and as to the best target-film distance to be used.

Full-spine radiography employing 14 × 36 inch exposure requires specific pieces of equipment not routinely found in many x-ray facilities (i.e., 14 × 36 inch grids and cassettes). Anteroposterior views of the spine on a 14 × 36 inch exposure can be produced with acceptable quality. Unnecessary exposure to areas not related to the spine should be a consideration. Lateral views of the entire spine create a more difficult task in producing an overall acceptable film quality. Again, unnecessary exposure to nonrelated areas should be considered. Endorsement of this type of radiation exposure for every patient seeking spinal manipulation cannot be given by this author.

Filtration at the collimator is recommended. Use of split-screen technology behind the patient, again results in excessive patient radiation. Therefore, the use of split-screen technology is not recommended.

In summary, many of the abovementioned conflicts have remained because no satisfactory resolution has been obtained. Excellent quality can be obtained using upright procedures. Postural evaluation without the effects of gravity can be obtained from recumbent procedures. Various positioning procedures are acceptable providing a knowledge of those procedures is taken into account when interpretation is in process. Use of positioning devices may be acceptable if their effects were accounted for in the interpretation process. Unnecessary patient exposure to ionizing radiation should be avoided where possible.

TABLE 1. **Studies of X-ray Differences in Leg Length**

Investigator	No. Cases	No. Cases with Short Leg	No. Cases with Short Right Leg	No. Cases with Short Left Leg
Bailey and Beckwith (1937)	610	610	288	322
Eggleston	465	338	186	152
Hobbs	307	257	141	116
Kerr et al.	150	137	71	66
Kraus	500	360	increased sacral-base plane	
Pearson	200	135	104	31
Rush and Steiner (1946)	1000	770	406	364
Schwab	540	345	—	—
Swift	90	62	29	33

From Beal (1950)

Structural Asymmetry

A critical area in the evaluation of spinal x-rays is the effect of structural asymmetry. When evaluating structural relationships of one side of the body to another, one must always be mindful that precise equality is probably a rarity. Relating this asymmetrical problem to structural interpretation Howe (1971) states, "Any method of spinographic interpretation which utilizes millimetric measurations from any set of preselected points is very likely to be faulty because structural asymmetry is universal in all vertebrae."

Many studies have been compiled to determine the incidence of anomalous development in the general population. For example, Beal (1950) compared the results of several studies evaluating differences in leg length.

From 65–91% of the people having low-back pain have a difference in leg length. Rush and Steiner statistics show that 77% of the group of soldiers who had symptoms of low-back pain had a difference in leg length. Of these, 37.5% had a difference in leg length over 5 mm. Among the controls, 71% showed a difference in the length of their lower extremities of which 33% had a difference of over 5 mm. Kerr and his associates found in their series of cases that 62% had a difference in leg length of over 5 mm. Schwab found that 64% of the cases he x-rayed had over 5 mm shortening.

Beal's summary (Table 1) certainly indicates that structural asymmetry occurs often enough for its effects to be considered in each radiographic evaluation.

To complete this subject justly, it must be pointed out that agreement does not exist with respect to the effects of asymmetry and its contribution to spinal pain syndromes.

In a comparative study of patients with and without backaches (Splithoff 1953), 100 patients with backache were compared with an equal number of persons who had never consulted with a physician or been disabled by backache. These findings are listed in Table 2 according to changes observed at the lumbosac-

TABLE 2. **Incidence of Changes Observed of Lumbrosacral Junction as Shown by Roentgenograms of 100 persons With and 100 Persons Without Backache**

Type of Change	Backache (%)	Normal (%)
Posterior displacehet of L5	14	16
Scoliosis or tilt, lumbar spine	9	16
Spina bifida occulta	6	4
Spondylolisthesis	3	2
Transitional vertebrae	10	10

From Splithoff: JAMA 152: 1610, 1953.

TABLE 3. **Position of Facets of the Lumbosacral Junction as Shown by Roentgenograms of 100 Persons With and 100 Persons Without Backache**

Type of Facet	Backache (%)	Normal (%)
Anterior-posterior-bilateral	59	55
Asymmetric	9	7
Left internal-exterior		
Right anterior-posterior		
Internal-external, bilateral	4	1
Oblique, bilateral or one	13	18
internal-external		
Rudimentary	4	0

From Splithoff: JAMA 152: 1610, 1953.

ral junction which include transitional vertebrae, spondylolisthesis, spina bifida occulta, posterior displacement of L5, scoliosis, and osteoarthritis. The facet relationships found at the lumbosacral junction in both groups by the author are listed in Table 3. Splithoff concludes by pointing out that radiographs of the lumbosacral region of normal persons and those with backache are quite similar: ". . . congenital anomalies and other anatomic details appear in close numerical sequence." (Splithoff 1953) This study suggests that developmental defects are not more common in people with backaches.

Since it is so common, structural asymmetry is an important factor in radiographic evaluations of spinal relationships.

Significance and Relevance

A presentation of standard procedures that are used to interpret radiographs for purposes of evaluating spinal posture and biomechanics has been offered. A comprehensive review of spinal biomechanics and related spinographic analysis has not been attempted.

Two points remain to be elaborated upon: the significance of these findings and their relevance to spinal manipulative therapy.

Significance

The use of radiography as a tool to aid in a postural and biomechanical evaluation of a patient is well accepted. The use of line-drawing procedures for evaluation is not as well accepted.

Three problems are present with line marking procedures.

Technical error may be present due to magnification and distortion. It has been discussed how proper patient positioning can *minimize* the introduction of errors.

Observer error is easy. Hinck and Hopkins (1960) concluded that the same observer could not measure the same particular interval on an x-ray film consistently. They found that, when observers measured the same area, the inconsistency increased over the single observer error. Inconsistency increased further when the films were of insufficient technical quality.

Tilley (1966) feels that there is an intrinsic mechanical ruling variation of 2 mm (SD 0.5 mm).

It has been shown that *various marking procedures* used on the same film do not indicate the same postural changes and can even contradict each other (Phillips 1975).

Relevance

The clinician employing spinal manipulative therapy should do so on the basis of all clinical findings. A knowledge of the radiographic depiction of the spinal structures should support other clinical data regarding the patient's complaint. Visualization of a spinal malalignment on the x-ray may give valuable information regarding the direction in which a spinal manipulation should be given.

Conclusions

Radiology has become a valuable and integral part of the evaluation of a patient needing spinal manipulative care. This chapter has dealt with the use of standard radiographic procedures. Radiology today is expanding to include the use of new techniques many of which have become extremely valuable in evaluating spinal pathology and biomechanics. These techniques include:

1. *Tomography*—a procedure used to give a radiograph of a specific level of body tissue, aids tremendously in describing anatomic detail (Reichmann, 1973).
2. *Fluoroscopy and cineradiography*—employed to further our understanding of the biomechanics of the spine (Howe 1972, 1975; Reichmann 1973).
3. *Computerized tomography and ultrasound*—beginning to make contributions to the field of biomechanics and postural analysis.

In conclusion, let us reemphasize that radiation exposure to the patient be held to an absolute minimum and film quality be at an absolute maximum. This will enable the clinician who employs manipulative technics, to gain information leading to a correct diagnosis and therapy, while ensuring the patient's safety.

REFERENCES

American Chiropractic Association: Basic Procedural Manual. ACA, Des Moines, IA, 1973

Bailey HW, Beckwith CG: Short leg and spinal anomalies. J Am Osteopath Assoc 36:39, 1937

Beal MC: A review of the short leg problem. J Am Osteopath Assoc 50:109, 1950

Beilke MC: Roentgenological spinal analysis and the technic for taking standing x-ray plates. J Am Osteopath Assoc 35:414, 1936

Cobb JF: Outline for the study of scoliosis. Instructional course lectures. Am Acad Orthop Surg 5:261, 1948

DeJarnette MB: The properly marked pelvis for determining pelvic subluxations. ACA J Chiropr 1:23, 1964

Denslow DO et al: Methods in taking and interpreting weightbearing x-ray films. J Am Osteopath Assoc 54:663, 1955

Department of Roentgenology, National College of Chiropractic: Outline for interpretation of a series of spinal x-rays. J Nat Chiropr Assoc 30:28, 1960

Fox EA: Roentgenological studies of lumbosacral distortion. J Nat Chiropr Assoc 24:24, 1954

Greenfield GB, Cooper SJ: A Manual of Radiographic Positioning. Philadelphia, Lippincott, 1973

Greenfield GB: Radiology of Bone Diseases. 2d ed. Philadelphia, Lippincott, 1975

Gonstead CS: Gonstead Chiropractic Science and Art. Mt. Horeb, WI, Sci-Chi, 1968

Hildebrandt RW: Synopsis of Chiropractic Postural Roentgenology, 2d ed., Lombard, IL, National-Lincoln School Postgraduate Chiropractic Education 1974 ,

Hinck VC, Hopkins CE: Measurement of the atlantodental interval in the adult. Am J Roent November 1960

Howe J: Some considerations in spinal x-ray interpretations. J Clin Chiropr Arch 1:75, 1971

Howe J: Facts and fallacies, myths and misconceptions in spinography. J Clin Chiropr Arch 2:34, 1972

Howe J: Cineradiography evaluation of normal and abnormal cervical spinal function. J Clin Chiropr Arch 2:76, 1972

Howe J: The role of x-ray findings in structural diagnosis. In Goldstein M (ed): The Research Status of Spinal Manipulation, National Institute of Health, Bethesda, MD, 1975

Janse J: Vertebral and pelvic subluxations and distortion-roentgenologically. J Nat Chiropr Assoc 33:31, 1963

Janse J: Measures entailing in postural and structural examination. J Nat Chiropr Assoc 24:9, 1954

Kapandjii JA: The Psychology of the Joints. vol 3. London, Churchill Livingstone, 1974

Levorone RA, Winterstein JF: Full spine radiography, its methods and value. Dig Chiropr Econ 17:26, 1974

Lind GAM: Auto-Traction Treatment of Low Back Pain and Sciatica. Linkoping, Sweden, 1974

Mehta MH: Radiographic estimation of vertebral rotation in scoliosis. J Bone Joint Surg 55B:513, 1973

Meschan I: An Atlas of Anatomy Basic To Radiology. Philadelphia, Saunders, 1975

Nash CL Jr, Moe J: A study of vertebral rotation. J Bone Joint Surg 51A:223, 1969

Pettibon BR: X-ray procedure. Dig Chiropr Econ 14:16, 1971

Phillips RB: An evaluation of the graphic analysis of the pelvis on the A-P full spine radiograph. ACA J Chiropr 12:12, 1975

Pruitt HW: Timely reflections on the need for spinal research. J. Nat Chiropr Assoc 23:28, 1953

Reichmann S: Radiography of the lumbar intervertebral joints. Acta Radiol [Diagn] (Stockh) 14:161, 1973

Rich EA: Roentgenological consideration of the spinal subluxation. J Nat Chiropr Assoc 33:33, 1963

Rush WA, Steiner HA: A study of lower extremity length inequality. Am J Roent 56:616, 1946

Santos NA: Highlights of Roentgenological Interpretation. ACA J Chiropr 2:8, 1965

Sausser WL: The spine viewed and recorded roent. in 4584 Cases. J Nat Chiropr Assoc 17:18, 1947

Solit M: A study in structural dynamics. J Am Osteopath Assoc 62:30, 1962

Splithoff CA: Lumbosacral junction: roentgenographic comparison of patients with and without backaches. JAMA 152:1610, 1953

Van Dusen LG: Chiropractic Relationship to Gravitational Forces. Sodus, NY, 1968

Vladeff T: A report on leg inequalities. J Nat Chiropr Assoc 17:n.p., 1948

Vladeff T: Findings in spinographic research. J Nat Chiropr Assoc 18:17, 1949

Winterstein JF: Chiropractic Spinography. Wheaton, IL, Kjellberg, 1970

CHAPTER ELEVEN
Spinal Radiographic Techniques, Quality Assurance, and Radiation Safety

LEON R. COELHO

In 1895 Wilhelm Roentgen, a German scientist, discovered the phenomenon of electromagnetic production of x-rays from the deceleration of accelerated electrons (Eastman Kodak 1968; Bushong 1975). The implications of penetration through matter by x-ray photons aroused the imagination of scientists around the world. Once photographic records of x-ray images become a reality their applications would absorb the concentration of researchers on a worldwide basis.

Dr. B.J. Palmer, one of the most prominent of the early chiropractors, adapted radiography to the study of the spine and the investigation of spinal vertebral misalignment—the "subluxation." In 1910 the Palmer School of Chiropractic introduced the x-ray as an integral component of the chiropractic examination and employed the "spinograph" as the instrument whereby spinal misalignments could be analyzed.

Through the years chiropractors have developed numerous spinographic analytical techniques resulting in extensive use of roentgenology in the practice of chiropractic. Not only was the subluxation a prime focus of roentgenological study but emphasis on hard and soft tissue pathology has been necessary to protect the patient from possible trauma which could result from certain methods of spinal adjustments.

Recent requirements that chiropractors appear in court as personal injury expert witnesses and malpractice defendants, and the inclusion of chiropractic in Letter Carrier insurance and Medicare coverage have resulted in the study of chiropractic x-ray techniques by third parties. Occasional inconsistency of image "quality" has led to some criticism of chiropractic x-ray technique by government agencies and individuals. This criticism has been compounded in recent years by the newly found radiation hazard.

Chiropractors are not alone as far as criticism of x-ray technique is concerned; all health professions have come under the scrutiny of government "radiation" agencies (Wochos 1977).

Through its Federation of State Licensing Boards, the chiropractic profession was the first health profession to establish a National Quality Assurance and Radiation Safety Program. The purpose of this program was to update chiropractic clinicians on matters regarding: 1) proper utilization and inclusion of safety procedures in x-ray production; 2) the monitoring of the quality of x-rays taken by chiropractors (Coelho 1976).

Radiographic Quality

Radiographic quality assurance, a subject which has gained the attention of both the government and private sector in the United States and abroad, covers a number of parameters. Each parameter is essential within itself, yet all the parameters have an accumulative impact on the outcome of x-ray film image quality.

Since the introduction of the x-ray to the chiropractic profession in 1910, utilization of ionizing radiation by chiropractors has continued at an ever increasing rate, both in x-ray exposure of patient and in the number of chiropractors purchasing their own radiographic systems. Instead of chiropractors utilizing the services of a specialist or diplomate for the taking and reading of x-rays thereby affording the x-ray diplomate the privilege of concentrating on his specialty and making it economically feasible to purchase reliable and suitable equipment, chiropractors have maintained their independence often using less efficient x-ray equipment which frequently resulted in less than optimum quality radiographs (Coelho 1977).

It is evident that a primary factor in the selection of appropriate radiographic equipment is the functional integrity of the equipment or system. However, such a factor becomes a consideration only if one is aware of the possibility of less than optimum performance in some x-ray systems. Until recently this has been the case when it was generally assumed that all x-ray systems, costly as they are, performed with the utmost accuracy required in radiographic applications (Coelho 1977). The radiographic market in the United States offers two basic categories of systems designed for private clinical use—an economical system and a sophisticated system—which possess performance standards consistent with cost.

Radiographic quality assurance, among other factors, is highly dependent upon the "performance" of a radiographic generator and imaging system. The degree of x-ray photon frequency and exposure reproducibility becomes critical in film contrast and exposure control. To demonstrate what is meant by performance, electronic performance data obtained from product data sheets of an economical system and from a sophisticated system are presented in Table 1, which illustrates the degree of functional integrity between economical radiographic systems and the more expensive and sophisticated systems. The question to be asked based on the foregoing statistics is whether one can get by in terms of x-ray quality assurance if one invests in an economical radiographic system. In the author's opinion the answer is no. The reasons for this negative answer are:

1. The economical system has an excessive error factor in all three exposure parameters: peak kilovolts (kVp), milliamperes, and time.
2. The maintenance of economical systems are generally carried out by untrained individuals.
3. Installations of economical systems are not accompanied by recalibration specific to the line voltages found in the practitioner's clinic. The exact opposite is true of the more expensive, sophisticated systems which are sold, backed, and maintained by company employees. Recourse to the x-ray company in the event of persistent or major problems with a system is easily available.

Quality Assurance Considerations

Quality assurance has been emphasized to a much lesser degree by the various healing professions. Unfortunately there is ample evidence (Wochos 1977) that carelessness and indifference to quality assurance has existed in all health professions utilizing radiography. The most serious breach in the caring of the patient is the apparent disregard of patient safety during radiographic exposure. Unnecessary patient radiographic exposure due to hospital or clinic policy, economic necessity, careless radiographic practices, or indifference for human welfare and safety probably constitutes one of the major problems in the American health delivery system.

Quality assurance begins with an awareness of radiographic problems and a desire to minimize the problems through control measures. To control potential problems, x-ray facilities, equipment, and procedures must be examined and must conform to certain criteria.

TABLE 1. **Performance Data for Two Commercially Available X-ray Systems**

Parameter	Product A* (expensive system)	Product B† (economic system)
kV(p) instability (range)	±1.5 kV(p)	±15kV(p)
Milliamperage instability (range ± 5 mamp)	±5 mamp	±20 mamp
Timer instability (accuracy)	4 msec at all timer settings	16 msec at 1/60 sec 60 msec at 3 sec
Approximate cost	$20,000	$15,000
Rating	300 mamp/125 kVp	300 mamp/125kVp

*Data from Picker Corp.; †Data from H.G. Fisher, Inc.

The X-ray Room

The x-ray facility in a private practice involves several rooms, one of which is the radiographic exposure room. In this facility the x-ray generator and the imaging system is housed (Coelho 1976). Either a radiographic table or upright bucky is utilized in most chiropractic facilities requiring a floor space of no less than 9 ft × 12 ft. The most economical location for such a room is usually in the corner of the building. Such a location helps eliminate lead lining of two walls unless the proximity of a neighbor requires shielding. Lead lining of the two inner walls is invariably required for patient and employee protection. Minimum shielding usually adequate for a 300 mamp/125 kV(p) system with moderate use, calls for ⅛-inch virgin lead on a primary barrier and 1/16-inch virgin lead on a secondary barrier. Lead lining may be covered with sheet rock, wallpaper, or paneling while leaded paneling may be obtained at a higher cost.

Floor coverings are mostly aesthetic in nature; however, if carpeting is included it should be grounded to eliminate the accumulation of static electricity during the winter months. If the radiographic facility is located above or below a business or private abode, the floor or ceiling may have to be covered with lead shielding to protect the inhabitants. A shielding equivalent comparable to virgin lead is reinforced concrete. One-eighth-inch virgin lead possesses the same x-ray absorption capability as 9 inches of reinforced concrete, while 1/16-inch virgin lead

corresponds to 5.5 inches of reinforced concrete (National Council on Radiation Protection and Measurements 1968). This amount of concrete in walls, floors, or ceilings may save the chiropractor from installing expensive lead lining. Equipment in the radiographic room should be limited to the x-ray tubestand, tube, tracks, transfer, buckies, and accessories such as lead aprons or lead coats. The control or generator should be located in a lead-lined operator booth, which affords the operator maximum shielding and protection.

X-ray Systems

Radiographic systems most suited for chiropractic applications should have a generating capacity of 300 mamp and 125 kV(p). This capacity allows for adequate penetration and exposure of both the axial and appendicular skeleton of the majority of patients. Obese patients may present an exposure problem. Several states have legislated a minimum generating capacity of 100 mamp and 100 kV(p) for chiropractic offices. Generators in excess of 300 mamp/125 kV(p) are very suitable; however, the cost of large systems becomes prohibitive for a private clinic.

Bucky Systems

The choice between vertical or horizontal bucky tables usually precipitates a debate as to the merits of each. Horizontal tables, which allow for patient immobilization along with gravity induced patient/bucky approximation offers superior film image resolution compared with vertical buckies. On the other hand the vertical bucky, which requires the patient to stand or sit, offers a structural view of the spinal column under a gravitational load and represents the patient's spinal column "at work." Occupational postures may then be evaluated. The presence or absence of the radiographic manifestation of the subluxation obtained in the vertical versus the horizontal position is an unknown factor at this time. Although opinions have been rendered, a conclusive study of vertical positioning compared to horizontal positioning is lacking at this time (Coelho 1977).

The Control Booth

The concept of a control booth, fully lead lined on three sides, stems from the necessity of protecting the x-ray operator. Traditional portable lead screens, popular because of cost and portability, have been used in private clinics; however, even though they may satisfy state minimum standards, these screens present a hazard to the operator largely due to the small and limited area of protection.

The control booth contains the generator or control panel. On federally certified systems (manufactured after August 1974) the exposure control is located directly on the control panel which requires the operator to remain at the panel when making an exposure thus ensuring his protection. A window installed with leaded glass enables the operator to view the patient during radiographic exposure.

The Darkroom

The darkroom is of utmost importance in the processing of carefully exposed films. Quality assurance procedures are critical in this area.

Layout is important for ease of movement and for establishing an expeditious flow of products. The darkroom should be divided into two halves or sides: the "wet side" and "dry side." The wet side is equipped with processing and wash tanks, dryers, sinks, and replenishment tanks. The dry side consists of counter tops for film loading, screen cleaning, and film and cassette storage.

The rationale in separating the darkroom is to separate the processing functions in such a manner that cross contamination between chemicals, films, and intensifying screens is avoided (Eastman Kodak 1968).

The three basic rules important in darkroom quality assurance are: 1) regulation of solutions; 2) cleanliness; and 3) safelight illumination.

Regulation of Solutions. Time-temperature processing is absolutely critical, and this applies to both manual and automatic processing. Manual systems must be controlled to stabilize temperatures. Refrigeration and heating systems operating off thermostats should be installed.

Solutions must be kept fresh at all times. A change of solutions every four weeks in manual tanks is highly recommended (Coelho 1975).

The reliability of a processor is related to its cost. Temperature control and replenishing rates depend on the hardware installed in the processor, and the degree of accuracy varies with various products. Processor function should be periodically checked with a sensitometer.

Cleanliness. X-ray film, which has a sensitive emulsion, cannot withstand physical abuse such as being exposed to dirt. Dust, chemicals, or fingerprints on the film or intensifying screens may manifest as artifacts on the exposed and processed film and should therefore be avoided.

Intensifying screens, which accumulate dust and dirt, should be periodically cleaned. Cleanliness regarding processing tanks and automatic processors extends the life of the metal hardware indefinitely if periodically wiped down and cleaned.

Safelight Illumination. The processing room should be equipped with both white light and safelight illumination. While white light is necessary to execute maintenance duties, the safelight allows for processing of x-ray film without undue exposure to the film (Eastman Kodak 1968).

Fast-speed films are highly sensitive to safelights; therefore, the light source of the latter should be restricted to 7.5 W at a minimum of 4 ft from the film-loading bench. Film fog occurs when film is unduly exposed to safelight.

Cassette Handling and Care

Radiographic detail and image resolution depend on the imaging system itself. Imaging systems, namely the cassette screen-film combination found in routine radiographic assemblies, eventually warp due to handling and use with resultant loss of film-screen contact. Loss of film-screen contact is accompanied by a loss of image resolution. To evaluate film-screen contact a special wire mesh is used. Radiographs of this precision mesh will reveal flaws in film-screen contact (Eastman Kodak 1968; Bushong 1975; Fuchs 1976).

Screens may lose their fluorescent property because of wear, loss of substance, and oxidation and should be replaced after five years of use.

X-ray Film Storage and Handling

From the time x-ray film comes off the production line it begins to deteriorate through oxidation; however, a one-year life expectancy may be expected for radiographic film under normal storage conditions. Normal storage conditions apply to a cool and dry storage area. Deterioration of x-ray film results in fogging of the film, or "base plus fog" (Bushong 1975).

Secondary Radiation. All exposed films should be protected from radiation preferably by storing the film behind a lead shield or in a lead-lined box. The darkroom where film is usually stored should therefore be radiation-proof. Cassettes placed in the x-ray room during exposure absorb secondary radiation resulting in film fog. Films to be exposed should be protected from radiation (Bushong 1975).

Chemical Fog. Depleted developing solution

results in precipitation of unexposed silver bromide and chemical fog. This activity is restrained by using fresh solutions. High-contrast imaging is therefore enhanced when developing solutions are replenished frequently and replaced monthly (Eastman Kodak 1968).

Light Fog. Stray light in the darkroom fogs radiographic film as does the safelight. The darkroom should be periodically checked for light leaks, particularly around the door and window frames as well as the air ducts (Eastman Kodak 1968).

Relative Film Speeds Versus Image Quality

Volumes have been written on x-ray films, maximum densities, response to exposure, grain, mottle, image clarity, and intensifying screens. Experience has demonstrated that films and intensifying screens offering the highest resolution are those requiring the highest radiation. Conversely, low-radiation film-screen combinations offer a lesser degree of image resolution (Coelho 1975).

The current trend in general roentgenology is the "compromise" between radiation levels and image quality. Such a compromise may be obtained by coupling a film of average speed with a relatively fast-speed intensifying screen. Photographic film speeds have been rated for many years. Photographers recognize relative film speeds by referring to the "ASA" indices supplied with each roll of film. This has not been the case with x-ray film to date. Relative x-ray film-speed factors have been obtained after inquiries into two major United States manufacturers. The relative film-speed factors of specific name-brand films are illustrated in Table 2. Numbers listed under the column "relative speed factor" indicate the degree of response to ionizing radiation. A speed factor of 180, as compared with one of 90 indicates that the film is twice as fast as the film of 90, thus requiring half as much radiation for full exposure as does the film rated at 90. Table 2 also illustrates the density (blackness) of certain name-brand films. Films with the high-

TABLE 2.   **Relative Film Speeds and Film Contrasts**

| | Kodak* | | | DuPont† | |
Film	Relative Speed Factor	D-Max	Film	Relative Speed Factor	D-Max
RP (X-Omat)	90	3.28	Cronex 2 DC	110	3.3
RP/L (X-Omat)	90	3.02	Cronex 4	100	3.3
RP/R (X-Omat)	180	3.20	Cronex 5	170	3.2
RP/S (X-Omat)	170	3.20	Cronex 6	110	3.0
Blue Brand	90	3.14	Cronex 6 plus	100	3.3
X-Omatic C with X-Omat screens	90	3.18			
X-Omatic H with X-Omat screens	180	3.32			
Ortho G with Lanex rare earth screens	360	3.40			

*Courtesy of Kodak Corp.   †Courtesy of DuPont Corp.

numbered densities are darker or have more contrast than those with lesser density numbers. A density factor of zero refers to a clear film which does not possess any silver after full processing.

The selection of films offering the highest degree of image quality for a particular procedure is left to the individual. However, it may be stated that films of high speed exhibit excessive grain from large silver crystals and are particularly sensitive to scatter radiation which results in a greater degree of fog. Maximum density selections vary with the type of radiographic study undertaken. Osseous structures, according to general opinion, are easier to perceive if the film exhibits a high contrast (a high maximum density) while the opposite is true of soft-tissue studies.

Principles of X-ray Generation and Recommended Exposures

X-ray Generation

X-ray energy, which is classified as electromagnetic radiation, is produced by the conversion of electrical energy to electromagnetic energy. This process is accomplished by three criteria: 1) a source of free electrons; 2) a means

of electron acceleration; and 3) a means of electron impact deceleration. The x-ray tube aided by elaborate electronic circuitry meets these criteria. Activation of the x-ray tube produces x-ray photons which are beamed at the object under study (Cullinan 1972).

Exposure

The art of executing the correct exposure on radiographic film relative to the object under study is most subtle. In view of the considerable number of variables inherent in any radiographic procedure, the technologist requires both a technique guide designed for the specific x-ray system and a sense of judgment which, when coupled with body measurements, makes the difference between an excellent radiographic exposure and an average, acceptable exposure. The subtleties of judgment come with experience. All radiographic procedures must follow those tried and proven parameters, determined empirically by the fathers of this art. The control of radiographic film contrast and exposure are found at the operator's fingertips. Radiographic quality assurance is intimately dependent upon these factors, namely, the measurements of kilovolt (peak) and milliampere-seconds.

TABLE 3. **Optimum kV(p) Settings for the Adult Spine**

Area	Average Thickness (cm)	Optimum kV(p)
Atlas/axis open mouth	17	88
Nasium	17	94
Base-posterior	23	100
Vertex	23	100
Cervical lateral	10	92
Cervical oblique	10	100
Lower cervical upper dorsal AP	12	98
Full spine AP	26	92
Cervical dorsal lateral	31	92
Lumbosacral lateral	31	100

Note: Recommended grid ratios, 10:1 or 12:1 (85 lines per inch); recommended film—DuPont Cronex 4; recommended screen—DuPont High

In an attempt to assist the practitioner by eliminating as many of the variables as possible, the following techniques are illustrated which represent the current trends in chiropractic x-ray.

Controlling Kilovolt Peaks [kV(p)]. The optimum kV(p) parameters recommended by the Palmer College of Chiropractic for the various views of the spine, coupled with a high density film are given in Table 3. Confining exposures to the following kV(p) settings helps eliminate one of the technique variables.

Controlling Milliampere-Seconds. Milliampere-seconds (mamp-sec) and the control of exposure will be discussed as a single function and as one of the variables. Traditionally milliampere-seconds has been considered as two separate entities, namely, milliamps and time expressed in seconds. To think of milliamperes and seconds as separate entities leads to confusion in calibrating an x-ray technique. Furthermore, milliamperage does not exist by itself; it must be accompanied by time. One may rearrange the milliamperes and seconds to come up with the same milliampere-seconds and there are certain preferences.

In selecting a given setting, several alternatives are possible on most control panels. A setting of 50 mamp-sec, for example, may be

TABLE 4. **Milliampere and Time Combinations**

mamp	sec	mamp-sec
50	1	50
100	1/2	50
200	1/4	50

From Coelho 1975

selected by any of the three combinations shown in Table 4. Of these choices one is preferred over the others, that is, 200 mamp at ¼ sec. This exposure is the shortest in terms of time, thereby reducing the chance of blurring the radiographic image caused by motion of the patient.

Exposure Guides

Selections for x-ray exposures may be computed by various calculators found on the market; however, a basic technique guide enables one to standardize exposure parameters thus providing expediency. Exposure guides suggest those parameters which may be used as a starting point in the development of a technique guide suitable for a specific x-ray system (Tables 5–8).

The techniques recommended in Tables 5, 6,

TABLE 5. **Cervical Spine Exposure Guide**

View	cm	mamp	sec	kV(p)	FFD (in)	mamp-sec	Film Size (in)
Open mouth	8–9	300	1/20	72	40	15	8 × 10
	10–11	300	1/20	74	40	15	8 × 10
	12–13	300	1/20	76	40	15	8 × 10
	14–15	300	1/20	78	40	15	8 × 10
	16–17	300	1/20	80	40	15	8 × 10
	18–19	300	1/20	84	40	15	8 × 10
AP Closed	8–9	300	1/20	62	40	15	8 × 10
	10–11	300	1/20	64	40	15	8 × 10
	12–13	300	1/20	68	40	15	8 × 10
	14–15	300	1/20	70	40	15	8 × 10
Lateral or oblique	8–9	300	1/10	74	72	30	10 × 12
nasium	10–11	300	1/10	76	72	30	10 × 12
	12–13	300	1/10	80	72	30	10 × 12
	16–17	100	1/2	74	40	50	8 × 10
	18–19	100	1/2	76	40	50	8 × 10
	20–21	100	1/2	80	40	50	8 × 10
Vertex or base	20–21	100	1/2	80	40	50	8 × 10
posterior	22–23	100	1/2	84	40	50	8 × 10
	24–25	100	1/2	90	40	50	8 × 10

TABLE 6. **Thoracic Spine Exposure Guide**

View	cm	mamp	sec	kV(p)	FFD (in)	mamp-sec	Film size (in)
A-P	16–17	200	3/10	68	40	60	14 × 17
	18–19	200	3/10	72	40	60	14 × 17
	20–21	200	3/10	76	40	60	14 × 17
	22–23	200	3/10	80	40	60	14 × 17
	24–25	200	2/5	76	40	80	14 × 17
	26–27	200	2/5	82	40	80	14 × 17
	28–29	200	2/5	86	40	80	14 × 17
	30–31	200	1/2	86	40	100	14 × 17
	32–33	200	1/2	90	40	100	14 × 17
Lateral	22–23	200	2/5	60	40	80	14 × 17
	24–25	200	2/5	64	40	80	14 × 17
	26–27	200	1/2	66	40	100	14 × 17
	28–29	200	1/2	70	40	100	14 × 17
	30–31	200	1/2	74	40	100	14 × 17
	32–33	200	1/2	76	40	100	14 × 17
	34–35	200	1/2	80	40	100	14 × 17
	36–37	200	1/2	84	40	100	14 × 17

TABLE 7. **Lumbosacral Spine Exposure Guide**

View	cm	mamp	sec	kV(p)	FFD (in)	mamp-sec	Film size (in)
Anteroposterior	16–17	200	3/10	76	40	60	14 × 17
	18–19	200	3/10	80	40	60	14 × 17
	20–21	200	2/5	74	40	80	14 × 17
	22–23	200	2/5	80	40	80	14 × 17
	24–25	200	2/5	84	40	80	14 × 17
	26–27	200	2/5	88	40	80	14 × 17
	28–29	200	7/10	88	40	100	14 × 17
	30–31	200	1	92	40	200	14 × 17
	32–33	200	1 1/2	86	40	300	14 × 17
Lateral	22–23	200	1/2	86	40	100	14 × 17
	24–25	200	1/2	90	40	100	14 × 17
	26–27	200	7/10	86	40	140	14 × 17
	28–29	200	7/10	90	40	140	14 × 17
	30–31	200	1	90	40	200	14 × 17
	32–33	200	1	92	40	200	14 × 17
	34–35	200	1 1/2	90	40	300	14 × 17
	36–37	200	1 1/2	94	40	300	14 × 17
	38–39	200	2	94	40	400	14 × 17
	40–41	200	2	98	40	400	14 × 17

Oblique: Add 6 to 8 kV(p) to AP lumbar technique.

TABLE 8. **Full Spine Exposure Guide**

View	cm	mamp	sec	kV(p)	FFD (in)	mamp-sec	Film size
Anteroposterior	18–19	200	3/10	82	72	60	14 × 36
	20–21	200	2/5	84	72	80	14 × 36
	22–23	200	2/5	88	72	80	14 × 30
	24–25	200	1/2	92	72	100	14 × 36
	26–27	200	7/10	94	72	140	14 × 36
	28–29	200	1	94	72	200	14 × 36
	30–31	200	1 1/2	94	72	300	14 × 36
	32–33	200	1 1/2	98	72	300	14 × 36
	34–35	200	1 1/2	102	72	300	14 × 36
	36–37	200	2	100	72	400	14 × 36

and 7 should be used with a reciprocating grid, 12:1 ratio and 85 lines per inch. The imaging system consists of DuPont Cronex 4 film and DuPont High-Plus intensifying screens.

The techniques shown in Table 8 should be used with a stationary grid, 8:1 ratio and 100 lines per inch. The imaging system consists of DuPont Cronex 4 film and DuPont High-Plus intensifying screens. A Sportelli or Baulan filter must be used to balance exposures of the thoracocervical spine with the lumbopelvic spine. The only modifications necessary would be in the milliampere-second settings.

Milliampere-Second Rules. To be visible on an x-ray film mamp-sec modifications must range between 35 and 50 percent. A 35 percent mamp-sec alteration is considered the minimum alteration necessary to effect a visible change of film exposure whereas a 50 percent change results in a marked difference in film exposure.

Routine Chiropractic Views

Principles of Patient Placement

Preparation and positioning of the patient for radiographic exposure necessitates a procedure which, if diligently followed, reduces the incidence of error and retakes.

Such a procedure should entail the following:

1. Complete disrobing of areas to be x-rayed. Gowning does not interfere with the radiographic procedure;
2. Removal of artifacts such as rings, watches, glasses, dentures, earnings, hearing aids, etc;
3. Mensuration of areas to be x-rayed;
4. Correlation of measurement to specific technique parameters;
5. Incorporation of film identification and appropriate markers;
6. Utilization of leaded aprons or gonad shielding, if possible;
7. Careful positioning of collimated x-ray beam, patient, and film alignment;
8. Rechecking of exposure settings.

Most Common Views

Most radiographic views employed in the practice of chiropractic encompass the spinal column. The following is a brief description of the most commonly utilized views (Palmer College of Chiropractic 1977; Hildebrandt 1977):

Lateral Cervical–Flexion and Extension

Film size: 10 in × 12 in vertical; identification and Mitchell marker
F.F.D.: 72 in
Patient placement: Sitting or standing at appropriate bucky, with cervical spine fully flexed or fully extended for appropriate view
Central ray: Perpendicular to center of the film
Structures necessary for analysis: The base of the skull and all cervical vertebrae
Purposes: Hyper/hypomobility, fixation, aberrant-movement subluxations; evaluation for possible pathological changes

Lateral Cervical

Projection: Longitudinal
Film size: 10 in × 12 in vertical; identification and Mitchell marker
F.F.D.: 72 in
Patient placement: Sitting with shoulder touching bucky
Central ray: Through C-1 transverse processes perpendicular to the film
Structures necessary for analysis: Floor of skull; cervical vertebrae C-1 through C-7
Purposes: Extension, flexion, anterolisthesis, retrolisthesis, and interosseous spacing subluxations; evaluation for possible pathological changes

Nasium

Projection: Horizontal
Film size: 8 in × 10 in vertical; identification and Mitchell marker
F.F.D.: 40 in
Patient placement: Sitting anteroposteriorly against the cervical bucky
Central ray: Caudal angle passing through a

point 1 in below the glabella through the level of the mastoid tip, to the center of the film

Structures necessary for analysis: Ocular orbits, medial inferior tips of the condyles, lateral inferior tips of lateral masses

Purposes: Lateral flexion, lateralisthesis subluxations of C-1; evaluation for possible pathological changes

Anteroposterior Open Mouth (Atlas-Axis)

Film size: 8 in × 10 in vertical; identification and Mitchell marker

F.F.D.: 40 in

Patient placement: Sitting or standing AP against the appropriate bucky

Central ray: Through the center of the mouth perpendicular to the center of the film

Structures necessary for analysis: C-1 and C-2

Purposes: Lateralisthesis, lateral flexion, and rotational subluxations of C-2; evaluation for possible pathological changes

Anteroposterior Cervical

Film size: 8 in × 10 in vertical; identification and Mitchell marker

F.F.D.: 40 in

Patient placement: Sitting or standing AP against the appropriate bucky with head tilted back against the bucky

Central ray: Angled 15° cephalad through the thyroid cartilage to the center of the film

Structures necessary for analysis: C-1 through T-1

Purposes: Lateralisthesis, lateral flexion, and rotational subluxations of C-3 through T-1; evaluation for possible pathological changes

Cervical Obliques

Film size: 8 in × 10 in vertical; identification and Mitchell marker

F.F.D.: 72 in

Patient placement: Sitting or standing at appropriate bucky, the patient at 45° angle to the film, the median sagittal plane of the skull is placed parallel to the plane of the bucky

Central ray: 15° cephalad through the level of the superior thyroid cartilage to the center of the film

Structures necessary for analysis: Diagnostic film only, not used for analysis

Purposes: Evaluation for pathological changes, especially of the intervertebral foramen and articular processes of the cervical spine

Vertex

Projection: Vertical

Film size: 8 in × 10 in vertical; identification and Mitchell marker

F.F.D.: Approximately 36 in

Patient placement: Sitting posteroanteriorally in front of the cervical bucky

Central ray: Enters the vertex of the skull

Structures necessary for analysis: Nasal spine and septum; basilar process; transverse foramen of atlas; odontoid process and interodontoid spaces

Purposes: Atlas rotational subluxation; evaluation for possible pathological changes

Base Posterior

Projection: Vertical

Film size: 8 in × 10 in vertical; identification and Mitchell marker

F.F.D.: Approximately 36 in

Patient placement: Sitting AP against the cervical bucky

Central ray: Enters 1 in posterior to symphysis menti passing through ½ in anterior to external auditory meatus to the center of the film

Structures necessary for analysis: Nasal spine and septum; basilar process; transverse foramen of atlas; odontoid process and interodontoid spaces

Purposes: Atlas rotational subluxation; evaluation for possible pathogical changes

Anteroposterior Thoracic Spine

Film size: 14 in × 17 in vertical; identification and Mitchell marker

F.F.D.: 40 in

Patient placement: Standing AP against the bucky

Central ray: Perpendicular to film center

Purposes: Lateralisthesis, lateral flexion, and rotational subluxations; evaluation for possible pathological changes

Lateral Thoracic Spine

Film size: 14 × 17 in vertical; identification and Mitchell marker

F.F.D.: 40 in

Patient placement: Standing laterally with the patient's shoulder against the bucky

Central ray: To film center

Measurement: Measure across lower axillary border

Purposes: Antero/retrolisthesis, extension, flexion, and interosseous spacing subluxations; evaluation for possible pathological changes

Lateral/Swimmer's View

Film size: 10 in × 12 in vertical; identification and Mitchell marker

F.F.D.: 40 in

Patient placement: Standing laterally against the bucky

Central ray: Perpendicular to the film to the level of T-1/T-2

Purposes: To visualize lower cervical and upper thoracic vertebrae

Anteroposterior Lumbo-Pelvic

Film size: 14 in × 17 in vertical; identification and Mitchell marker

F.F.D.: 40 in

Patient placement: Standing against the bucky

Central ray: Perpendicular to a point one inch below the level of the iliac crests

Purposes: Lateralisthesis, lateral flexion, rotational and sacroiliac subluxations; evaluation for possible pathological changes

Lateral Lumbar

Film size: 14 in × 17 in vertical; identification and Mitchell marker

F.F.D.: 40 in

Patient placement: Standing laterally with hip against the bucky

Central ray: Perpendicular to a point 1 in above

the level of the iliac crest to the center of the film

Purposes: Antero/retrolisthesis, flexion, extension, and interosseous spacing subluxations; evaluation for possible pathological changes

Lumbar Obliques

Film size: 14 in × 17 in vertical; identification and Mitchell marker

F.F.D.: 40 in

Patient placement: 25 to 45° angle to bucky with right gluteal touching bucky

Left posterior oblique: 25 to 45° angle to bucky with left gluteal touching bucky

Right anterior oblique: 25 to 45° angle to bucky with the right anterior iliac crest touching bucky

Left anterior oblique: 25 to 45° angle to bucky with left anterior iliac crest touching bucky

Central ray: Perpendicular to the level of the iliac crest to the center of the film

Purposes: Diagnostic evaluation, especially of the intervertebral foramen, articular processes and pars interarticularis of the lumbar vertebrae

Anteroposterior Full Spine

Film size: 14 in × 36 in vertical; identification and Mitchell marker

F.F.D.: 72 in

Patient placement: Standing AP against full spine bucky

Central ray: Perpendicular to the center of the film

Measurement: Measure patient at sternum and umbilicus; take thickest measurement

Structures necessary for analysis: Full spine to include ischial tuberosities to occular orbits

Purpose: Lateralisthesis, lateral flexion, rotational subluxations, and scoliosis; evaluation for possible pathological changes

Radiation Protection

"The fact that ionizing radiation produces biological damage has been known for many years. The first case of human injury was reported in the literature just a few months following Roentgen's original paper in 1895 announcing the discovery of x-rays. As early as 1902, the first case of x-ray induced cancer was reported in literature." (Barnett 1976) In the 1920s and 1930s evidence regarding the harmful effects of radiation on humans existed. This evidence was based upon clinical experience gained from early radiologists, underground miners who were exposed to airborne radioactive materials, radium watch dial painters, and other special occupational groups that were exposed to excessive amounts of radiation. The long-term biological significance of smaller, chronic doses of radiation, however, was not widely publicized or known until recent years. For that matter, it was not until after the atomic bombings of Hiroshima and Nagasaki that significant knowledge of the biological effects of radiation was obtained (Barnett 1976).

In reviewing the various studies, it becomes apparent that diagnostic x-rays may be harmful. Studies on DNA structures of drosophila have demonstrated a high probability of chromosomal chain damage as well as possible translocation of nucleotides resulting from exposure to ionizing radiation (The Advisory Committee on the Biological Effects of Ionizing Radiation 1976). These changes may result in cellular mutations due to alteration of transfer and messenger RNA affecting protein synthesis (The Advisory Committee on the Biological Effects of Ionizing Radiations 1976). This study raises the question of the effects on future generations of human populations if exposure to x-ray occurs and is repeated with each generation. The drosophila studies indicated a lingering effect in several generations from a single exposure (The Advisory Committee on the Biological Effects of Ionizing Radiations 1976).

In view of the fact that most Americans are exposed periodically in one lifetime, mutations may become compounded over several generations. Several conditions have been correlated with x-ray exposures, both intero and extero, and have been manifest during prenatal as well as postnatal life (The Advisory Committee on the Biological Effects of Ionizing Radiations 1976; Bushong 1975). Such disorders include:

Leukemia
Cataracts
Microcephaly
Growth impairment
Mental retardation
Benign brain and scalp tumors
Cancers (lung, breast, stomach, thyroid)

The government's interest in x-ray exposures on humans is triggered by two considerations. One deals with the effects on humans from radiation exposure, as illustrated in a compilation of studies assembled by the National Academy of Sciences (National Research Council) in a text entitled *The Effects on Populations of Exposure to Low Levels of Ionizing Radiation* (Advisory Committee on the Biological Effects of Ionizing Radiations 1976). The other deals with the range of radiographic exposure a patient may experience between different radiographic facilities for the same examinations. These statistics are compiled under a program known as N.E.X.T. (National Evaluation of X-ray Trends) (Wochos 1977).

Statistical profiles compiled by the Bureau of Radiological Health, Food and Drug Administration of the Department of Health, Education and Welfare imply that radiation levels imposed on patients during routine x-ray examinations may vary considerably as different radiological facilities are used.

For example, the organ-dose index system (ODIS) is used to demonstrate the variations of organ doses delivered to a standard patient and the varieties of exposure techniques which produce these variations. An example of the potential ODIS was presented in a pilot study conducted by five states and the District of Columbia in 1972 (Bureau of Radiological Health, FDA 1973). Data for 42 lumbosacral examinations were collected in this pilot. For these 42 cases the:

1. Mean ovarian dose index varied from 11 to 660 mrad;
2. Testicular dose index varied from 0.5 to 1,000 mrad;
3. Source to film distance varied from 30 to 72 in;

4. Milliamperage/seconds used varied from 21 to more than 200;
5. X-ray-beam size varied from 13 to 38 in or a diagonal measurement;
6. Entrance radiation exposure varied from 100 to over 1,500 mrad.

Furthermore, excerpts from the N.E.X.T. program in Kentucky illustrate the range of radiation levels a patient may be exposed to for any one given examination. Comparisons of radiation levels are made by considering the full-spine anteroposterior, the lumbosacral spine, and a dental x-ray known as the "bitewing posterior." Three parameters are measured: skin entrance exposure, testicular absorbed dose, and ovarian absorbed dose.

N.E.X.T. Statistics from Kentucky

Full-spine anteroposterior
    (22 surveys)

Skin entrance exposure	48 to 673 mrad
Testicular dose	Less than 0.5 to 367 mrad
Ovarian dose	Less than 0.5 to 107 mrad

Lumbosacral spine
    (409 surveys)

Skin entrance exposure	41.0 to 372 mrad
Testicular dose	Less than 0.5 to 4105 mrad
Ovarian dose	4.0 to 293 mrad

Dental bitewing post
    (886 surveys)

Skin entrance exposure	62 to 6771 mrad

Federal Controls

Since radiation is harmful to the population and exposure varies considerably, guidelines and restrictions have been considered essential. For these reasons, the federal government has implemented controls on the performance of diagnostic x-ray equipment (Advisory Committee . . . 1976).

The following is a summary of the "federal diagnostic x-ray equipment standard" as published by the U.S. Department of Health, Education and Welfare (1974).

Diagnostic X-Ray Equipment Standard. The purpose of the federal diagnostic x-ray equipment standard is aimed at reduction of patient radiation exposure during x-ray examinations. Ninety percent of the exposures to the United States population from artificial radiation sources is attributed to the diagnostic use of x-rays. More than 130 million people are estimated to receive some kind of x-ray examination each year in the United States.

Major Provisions of the Standard. The federal diagnostic x-ray equipment standard may be viewed under two general points. First, it is an equipment performance standard. It cannot regulate equipment design features, neither can it stipulate components. A certain type of beam-limiting device (collimator), for example, cannot be stipulated. It is up to the manufacturer to determine how to achieve levels of equipment performance mandated by the standard.

The other point is that the standard does not regulate diagnostic x-ray equipment users. It neither requires health professionals to practice radiology in certain ways nor prohibits them from using x-ray equipment for a desired purpose.

The standard applies to major components and complete systems manufactured after August 1, 1974. With respect to systems in use prior to the effective date, the standard in no way requires or implies that these units must be modified, upgraded, or discarded.

Components covered by the standard are tube-housing assemblies, x-ray controls, x-ray high-voltage generators, fluoroscopic-imaging assemblies, tables, cradles, film changers, cassette holders, and beam-limiting devices. All components made after the August 1, 1974 effective date of the standard must be certified by manufacturers for compliance with its provisions. All components must bear permanent certification labels, which are readily visible after component assembly.

The Practitioner's Responsibility. Federal controls on diagnostic x-ray equipment may restrict the amount of radiation per patient exposure; however, the only control on those

TABLE 9. **Effect of Filtration Added at X-Ray Tube on Patient Dosage**

	Filter	kV(p)	Mamp-sec	Entrance Exposure (rad)	Comments
Film #1	None	60	75	3.1 rad	Patient receives heavy skin dose
Film #2	1 mm Al	60	80	1.4 rad	Reduces entrance dose by more than 50%, despite increase in mamp-sec
Film #3	2 mm Al	60	88	0.95 rad	Increases mamp-sec but decreases skin dose by a further 35%.
Film #4	3 mm Al	60	98.5	0.80 rad	Mamp-sec again increased, but patient dose decreased by another 16%; total entrance dose reduced by 74% with 3 mm Al filtration

From Indiana Board of Health 1964

parameters which accumulatively will drastically reduce patient exposure are those which the doctor places on his own x-ray facility. By demanding certain techniques and certain products, the doctor can ensure patients a minimum of radiation exposure. These controls or considerations may be listed as follows:

1. Avoid x-raying a pregnant patient;
2. Determine the date of last menstrual period of all female patients of child-bearing age and capability;
3. Restrict x-ray exposures on children;
4. Protect the gonads of the present "genetic pool";
5. Use low dosage exposure techniques whenever possible;
6. Use modern, reliable equipment;
7. Protect the doctor and staff.

The Technology of Low-Radiation Exposures

Radiation control technology is the implementation of those factors which singularly or cumulatively reduce the patient radiation exposure, while at the same time producing a radiograph of acceptable quality.

Filtration. Filtration deals with x-ray primary-beam attenuation for the purpose of modifying the primary beam in such a manner that the x-ray photons of low frequency and limited penetration may be absorbed. This re-

sults in the protection of the patient from possible tissue injury due to ionization (Bushong 1975).

Permanent filtration, utilizing aluminum alloy—type 1100—permanently installed to attenuate the entire primary beam, is required by most states. Effects of aluminum filters in x-ray beam attenuation are illustrated in Table 9.

Reducing Input Radiation to Patient. Increased filtration at the tube head amounting to 2–3 mm of aluminum in the low-voltage range will reduce the entry dose to the patient by 50 to 75 percent.

Beam attenuation in addition to regulation filters should be of vital interest to every chiropractor employing radiographic studies.

The Radiation Control Commission of the International Chiropractor Association has for many years made patient safety one of its prime concerns. The commission continues to develop and adopt radiographic technologies that lower patients' radiation levels.

During the last few years the commission has encouraged the utilization of certain radiographic accessories which significantly reduce patient radiation. The full-spine radiographic projection has become popular in the practice of chiropractic and is heavily promoted by certain segments of the profession. This was made possible by a variable (split) intensifying screen technique allowing radiographs of the entire spine. Even though such a technique accomplishes the objectives of obtaining a full-spine radiograph, undesirable factors such as split-screen artifacts and excessive patient radiation tend to negate the advantages of these films.

Furthermore, the utilization of split-screens to compensate for anatomical variations resulted in greater body entrance exposures than would be expected if the axial skeleton were radiographed sectionally.

The development and subsequent adoption of the Sportelli-Winterstein supplemental filter offered an alternative to split-screen technology at a lower radiation level. Even though this new technique has been highly publicized, some resistance to the adoption of the wedged filter persists. Even though the Sportelli-Winterstein filter may attentuate the primary beam, secondary radiation produced by the filter far exceeds the radiation levels encountered with the split-screen technique.

The Department of Roentgenology of the Palmer College of Chiropractic conducted studies regarding patient entrance exposure encountered by both the split-screen and Sportelli-Winterstein filter techniques (Coelho 1977). A study of the techniques necessitated a comparison of screen speeds, film speeds, and x-ray techniques on an average-sized patient.

Anteroposterior Technique. The calibration for the AP full spine was based on an average-sized patient for both the split-screen and Sportelli-Winterstein filter techniques, yielding an AP measurement of 22 cm.

Lateral Technique. Measurements for the split-screen technique were based on an average-sized patient. The thoracic lateral measurement averaged 31 cm while the pelvic lateral measurement was 35 cm.

A measurement of 33 cm was used for the Sportelli-Winterstein filter technique in obtaining the single, full-spine, lateral exposure. Tests were performed by duplicating each radiographic technique according to the criteria of that technique. The AP split-screen technique required a tube-to-film distance of 72 inches on a single exposure and the lateral full spine was obtained by making two separate exposures on a 14 inch × 36 inch film at 72 inches resulting in an overlap of exposures at the twelfth

thoracic vertebral level. Each exposure was collimated to a 14 inch × 18 inch projection.

The split-screen technique required intensifying screens of three different speeds in cassettes used for AP and lateral projections; hence the name "split-screen." A medium-speed screen was used to radiograph the cervical spine—the thoracic screen being slightly faster. At the lumbopelvic spine a high speed screen was used.

The Sportelli-Winterstein beam attenuation technique requires a 14 inch × 26 inch cassette for the full-spine projection in which a pair of single-speed screens were mounted. The specific screen used was DuPont's High Plus screen. The AP projection was made at 72 inches with a single exposure and the filter attenuated the beam across the skull, cervical spine, and upper thoracic spine. The lateral projection was obtained with a single exposure utilizing a pair of single-speed screens (DuPont High Plus) and a tube to film a distance of 72 inches. The Sportelli-Winterstein filter was again employed to attenuate the beam over the skull, cervical spine, and upper thoracic spine (Coelho 1977).

The entrance exposures measured in this study are listed in Tables 10 and 11. The specific radiographic techniques including the grid characteristics and film types used in the study are shown in Table 12.

The preceding charts strongly suggest the direction every chiropractor should follow. A radiograph of acceptable quality, compatible with chiropractic analytical criteria, and obtained at the lowest radiation level possible is a goal worth striving for. The above techniques are by no means optimum. Even lower exposure levels are possible.

Certain limitations of the Sportelli-Winterstein filter may be averted with the Bauer-Nolan multiple filtration system, which is highly versatile and, as in the case of the Sportelli-Winterstein filter, may be used on a radiograph of any size.

Peak Kilovolts Versus Milliampere-Seconds Versus Patient Exposure. Patient exposure levels may be modified by selecting various kV(p)/mamp-sec combinations, all of which

TABLE 10. **Entrance Exposures: Full Spine A-P (mR)**

Anatomical Location	Split-Screen Technique	Sportelli Filter Technique
Eyes	92.0	7.5
Thyroid	131.0	20.0
Zyphoid process	120.0	100.0
Umbilicus	140.0	110.0
Symphsis pubis	95.0	50.0

From Coelho (1977)

TABLE 11. **Entrance Exposures: Full Spine Lateral (mR)**

Anatomical Location	Split-Screen Technique			Sportelli Filter Technique
	Upper Spine	Lower Spine	Total	
Eyes	160.0	1.2	161.2	21.0
Thyroid	160.0	2.0	162.0	110.0
Zyphoid process	120.0	420.0	540.0	340.0
Umbilicus	1.0	440.0	441.0	330.0
Symphysis pubis	0.2	430.0	430.2	360.0

From Coelho (1977)

TABLE 12. **Radiographic Parameters**

Parameters	Split-Screen Technique			Sportelli Wedge Technique	
	AP	Lateral Upper	Lateral Lower	AP	Lateral
Centimeters	22	31	35	22	35
Kilovolt peak	80	90	90	106	100
Milliampere-seconds	180	150	375	60	160
Tube distance	72	72	72	72	72
Film	DuPont Cronex 6 Plus			DuPont Cronex 4	
Grid ratio	10:1	10:1	10:1	10:1	10:1
Grid (lines/inch)	60	60	60	60	60
Grid	Reciprocating			Reciprocating	
Collimation	14 × 36	14 × 18	14 × 18	14 × 36	14 × 36
Permanent total filtration (mmAl)	3.0	3.0	3.0	3.0	3.0

From Coelho (1977)

TABLE 13. **Effects of Kilovolt Peak on Patient Exposure**

	kV(p)	Grid	mamp-sec	Entrance Exposure
Film 1	60	8:1	50	440 mR
Film 2	80	8:1	16.1	250 mR
Film 3	100	8:1	5.0	110 mR
Film 4	120	8:1	3.3	100 mR

From Indiana State Board of Health (1964)

could produce an x-ray film of acceptable quality. The only visible changes to the film would affect contrast. Table 13 illustrates the differences in patient entrance exposures when the kilovolt peak is changed and milliampere-seconds are accordingly modified to balance the peak in obtaining an acceptable exposure. Reduction of patient entrance exposure is accomplished when increases in the kilovolt peak are made with reductions of the milliampere-seconds. Essentially, increased kV(p) settings increase photon frequency and hence penetration. Increased penetration allows for fewer photons necessary for adequate exposure, and milliampere-seconds are therefore reduced, lessening the number of photons produced. The end result is a more efficient beam and reduced exposure to the patient.

The Effect of Grids on Patient Exposure.

Grids, essential in radiographing an anatomical part measuring in excess of 12 cm, present a negative factor in patient radiation control or reduction. Due to the physical characteristics of the grid (lead strips interspaced with a radioluscent substance such as aluminum) additional exposure levels are necessary to compensate for the absorption of photons by the grid. This exposes the patient to higher levels of radiation.

The benefit of a grid in x-raying structures larger than 12 cm is a film lacking large amounts of secondary radiation which would otherwise result in a poor image due to film fog.

Grid ratios control secondary radiation exposure on a film in varying degrees. The ranges of patient exposure due to different grid ratios are shown in Table 14.

Reduction of Patient Radiation: Film/Screen Selections. Whenever a radiographic image is obtained by means of high-speed films and screens, the patient dose is correspondingly reduced as compared with conventional films and screens. This is the most effective way of accomplishing dose reduction in diagnostic roentgenography because it significantly decreases the amount of skin, volume, and gonadal irradiation. Certain technical factors influence the amount of exit radiation required by the recording film (Indiana State Board of Health 1964).

Intensifying Screen. The use of high-speed intensifying screens compared with par or slow-speed screens reduces the radiation necessitated by the film for adequate exposure by approximately 40 percent.

Film Speed. Ultrafast film emulsion reduces the film radiation requirement by about 35 percent over fast film and by about 65 percent over some regular emulsions.

Developer. The radiation dose necessary to fully expose the film emulsion is dependent both on the development time and temperature as well as upon the type of active ingredient used as the silver-reducing agent in the developer itself. At a temperature of 68 F using metolhydroquinone developer, an increase of development time from 3 to 5 minutes reduces the necessary film radiation requirement by 33 percent. If phenidone hydroquinone developer is used, a further 25 percent reduction is achieved in necessary radiation exposure (Indiana State Board of Health 1964).

Collimation. The single, most effective means of reducing patient radiation exposure is by means of positive beam limitation, i.e., collimation. The concept behind automatic collimation is to ensure that the size of the primary beam is restricted to the actual area occupied by the x-ray film.

A primary beam larger than the film size subjects the patient to unnecessary primary and secondary radiation without contributing to the information sought by the procedure.

TABLE 14. **Effects of Grids on Patient Exposure**

	Grid	kV(p)	mamp-sec	Entrance Exposure(R)	Comments
Film 1	16:1	70	1000	18.9	High-ratio 16:1 grid, used at conventional kV level, needs high mamp-sec and delivers high entrance dose.
Film 2	8:1	70	500	9.5	Lower ratio 8:1 grid (same kV as film 1): slightly lower radiographic contrast but entrance dose reduces by 50 percent.
Film 3	16:1	100	160	5.9	Regardless of ratio of grid used, high kV(p) results in lower patient dosage. In the case of the 16:1 grid, high kV(p) lowers dosages 69 percent.
Film 4	8:1	100	120	4.5	Even with high kV(p) the 8:1 grid shows an advantage of 24 percent less patient dosage compared with 16:1 grid.

From Indiana State Board of Health (1964)

In fact, additional primary and secondary exposures subject the film to higher levels of scatter radiation thereby increasing the radiographic fog on the film and reducing the film contrast levels.

Darkroom Chemicals. The importance of fresh chemicals becomes evident when an exposure comparison is made between old chemicals and fresh chemicals. Exhausted chemicals require increased exposure to the film in order to secure a visible radiographic image. The patient is then subjected to increased and unnecessary exposures. Table 15 compares patient exposures between a procedure utilizing fresh chemicals and one utilizing exhausted chemicals (see also Morgan 1965).

A Summary of Technical Factors and Exposure Levels. Table 16 illustrates exposure differences between two techniques; the resultant patient exposures speak for themselves. The techniques selected, although extreme when compared with normal techniques, offer films with good and comparable quality.

Patient Protection

The Leaded Coat. Traditionally, lead aprons have been utilized for patient protection against primary beam exposure as well as from secondary radiation. Unfortunately, the lead apron is inadequate in the protection against secondary radiation. The lead coat, a garment manufactured of lead impregnated PVC (polyvinylchloride) offers protection to both the front and back of a patient's body. In the radiographic procedure, a patient receives secondary radiation from the image receptor (bucky) as well as from other sources and adequate protection from this source of radiation may be had by utilizing a leaded coat.

Consider the typical upper cervical chiropractic radiographic procedure where only a minimal portion of the patient's anatomy is exposed. The intensity of the beam produces a considerable amount of secondary radiation from the patient, the bucky, the collimator, and the additional aluminum filtration on the collimator. Tube-house leakage at 42 in is an additional factor. By wearing a leaded coat, the patient is protected both anteriorly and pos-

TABLE 15. **Effect of Processing on Dosage in Radiography**

	Technique A	Technique B
Processing Data		
Developer	Exhausted (Phenidone)	Fresh (Phenidone)
Age of developer	5 mo	2 weeks
Developing time (min)	3	3
Exposure Data		
Kilovolts	100	100
Milliampere-seconds	10	1.6
	(100 mamp × 1/10 sec)	(100 mamp × 1/60 sec)
Radiation Doses		
Skin entrance exposure (mR)	28	18
Gonadal		
Male (mR)	<0.02	<0.02
Female (mR)	<0.025	<0.02
Volume (gm/rad)	164	64.6
Film (mR)	2.4	1.8

From Indiana State Board of Health (1964)

TABLE 16. **Anteroposterior Lumbar Exposure Guide**

	Technique A	Technique B
Parameters		
Kilovolts	75	115
Distance (in)	40	40
Milliampere-seconds	75	3.3
	(300 mamp × 1/4 sec)	(100 mamp × 1/30 sec)
Grid	12:1	12:1
Screens	Slow detail	High speed
Processing		
Film	Regular	Extra fast
Developer	Metol	Phenidone
Filter (mm Al)	0.5	4.5
Collimation	Wide open	8 × 12
Radiation shielding	None	Gonadal
Radiation Doses		
Skin entrance exposure (mR)	1160	60
Gonadal		
Male (mR)	108	0.49
Female (mR)	100	9
Volume (gm/rad)	7183	610
Film (mR)	18	1.8

From Indiana State Board of Health (1964)

teriorly. The lead coat should, therefore, be worn during all x-ray exposures, providing it does not interfere with the analytical diagnostic procedure.

Gonad Shielding. Full-spine radiography makes a leaded coat difficult to use and the question is raised regarding the necessity of protection during full-spine exposures. The gonads should always receive protection from ionizing radiation. The ovaries are virtually impossible to protect because their protection in full-spine radiography interferes with the analytical process. Fortunately, the ovaries receive lower levels of exposure relative to the levels received by the testicles because of their location.

Testicular protection has traditionally presented a problem. Devices worn by the male usually blocked the symphysis pubis and at times the ischial tuberosities. These structures, necessary for the analysis, must be visible on the x-ray.

An effective and acceptable male gonad cup is currently available. This shield, constructed of polyvinylchloride is impregnated with an equivalency of 0.5-mm virgin lead. It adequately covers the testes without obstructing the osseous structures in the area. The cup-shaped shield protects the testes from both primary and secondary radiation by virtue of offering protection anteriorly, laterally, inferiorly, and posteriorly.

REFERENCES

Advisory Committee on the Biological Effects of Ionizing Radiations: The Effects on Populations of Exposure to Low Levels of Ionizing Radiation. Division of Medical Sciences of the National Research Council, Washington, 1976

Barnett MH: The Biological Effects of Ionizing Radiation: An Over-View DHEW Publication (FDA) 77-8004. Washington, U.S. Government Printing Office, 1976

Bureau of Radiological Health: Medical X-Ray Protection Seminar. Rockville, MD, FDA, Division of Training and Medical Applications, 1973

Bushong SC: Radiologic Science for Technologists. St. Louis, Mosby, 1975

Coelho LR: Quality Control in Chiropractic X-Ray. Davenport, IA, Palmer College of Chiropractic, 1975

Coelho LR: X-ray forum. Int Rev Chiropr 29, 5:10, 1975

Coelho LR: X-ray forum. Int Rev Chiropr 30, 5:6, 1976

Coelho LR: X-ray forum. Int Rev Chiropr 31, 4:8, 1977

Coelho LR: X-ray forum. Int Rev Chiropr 31, 2:12, 1977

Coelho LR: X-ray forum. Int Rev Chiropr 31:7, 1977

Commonwealth of Kentucky: N.E.X.T. Data. Frankfort, Kentucky Department of Health, 1973

Cullinan JE: Illustrated Guide to X-Ray Technics. Philadelphia, Lippincott, 1972

Eastman Kodak: The Fundamentals of Radiography. 11th ed. Rochester, NY, Radiography Markets Division of the Eastman Kodak Company, 1968

Fuchs AW: Principles of Radiographic Exposure and Processing, 2nd ed. Springfield, IL, Thomas, 1976

H.G. Fischer, Inc: Operator's Manual: Fischer 125 kV(p)/300 mA Radiographic System. Franklin Park, IL, 1974

Hildebrandt RW: Chiropractic Spinography. Des Plaines, IL, Hilmark, 1977

Indiana State Board of Health: Low Dosage Medical Roentgenography. Indianapolis, Commission on Radiation Control, Indiana University Medical Center, 1964

Morgan RH, Chaney HE: Darkroom practice and unnecessary patient exposure. Am J Roentgenol 94:236, 1965

National Council on Radiation Protection and Measurements: Medical X-ray and Gamma Ray Protection. NCRP Report no. 34. Washington DC, 1968

Palmer College of Chiropractic, Department of Roentgenology: X-Ray Positioning Manual. Des Plaines, IL, Palmer College of Chiropractic, 1977

Picker Corporation: GX 325 X-Ray Generator. Cincinnati

U.S. Department of Health, Education and Welfare: A Practitioner's Guide to the Diagnostic X-Ray Equipment Standard. DHEW Publication (FDA) 75-8005. Washington, U.S. Government Printing Office, 1974

Wochos JF, Cameron JR: Patient Exposure from Diagnostic X-Rays. An Analysis of 1972–1974, N.E.X.T. Data. DHEW Publication (FDA) 77-8020. Washington, U.S. Government Printing Office, 1977

CHAPTER TWELVE

The Use of Instrumentation and Laboratory Examination Procedures by the Chiropractor

JOHN J. TRIANO

The vertebral motion segment is defined as the smallest functional component of the spine composed of two adjacent vertebrae with their interposed discs. With its inadequately understood biomechanics, the motion segment presents the clinician with several significant problems of differential diagnosis. Each unit is acted upon by a minimum of 24 ligamentous and muscular elements which are responsible for the initiation and guidance of osseous movement. The effect of the myriad combinations of force vectors capable of being simultaneously generated on any given vertebral joint are beyond our comprehension. The simplistic motions of flexion, extension, rotation, and lateral flexion are a consequence of the unhindered function of these multiple factors. With the available state of knowledge of spinal mobility and pathomechanics, accurate diagnosis of functional and organic lesions of the spine can be difficult. Problems that must be addressed for each patient include the identification of the source of symptoms as arising from 1) joint irritation and referred pain; 2) muscle strain and inflammation; 3) nerve irritation with radiation, somatically or viscerally; or 4) somatic pain referred from internal structures.

Controversy as to the factors involved in the causation of spinal pain and radiating syndromes has continued for years. Discussion of the role of postural "biomechanics," anomalous bone structure, aberrant mobility, subluxation, muscle spasm, and nerve irritation persists (Grice 1970, 1973; Illi 1965; Pettibon and Loomis 1973; Evans and Lissner 1959; Jaquet 1976; Coggins 1975; Hildebrandt 1977; Schafer et al. 1978).

The broad ramifications of spinal lesions causing root and cord compression have been well documented; however, the precise nature of less severe vertebral aberrations remains relatively unknown. It is generally accepted throughout the chiropractic and osteopathic professions that many forms of functional internal disturbances may result. It is not uncommon for the clinician to witness apparent improvement in disorders of the cardiovascular, gastrointestinal, genitourinary, endocrine, and immunological systems follow the treatment of spinal lesions (Haldeman 1978). Over the years these experiences have molded the clinical impressions of clinicians who must now contend with the differentiation of spinal, visceral, and spinovisceral disorders.

Herein lies the enigma facing the practitioner who is presented with the individual patient who seeks relief—how to objectively identify and quantify the lesion as well as to determine the presence and degree of visceral involvement. Unfortunately, no concise answers are available. Recent work using various instrumentation and laboratory data when added to physical examination findings is very helpful in confirming a diagnosis.

Many methods of investigation of spinal lesions have been attempted with varying degrees

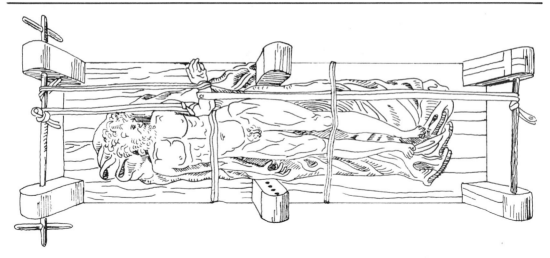

FIG. 1. **Spinal distractor used during the time of Hippocrates. (From Moe et al. 1978)**

of success and our knowledge remains fragmented. As in most other body systems frank pathology, both congenital and acquired, has yielded its secrets more readily to our current methods of evaluation than have functional disorders. These are defined as abnormalities in function that do not demonstrate morphologic changes but may lead to structural lesions if not corrected. The primary tools of diagnosis at the disposal of the clinician include physical, radiographic, and laboratory examination along with thermographic, electromyographic and electrocardiographic analysis. The status and history of these and other forms of instrumentation used by the chiropractic profession will be reviewed.

Postural Analysis

Historically, man has claimed that normal "healthy" posture was achieved when the spine assumed as vertical a position as possible, as seen from the posterior. The normal lateral view of the spine includes primary and secondary anteroposterior curvatures with cervical and lumbar lordosis of 30 to 45° and thoracic kyphosis of less than 55° (Mac Rae 1974). The earliest and simplest evaluation of posture was through observation of anatomical landmarks.

Based on these factors, Hippocrates (Moe et al. 1978; Fig. 1) developed a torso distractor in an attempt to induce anteroposterior spinal straightness in compliance with "normal posture." Good posture has long been evaluated by comparison of the stance to a hypothetical "gravity line." This was described from a lateral view by envisioning a line drawn from the external auditory meatus vertically downward to the floor (Fig. 2). If this line intersected the tip of the shoulder, passed just anterior to the anticubital fossa, bisected the thigh, passed posterior to the center of the knee, and ended at the dorsal surface of the arch of the foot anterior to the ankle, the patient was considered to have good posture. From the anterior, the gravity line was simply defined as a midsagittal bisection passing from the external occipital protuberance through the gluteal cleft and ending equidistant from each foot. The center of gravity of such an individual would be located at the second sacral segment (Daniels and Worthingham 1977).

Plumbline Analysis

One of the first tools to be utilized by the clinician to assist in analyzing posture was the plumbline. Used as a visual comparator for the gravity line, it accentuated any deviations noted during the observational examination. Kouval-

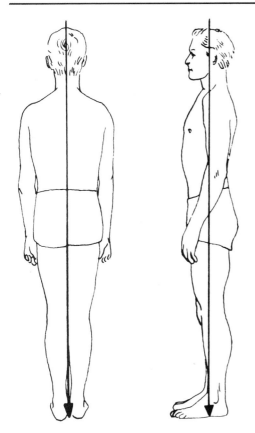

FIG. 2. Normal gravity line. Posteroanterior and lateral view.

chouk (1971) and Jaquet (1976) felt that the plumbline comparison is an effective determination for differentiating compensated asymptomatic scoliosis from the compensated symptomatic scoliosis. With the plumbline centered over the first sacral tubercle in a compensated scoliosis, it should extend superiorly, passing through the external occipital protuberance. If it were to pass laterally to the external occipital protuberance, the scoliosis would be considered decompensated, thus symptom producing. Logan (Coggins 1975) and Mitchel (1971) concur with this viewpoint and believe that balance of the head and shoulder girdle over the pelvis may, in fact, be more important than actual degree of curvature.

Coupled with the findings of gravity-line comparison, the clinician has utilized other tools of physical examination to bolster his diagnosis. A few of the most frequently used indicators would include the findings of pelvic rotation and tilt, shoulder and mastoid levels, rib deformation, knee flexion, joint mobility or fixation, pedal pronation, supination, eversion or inversion, muscular spasm, tenderness, and muscle strength testing (Coggins 1975; Jaquet 1976; Stoddard 1969; Walther 1976).

Scoliometer

Plumbline evaluation has since been modified with several devices designed to provide further visual accentuation of posture deviation from the gravity line. In 1906 the scoliometer, developed by Fipps, provided a grid system for the actual plotting of spinal deformity and postural changes. Consisting of a celluloid sheet with scaled grid lines, the ambitious clinician could record a subject's deformity by plotting anatomical landmarks. Further modification was achieved by the movement of the plumbline into two laterally placed, vertical, tubular frames constructed and set on a base that stabilized the position of the patient by means of a foot plate (Fig. 3). This arrangement was an attempt to afford comparable subsequent evaluations. Movable cords were stretched between the upright supports and, by means of magnets, could be placed parallel to shoulder and pelvic levels. Thus, in both instances, these instruments provided a greater degree of visual accentuation of deviations from the normal gravity line. Neither system, however, provided a practical means of quantifying or recording the actual deviations for later comparison. Current systems providing some degree of measurement of deviation from the normal gravity line are likely to have been derived from this type of system.

Bubble levels have been developed which can be placed by the clinician across the shoulder and pelvic girdle at specific vertebral levels, and a vertical centimeter rule has been used to measure the shoulder or pelvic height above the horizontal line. Even with this device, which is an improvement in quantification, it is still difficult to reproduce comparable results at separate examinations since there is variation in the

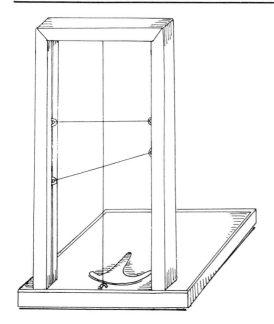

FIG. 3. **Modified plumbline and scoliometer device for clinical postural analysis.**

exact positioning of the horizontal relative to the vertebral segments.

Silhouettograph

Fradd (1923) searching for a more rapid and versatile screening method introduced the silhouettograph, a simple use of light and dark contrast on photographic film to evaluate general postural patterns. Needing to evaluate large numbers of matriculating students, he utilized a linen sheet lit from behind by a bright light source. The subject would then stand between the light source and the sheet. The shadow cast was photographically recorded for both the anteroposterior and lateral stances. Effective as a gross postural screening method, it held obvious drawbacks as a diagnostic technique.

Bilateral Weight Distribution

These simple means of evaluating the body's posture relative to the gravity line do not demonstrate functional changes of weight bearing.

Although most logical concepts assume a shift in loading of the lower extremity concurrent with spinal deviation, none had actually recorded it. The simplest means employed to measure that shift was the use of two scales (Coggins 1975; Hoppenfeld 1965). With the patient standing, each foot on a separate scale (Fig. 4), the clinician could directly record unilateral loads imposed upon the pelvis. Such imbalance has been proposed (Hildebrandt 1977; Mitchel 1971; Coggins 1975; Fisk 1977; Illi 1965) to be responsible for increased incidence of degenerative joint disease, sacroiliac instability, chronic lumbar strain, and other conditions related to asymmetrical weight bearing. Such claims have been more often based on clinical impression from empirical data rather than actual prospective or retrospective study. Care in patient positioning astride the scales is

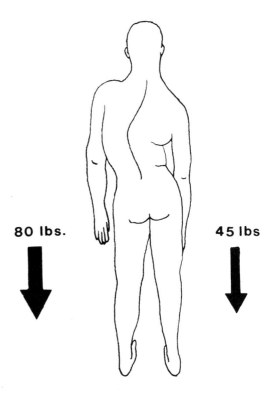

80 lbs.   **45 lbs**

FIG. 4. **Functional shift in weight-bearing load of each lower extremity occurring with the development of scoliosis.**

extremely important so as to avoid transposition of weight forward, back, or laterally due to stance.

Conformateur Analysis

More sophisticated measurement systems have been devised but most have been too cumbersome for routine use in practice. The conformateur was first described by Reynolds and Levitt in 1909 in an effort to establish the erect center of gravity. Jenness et al. (1974) tried to use the conformateur as a means of refining postural measurement. Two upright steel poles were constructed with holes match-drilled to accept freely movable push rods. Placement of the patient between the posts allowed the push rods to be extended to contact the spine. With standardized foot placement, a high test-retest correlation of .93 was found. Thus, the conformateur appears to be an effective instrument for the evaluation of anteroposterior curvature. However, further modification of the instrument is needed before it can be used as a rapid, clear, clinical means of evaluating spinal curvatures.

Moiré Topography

A recent postural evaluation technique that has achieved a much broader clinical acceptance is that of Moiré topography (Speijers 1975; Free 1975). A much simpler system, the topography evaluation is similar to radiographic analysis in terms of time requirements and interpretation. Moiré topography is a contour evaluation system that detects relative posteriority of structures in the back. It is based on optical principles reported originally by Meadows et al. (1970) in which a grid is placed between an angled light source and the object being analyzed. The investigator, standing directly in line with the subject and grid, photographs the pattern created by the visual overlap of the shadow cast by the grid and the grid itself. The Moiré effect on postural analysis is shown in Figure 5. This was first used effectively in a biological system by Terada and Kamazawa (1974) to analyze the euryon of the human skull. The Moiré analysis has an impressive potential but awaits good cor-

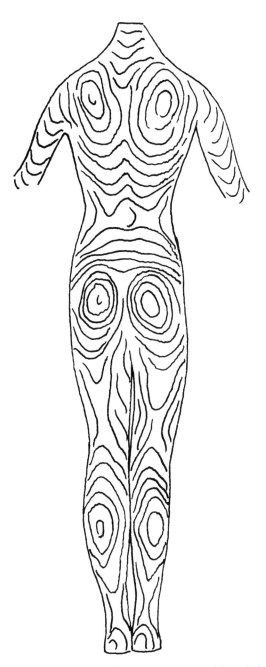

FIG. 5. **Contour analysis pattern seen with Moiré topography. Shadows are on optical effect of a grid superimposed on its own shadow created by an angled light source.**

relative studies relating specific patterns with physical findings.

First reported as a spinal analysis technique by Free (1975), the concentric contours relate to the degree of relative posteriority of specific anatomical landmarks of the back, each line is said to represent 6 mm of difference in elevation. Contour patterns have been found for the scapula, thoracic spine, lumbar spine, gluteals, and erector spinae. Patient positioning is extremely important with this analysis as the grid-patient distance relationship must be constant for bilateral symmetrical points in order to achieve accurate follow-up evaluation. This constancy is easily established by use of a stationary foot plate and by standardizing body position with the arms at the sides to avoid artifact produced by scapular rotation or shoulder elevation. Free (1975) reported elaborate interpretations of these patterns and stated that a high correlation with x-ray findings existed. Unfortunately, neither the x-ray findings nor the interpretations were quantified or statistically analyzed.

Speijers et al. (1975), seeking to validate the Moiré effect as a tool of postural analysis, took simultaneous photographs from the anterior through the grid and perpendicularly from the side of the patient. Careful repetitive measurements were made of the distance of selected landmarks from the grid. These were then used to develop a geometric equation to describe the depth of difference between adjacent shadow lines:

$$\Delta = \frac{a \ (\cos \alpha) \ (\cos \beta)}{\sin \ (\alpha + \beta)}$$

where Δ is the depth difference between shadow lines; α is the angle of light beam creating the shadow; β is the line of sight of camera; a is the distance between grid lines. Assuming a camera angle of zero degrees and light rays that are parallel. This can be simplified to

$$\delta = a \ (\cot \alpha)$$

Speijer's system may be useful as a research tool, but clinically it is again time consuming and burdensome. Contour analysis alone seems to fulfill clinical criteria for being quickly performed, reproducible, and reliable. What is now needed is good correlation to physical findings in order to develop adequate interpretation.

Functional Short-Leg Measurement

Throughout the development of the chiropractic profession, with its interest in spinal structure and dynamics, a preponderance of concern has been placed on anatomical and functional leg-length discrepancies. Of the various schools of thought that have existed within the profession, all have at one time or another addressed this concept with marked controversy existing both as to significance and correction of leg deficiency. Pry (1947) and Gonstead (Hildebrandt 1977) developed mathematical correction factors to be used with the 14 × 16 inch postural radiograph. These techniques attempted to neutralize the distortional effects of x-radiation in order to accurately evaluate the magnitude of leg deficiencies. Studies on the Pry off-centering rule suggested an accuracy approximating 75 percent. Recent comparative structural studies and a statistical analysis by Rozeboom and Davis (1977) comparing Pry and Gonstead methods versus a 14 × 17 x-ray at the femur head level suggest that these factors may perform only at a 50 to 75 percent accuracy.

Controversy continues as to the degree of leg-length discrepancy necessary to cause or aggravate spinal symptoms, as well as effective therapeutic measures of correction. Judovick and Bates (1949) in a fluroscopic study of leg length, concluded that a leg deficiency of ⅜ inch or more could cause chronic back pain and that raising the leg would aggravate the pain. Stoddard (1952) and Nichols (1960) agreed that approximately 10 mm of asymmetry was necessary to induce symptoms. More recently, Gregory and Seeman (1978) have published a study in which they report the concensus of one group within the profession that a 3.25-mm leg deficiency may be an adequate discrepancy. The influence of such a minimal difference may not be a causitive factor but rather an aggravating co-contributing component of symptoms. Logan (Coggins 1975), Gregory and Seeman (1978), Bailey (1978), and Fisk (1977) felt that the pelvis and leg length should be balanced to achieve relief of structural strain and resulting symptoms.

A most extensive survey of length inequality was performed by Bailey and Beckwith (1937). Using carefully positioned 14 × 17 pelvic radiographic evaluations, they examined a series of 432 short legs. Of these subjects an approximate equal distribution of sides was involved with 53 percent occurring on the right and 47 percent on the left. The average discrepancy noted was 8.8 mm. Effects of this asymmetry on standing spinal mechanics were carefully noted. In 88 percent of the cases the innominate ipsilateral to the short leg was found to be low as was the sacrum 72 percent of the time. Such a clear correlation was not seen, however, in convexity of any lumbar curvature which tended to develop. In 45 percent of the cases, convexity was directed to the short-leg side and in 32 percent of the cases to the long-leg side. No lateral deviation occurred in 23 percent of the cases. This would seem to suggest that the principal mechanisms of accommodation to a short leg are more dependent on lumbar mechanics than on the pelvis.

Clinically, both improvement and exacerbation have been seen on the occasion of trying to correct leg deficiency. This would seem to suggest that a more rigid criteria is needed for the identification of the patient needing correction versus the one that would be best left alone.

As in most clinical areas, several methods of measurement for vertical symmetry of the lower extremities have been utilized. Clark (1972) performed a reliability study on two of the more commonly used methods. He compared results in palpation and leg measurement to those of a standing 14 × 17 inch radiograph with the central ray positioned at the level of the femoral heads. He considered agreement to exist between methods of measurement when the system being evaluated yielded a value within a tolerance of 5 mm of the x-ray findings. On this basis he determined that palpation

of the femoral trochantor agreed 32 percent of the time and the measurement of the iliac crest-internal maleolus distance was accurate in 40 percent of the measurements. Such poor performance as this is unacceptable when the standard used for determining accuracy of technique allows for a variance equaling 50 percent of the 10-mm maximum deficiency considered clinically significant.

Anatometer

Gregory and Seeman (1978) have reported the development and preliminary testing of the anatometer, an instrument designed to measure pelvic and lower-extremity symmetry. The instrument consists of a variable level platform which provides separate support for each extremity (Fig. 6). Pedal positioning is standardized by setting the distance between the calcanei equal to that at the widest portion to the iliac crests. Relative pelvic rotation and tilt is measured by adjustable horizontal arms supported by a vertically adjustable post situated behind the patient. Pelvic rotation and tilt are noted and brought into symmetry by adjusting unilateral pedal levels. Assuming basic biomechanical theories of pelvic rotation, partially supported by the results of Gregory and Seeman, additional validation studies may prove this instrument useful as a noninvasive, nonionizing mode of evaluation.

Computer-Aided X-ray Analysis

The most advanced and sophisticated methods of evaluation currently being refined for determination of spinal mechanics and measurement are those of computer-aided x-ray analysis initiated by Suh (Suh and West 1974). Using a reference-frame system worn by the patient, anteroposterior and lateral radiographs are taken. Computer measurement of x-ray distortion and magnification of the reference frame is made. Compensation for computed distortion allows for fractional millimeter accuracy determinations of vertebral position and attitude. Thus far this system has been primarily used as a research tool. The computer language and

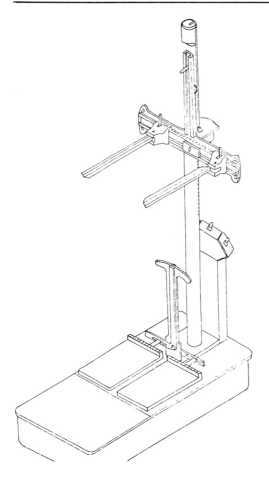

FIG. 6. **Anatometer designed to evaluate pelvic symmetry and leg-length discrepancies. (Courtesy of DC Seeman and RR Gregory)**

program is standard and could easily be adapted to any of the several small business computers that are finding their way into larger clinics. It is hoped that this technique will begin to spread into the general clinical practice.

The apparently simple clinical problem of postural analysis is fraught with many ambiguities. More recent technological tools promise to help alleviate these gray areas, but simultaneously there are obstacles of expense and gaps in technical expertise at the practitioner level. The reliability of individual postural and biomechanical analysis which should theoreti-

cally dictate the therapeutic regimen has remained a matter of clinical experience and judgment.

There are, then, most promising methods available to assist in spinopostural analysis that do provide some measure of objectification of data. The most reliable at this time include bilateral weight determination, plumbline analysis, Moiré topography, anatometer analysis, radiographic evaluation of leg deficiency, and computer-aided x-ray analysis (Table 1).

Thermography

Temperature Regulation and Heat Loss

The role of the thermogram in musculoskeletal diagnosis is a relatively new field of investigation. A promising area of clinical application—the measurement of temperature differentials of the torso, extremities, and head—provides a means of evaluating functional changes resulting from somatic lesions. Thermograms have taken many forms as the study of somatic temperature patterns have progressed. Instruments range from thermocouples which measure heat conduction of local skin areas to infrared radiation detectors that are capable of mapping the entire torso at one time.

Local temperature regulation is a summation of the combined interaction of central autonomic control mechanisms (Ruch et al. 1965) as well as multilevel spinal reflexes (Fuhrer 1975). The hypothalamus contains two reciprocally acting and opposing thermoregulatory centers that coordinate and integrate neural discharges to structures that are involved with temperature regulation. Lesions of the rostral hypothalamus in man (Davison 1940; Zimmerman 1949) have been shown to affect heat loss mechanisms; principally those of cutaneous vasodilation causing increased radiant and evaporative loss. Caudal lesions result in poikilothermia as a consequence of elimination of normal vasoconstrictive, shivering, and epinepherine secretion responses. Afferent thermal impulses derived from both cutaneous

TABLE 1. **Methods for Analyzing the Spinopostural Condition**

Technique	Precautions	Normals
Bilateral weight scales	Standard foot position	Equal weight carried bilaterally
Moiré topography	Standard foot position	Symmetrical contours over scapula, thoracic spine, lumbar spine, gluteals, and erector spinae
Anatometer	Heel distance equal to the widest part of iliac crests	Symmetrical crest and foot levels; no pelvic rotation
X-ray analysis of "short leg"	Central ray at level of femur heads	Femur head levels equal
Computer-aided x-ray	Use reference frame; two x-rays at 90°	Removes distortion effect of x-ray; gives true position of vertebrae

and centrally located thermal receptors are presumed to reach hypothalamic centers and initiate appropriate reciprocal responses.

Spinal segmental influence on the thermal regulatory system consists of extensive integration of vasomotor reflexes that are multisegmental. Basic responses in vasoconstrictive sympathetic action mediated for both upper and lower extremities have been measured in the cervically transected human spinal cord. These reflexes provide the individual with a more localized protective response that appears not to work independently of the hypothalamus; rather it is capable of locally modifying control messages. Overall the body is consistently regulated; however, this is not true from region to region.

Heat loss by the body occurs through various routes. Primarily, the greatest heat exchange is via radiation and evaporation with a secondary loss through respiratory evaporation. Overall heat exchange may be described by a general equation of body heat balance (Stolwijk 1974):

$$S = M \pm (W) - E - R - C$$

expressed in watts per meter of body surface, where S is the rate of heat storage in watts; M is the metabolic heat production; W is the mechanical work accomplished; E is the evaporation loss; R is the net radiant loss; and C is the convective loss.

Exchange rate is influenced by absolute temperature and shape of the surface area in addition to radiant activity. Heat traps are created by the complex shapes and multiple folds of human skin e.g., the axilla. Together with regional variations of sympathetic thermoregulation, a complex pattern of temperature distribution can be developed. To clearly understand the variables and limitations of thermographic instrumentation, a brief review of cutaneous structure and thermal conductivity will be presented.

The skin has been described as a thermal "black body" which neither gives up nor absorbs heat from normal environmental temperatures (Stolwijk 1974). However, skin does have a 5 percent reflectance of any temperature which is substantially different from skin temperature. This can result in a significant absolute measurement error of 0.5 F should ambient room temperature not be accounted for.

Skin is roughly divided into an outer layer with negligible circulation and an inner layer consisting of fatty tissue and a variable circulation. Heat transfer between the vascular compartment and interstices occurs primarily at a capillary level where it is presumed to be perfect (Van den Burg 1974). Figure 7 demonstrates a model of skin similar to that proposed by Atkins and Wyndham (1960) for the study of heat transmission. Various difficulties become obvious when trying to model this system. Thickness, heat conductivity, capillary bed activity, and thermal resistivity of skin all enter into the significance of absolute temperature evaluations. For these reasons, thermography

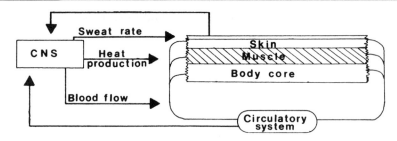

FIG. 7. **Model of heat loss through the skin. Accuracy depends on skin thickness and thermal conductivity variables. (After Atkins and Wyndham 1960)**

should be considered a qualitative, not a quantitative, measure when used for clinical study. As such, simultaneous comparison of anatomically symmetrical points yields useful information relative to distribution of circulation to the parts.

Both the principles of conduction and radiant emission of heat energy have been used to develop measuring instruments for skin temperature. Based on heat of molecular vibration, thermocouple devices have been developed to detect skin temperature via conduction. Similarly, infrared emission accounting for 66 percent of heat loss (DeBois 1937) has been measured by several methods. The total amount of energy detected from the skin depends primarily on two factors—the emissivity of the skin and the Stephen-Baltzman law (Poole 1974; Houdas and Guieu 1974) which is defined as radiant-heat loss proportional to the fourth power of the absolute temperature of the skin. Therefore, although the skin is considered a black body with an emissivity of 1, a negative load may be imposed with resultant drop in skin temperature when the environment changes. Such environmental change would include ambient air changes, contact with a cold treatment table, and radiant loss from the unclothed subject (Jones 1979; Stolwijk 1974).

Normal body temperature varies in a cephalocaudal pattern. The forehead mean temperature is 34.8 C, while the feet record a mean of 31.6 C. The nude subject will elicit no thermoregulatory activity of his own and thus be considered neutral if the mean radiant temperature is controlled externally at a level of 33.5 to 34 C (Houdas and Guieu 1974). Simply removing the clothes results in an abrupt drop toward environmental temperature with a time constant averaging 8 minutes (Fig. 8). An arbitrary equilibration period threefold of the time constant has been proposed prior to recording to ensure a sufficiently representative steady state for the skin temperature.

Various other factors should be noted. Halberg et al. (1969) have observed circulation changes in both skin and core temperatures that cycle regularly on 24-hour, 7-day, 30-day, and annual periods. The primary influence of importance to the clinical use of thermography is that of synchronizing patterns of work and rest and establishing a constant sample period within the patient's schedule. The acrophase of body temperature in the average individual working on a regular day shift schedule occurs at approximately 3:00 to 4:00 P.M. (Reinberg 1974). Desynchronization of these patterns may be seen in the chronically ill patient suffering from such diseases as cancer, epilepsy, mental retardation, etc. (Halberg 1960) and thus distorts the findings. This is of particular value to those who may be interested in absolute-temperature measurements.

A forerunner of thermography was the visual spinal analysis system called the *analyte* (Adelman 1963; Kimmel 1966). Based on the observations of Weiant and Adelman (1952) that paraspinal discoloration may occur in an area coinciding with tenderness over a subluxated vertebra, microscopic transcutaneous examination revealed the mechanism to be capillary dilation. Using monochromatic light of the

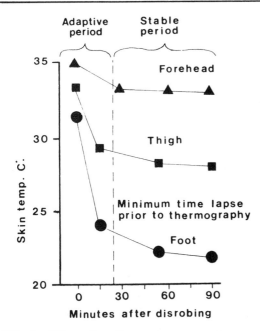

FIG. 8. Effect of ambient room temperature on skin temperature of the unclothed subject. (After Houdas and Guieu 1974)

wavelength of hemoglobin, the analyte was used to evaluate reflection from the engorged vascular beds. Little has been found in the available literature to substantiate the reliability or usefulness of this instrument.

Normal Thermographic Pattern

Of the greatest significance to the clinician is the establishment of the normal thermographic pattern and the interpretation of variance from that pattern. Several possible interpretations can be made depending upon the mechanism causing the temperature changes. Increased heat in an area has been ascribed to vasodilation as in migraine (Walshe 1973), inflammation (Duensing et al. 1973; Agar Wol et al. 1970; Owen et al. 1973; Huskisson et al. 1973; Kimmel 1966), or muscular spasm (Dudley 1978; Cooper 1959; Hartman et al. 1970). Decreased cutaneous temperature may reflect vasoconstriction, vascular obstruction, or fibrous and fatty replacement (Jones 1974). Some have

suggested that the magnitude of temperature differential of the paraspinal tissues indicates the severity of subluxation (Electronic Development Laboratories n.d.). Recent work by Triano and Luttges (1978) on nerve inflammation suggests this view to be too simplistic. Such differences might conceivably reflect the duration of the supposed lesion.

Thermocouple Devices

Several thermocouple devices have been designed (Table 2) for manual determination of paraspinal temperature variations. Used with either unilateral or bilateral probes, these devices all operate similarly and only one will be described.

An example of early hand-held instruments was the nervoscope. A dual thermocouple device, the nervoscope provided a limited simultaneous evaluation of skin temperature bilaterally and was used to scan the entire spine (Electronic Development Laboratories n.d.; Pulella 1974, Trott et al. 1972). With the patient seated, the probes are placed astride the spinous processes and allowed to equilibrate to the body temperature for 5 seconds. With a smooth gliding motion the clinician scanned the length of the spine. The temperature differential which was detected was displayed by a calibrated galvanometer that caused the needle to indicate the relatively warmer side.

Sample plottings from the nervoscope of an

TABLE 2. Thermocouple and Thermistor Instruments Used for Recording Variance in Skin Temperature

Instrument	Probe	Graphic Record
Neurocalometer	Bilateral	No
Neurocalograph	Bilateral	Yes
Neurotempometer	Bilateral	No
Nervoscope	Bilateral	No
Thermoscribe	Unilateral	Yes
Derma thermograph	Unilateral	Yes
Chirometer	Unilateral	No
Synchrotherm	Bilateral	Yes

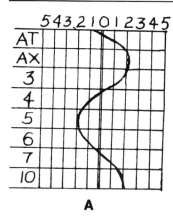 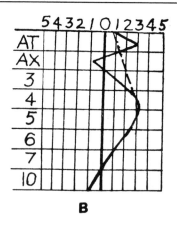

FIG. 9. **Plotted nervoscope readings from an asymptomatic (A) and a symptomatic (B) patient.**

A   B

asymptomatic and symptomatic patient are shown in Figure 9. Sharp deflections were interpreted as being indicative of lesions causing localized changes in vasoconstriction or vasodilation.

Gradual wandering of the needle was considered insignificant but created a high signal-to-noise ratio and raises questions about the sensitivity of the instrument. In very skilled hands, this instrument may have been useful as a qualitative analysis. However, several significant variables caused great difficulty in assuming reliability between operators. Pressure and angle of probe contact with skin as well as glide rates could not be readily standardized. Further, absence of graphic display prevented ready comparison of sequential test results, a problem solved later with the dermathermograph (Kimmel 1971). Zeroing the nervoscope was not possible by a direct adjustment and data-sheet patterns of nonsymptomatic patients do not agree well with infrared thermographs developed later.

Trott and co-workers (1972) evaluated the neurocalometer (NCM) and considered it to be most accurate in the lumbar-spine region. Of 12 subjects with other evidence of neurologic involvement, 67 percent showed positive NCM findings. However, in the thoracic spine the correlation was much less reliable with only 21 percent of the NCM findings agreeing with other physical signs.

Infrared Thermography

Infrared thermography is a measure of the radiant heat loss of the body which occurs in the infrared ranges. DeBois (1937) described the range of body emissions ranging from 5 to 20μ with an average of approximately 9μ. With infrared-sensitive film, a simultaneous evaluation of all areas of the spine can be made. Using the principles of body heat loss described earlier, a simple procedure can be designed that will allow for accurate evaluation of mean radiant temperature of body surface. Allowing for adequate stabilization of body temperature after disrobing the patient and avoiding ambient drafts, fairly characteristic patterns have been described (Dudley 1978; Raskin 1959; Goldberg 1966; Edeiken et al. 1970; Owen et al. 1973; Hartman et al. 1970) which provide the first reliable and objective method for clinical evaluation of muscular ligamentous injuries.

Raskin (1959) reported a comparative study between the results of myelography and thermography in 82 patients (Table 3). Of the patients with surgically verified disc compression of the nerve root, 88 percent demonstrated a positive myelogram while 71 percent showed a positive thermogram. This would suggest that a positive thermogram is a reliable noninvasive method of evaluating compression nerve injury, whereas a negative thermogram remains suspect (Raskin 1959; Duensing 1972). In acute

TABLE 3. **Positive Myelograms Versus Positive Thermograms in Surgically Confirmed Cases of Lumbar Disc Herniation**

Number of Patients	Positive Myelogram (%)	Positive Thermogram (%)
Surgically treated (38)	31–79	20–46
Confirmed disc (24)	21–88	17–71
Confirmed spinal stenosis (14)	10–71	3–21

From Raskin (1959)

injuries with normal radiographs, this technique provides functional evidence of the lesion which might otherwise be masked (Hartman 1970).

Agar Wol et al. (1970) and Owen et al. (1973) have presented studies that show the heat changes of the lumbar spine associated with ankylosing spondylitis, resulting from localized hyperemia (Connel et al. 1964). Both here and in chronic musculoligamentous injuries, serial studies may provide the greatest value in low-back-pain evaluation when correlated with clinical findings (Hartman 1970). Although there is some disagreement as to the constituency of a normal thermogram of the back (Heines 1964; Lebkowski 1973; Jenness 1975), several authors have presented findings that appear to provide a basis for clinical use.

The erect posture thermogram presents three bilaterally symmetrical areas of increased heat in the lumbar region of the spine (Fig. 10). A central vertical strip that begins somewhat wider at the thoracolumbar area extends down immediately over the spine. Areas overlying the upper third of both sacroiliac joints and the gluteal cleft form the remaining distributions of heat (Edeiken et al. 1968). Dudley (1978) observed that it is uncommon to find no variable in the pattern and thus integration of all clinical findings are important. However, basic symmetry can be expected in the normal subject.

Findings associated with lesions of the L4/5, L5/S1 disc have been best reported by Edeiken, Wallace, and Curley (1968). Central herniation of an L4/5 disc produces a bilaterally warm region between the normal lower lumbar and sac-

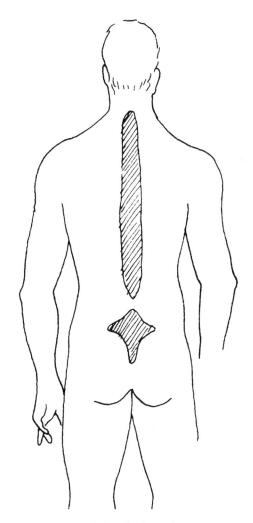

FIG. 10. **Normal distribution of heat areas on a thermogram of the lumbar spine.**

roiliac areas. If laterally placed, the area of heat will be unilateral. The lesion of L5/S1, when centrally placed, obliterates the normally cool region at the lumbosacral area. If laterally positioned, the disc will cause a focal area of warmth at the level of and slightly medial to the normal sacroiliac area.

Judovick and Bates (1949) investigated skin temperatures associated with tender areas and found as much as 5 F reduction. They attributed this to vasoconstriction and felt this to be good objective evidence of the patient's complaints.

Infrared emissions of spondylitis and sacroilitis are much less localized but remain characteristic (Agar Wol 1970; Owen and Holt, 1973). Active disease causes a diffuse irregularity over the involved areas. Late quiescent disease following ankylosis results in a cooling down with a return to the normal pattern.

From data reported, it would seem difficult to mistake a spinal strain/sprain injury with disc involvement as cause for back pain or radiculitis. The diffuse areas of spasm and heat associated with these lesions are quite large and persist longer than disc lesion patterns (Hartman et al. 1970). Individual patterns of hypertonus, thought to be associated with subluxation, also produce broad patterns (Dudley 1978) that form a silhouette of the muscle responsible. Although both of these circumstances could mimic the pattern of a sacroilitis or spondylitis just described, the correlation of history and physiological findings should be adequate to give a differential diagnosis.

Much more work is needed in this area in order to clearly delineate normal variants of infrared emissions. Correlation directly with the findings of subluxation would then provide an even greater reliability for the chiropractic practitioner.

Millimeter Wavelength Thermography

A variation of the radiant thermograph has been promoted by Toftness for several years and more recently by Edritch. The use of millimeter-wavelength thermography produces a graphic display of emitted electromagnetic radiation the intensity of which is described by the Raleigh-Jeans expression of thermal motion:

$$1(f) = \frac{4\,E(f)\,KVTf^2}{c^2}$$

where $1(f)$ is the radiant power/area and frequency band width; c is the speed of light; K is Boltzman's constant; T is the absolute temperature; and $E(f)$ is emissivity.

Emissions of approximately 69.5 GHz are collected by a lens system and passed to a mixer preamplifier which converts the signal to an intermediate frequency of 1.5 GHz which is then amplified. Since $E(f)$ approaches unity for frequencies above 40 GHz, the air–skin interface does not interfere significantly with transmission and a reliable index can be assumed. With a resolution of 0.12 C the motorized unit scans the spine at a rate of several centimeters per minute.

The presence of this "critical" radiation is thought to denote a subluxation lesion. As focal range of the lens system bears a direct relationship to intensity, Jenness et al. (1977) reported that subjects previously being followed had an increase in the focusing range following a traumatic incident. Unfortunately, no statistics were reported. This system has attained a high degree of sophistication and deserves a well-defined double-blind study for validation.

Galvanic Skin Response

Utilizing the premise of neurovisceral response to subluxation lesions, several attempts have been made to evaluate galvanic skin responses (GSR) in subluxated areas. Two types of technique can be used to elicit the GSR: an external voltage source or exosomatic technique and an inherent somatic voltage source or endosomatic technique. Exosomatic GSR has also been used as an hypothesized indicator for acupuncture diagnosis and therapy points. Most endosomatic galvanic instruments are difficult to utilize routinely for long-term recordings because of their tendency for baseline drift (Schneider 1978).

Galvanic skin response is a measure of the cutaneous conductivity or resistivity, which are known to fluctuate with the level of perspiration. Conductance follows Ohm's law and is more physiologically expressive than resistivity since it has been shown that the conductance has a direct positive correlation with the number of active sweat glands (Thomas and Korr 1957). That glandular activity is controlled by cholinergic postganglionic sympathetic fibers has been substantiated by atropine studies showing effective abolition of gland activity (Lader and Montague 1962). Both central and spinal mechanisms are responsible for the overall control of perspiration which has the primary purposes of waste elimination, evaporative heat loss, and maintenance of the cutaneous acid mantle layer (Fuhrer 1975).

Endosomatic and exosomatic techniques have been used to record GSR. The endosomatic method uses a highly sensitive voltmeter to measure endogenous electromotive force between skin points. The exosomatic method used DC/AC current passed through the skin with a direct galvanometer reading of skin conductance. Exosomatic recordings are typically monophasic while endosomatic are biphasic (Fuhrer 1978). Endosomatic responses proceed cephalocaudally with a predictable time lag for conduction to the feet as opposed to the hands. Fuhrer has studied these traveling waves and has reported statistical reliability across four consecutive days of recording sessions.

The effects of increased sympathetic stimulus as seen on GSR have been exploited in forensic medicine for years. Increased amplitude leaves the telltale response of the fight-flight mechanism with increased amplitude of the galvanic response. Conversely, areas of decreased stimulation due to denervation show a reduced skin conductance while cord transection produces an asynchrony of nonspecific GSRs. Regional alterations within the normally symmetrical pattern is one of several factors which are likely to change galvanic resistance records. These include time of day, temperature changes and humidity, substances ingested, blood pressure, heart rate, emotional state, and amount of current introduced into the body (Kimmel 1966, 1972). A standard testing schedule should be utilized to minimize anxiety and emotional influence by reducing the likelihood of occupational stress at the end of the patient's busy workday.

The very nature of GSR sensitivity to temperature change is an additional argument used for its application to the detection of effects of subluxation. As cutaneous vascular and sebaceous gland responses are both sympathetically controlled and often coincidentally responsive in local areas, some have felt that an increased gain is achieved by this measurement. Studies have been reported suggesting that a 1 mV increase occurs for every degree of skin temperature change. Coupled with the electrochemical changes known to occur with sweat gland activity, a hypothetical dual measurement can be made.

Such an instrument, the electrodermometer, was developed by Ishikawa and Tachio (1960) and used to detect presumed viscerosomatic reflexes emanating from internal diseases (Naito and Morisue 1962). This consisted of a hand-held reference and a second electrode in the form of a probe that was moved slowly along the spine.

It would appear, then, that neurologic malfunction may result in either an increased or decreased GSR. If the lesion is irritative, as in a sympathetic neurodystrophy resulting in augmented peripheral autonomic action, the skin conductance may be increased. If the injury is inhibitory in nature, as in brachial plexus avulsion, a decreased conductance can be anticipated. The difficulty with this concept as well as others involving instrumentation is that the pathophysiologic factors of subluxation have not been clearly delineated (Haldeman 1975; Triano and Luttges 1978). Clinical evidence does point in both directions suggesting that subluxation may have both effects dependent upon its severity and duration.

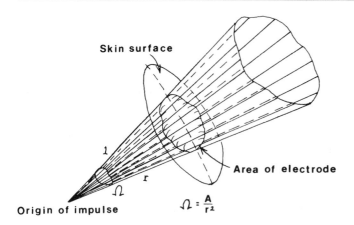

Skin surface

Area of electrode

Origin of impulse

$$\Omega = \frac{A}{r^2}$$

FIG. 11. **The surface potential recorded is proportional to the amplitudes of the membrane potential and the solid angle formed at the surface. (From Ruch et al. 1965)**

Electrophysiologic Recording

Although clinical electrocardiography began in 1901 and electromyography in 1938, the potential of electrophysiologic recording of various excitable tissues as a clinical technique within the chiropractic profession has hardly been approached. Recent data suggest that this, in fact, may be most valuable for reliable objective evidence of neural dysfunction accompanying the acute subluxation complex.

The generation of a membrane potential, regardless of the type of excitable cell, is based upon transmembrane electrochemical gradient, theoretically described by the Goldman equation (Ruch et al. 1965). Transmission characteristics of the impulse leading to propagation are defined by cable properties of long thin cells. The resulting resistance produced by the high length to diameter ratio provides for a

leakage of current into the surrounding less resistant interstices. By this leakage, called volume conduction (Fig. 11), a sensing electrode placed on the skin surface or inserted adjacent to the muscle or nerve can sense a passing action potential. In general, the compared potential will appear as a biphasic deflexion indicating the approach and recession of the impulse relative to the recording electrode (Fig. 12).

Different tissues (e.g., fat as opposed to muscle as opposed to skin) produce different electrical resistances. As a result, the potential actually recorded by a surface electrode represents a summation of these various resistivities (Remond 1973). Furthermore, a decrease in amplitude can be expected as a consequence of simple voltage drop over the distance between the electrode and the source of the impulse. Other factors that alter the shape of the recording, such as size and location of the recording electrode and configuration of the electrode

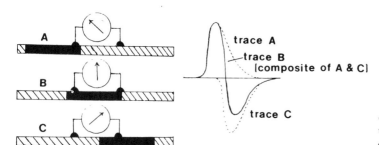

trace A

trace B [composite of A & C]

trace C

FIG. 12. **Mechanism of polarity change produced by an action potential passing a bipolar recording electrode. (From Ruch et al. 1965)**

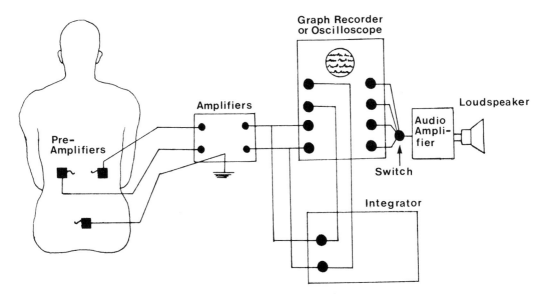

FIG. 13. Sample electrode and recording configuration for bilateral recording of paraspinal muscles.

position relative to the structure being recorded, are beyond the scope of this chapter. However, just such alterations can bring out changes in shape or polarity of the impulse. In most instances this dictates the selection of a recording point as close as anatomically possible to the source. In the field of electrocardiography, changes such as this have been exploited by the use of multiple locations for a more precise interpretation of the findings. This, of course, could only have been achieved after extensive ongoing correlative study. The optimal location for electrode positioning for electrocardiography, electroencephalography, electromyography, and electroneurography are well described in standard clinical handbooks on each topic.

Electromyography

A sample setup for bilateral recording of paraspinal musculature is shown in Figure 13. Obviously many variations or adaptations may

be made to meet the individual experimental needs.

Although the sample area being recorded is small and only a portion of the cummulative muscle action, it is considered representative of the whole muscle. The overlapping and interdigitating nature of neuromuscular motor units throughout the muscle belly allows this to be true. Each motor unit consists of a single motor nerve and up to 200 separate muscle fibers which are interposed between fibers from other motor units. Quantification of muscular performance is much more reliable when integration of the responses is utilized. Calculation of the integral of recruitment and frequency of muscle fiber activation is directly proportional to the isometric force exerted. Use of the muscle through a range of motion, however, causes a curvilinear relationship that is less well defined (Basmajian 1974; Missiuro et al. 1962; Eason 1960).

Dynamic isotonic contraction, stationary isometric contraction, and evoked potentials may all be used to evaluate neuromuscular performance. Some of the standard tools of the

TABLE 4. **Basic Electromyographic Test Procedures With Indications for Testing**

Test	Structure Tested	Indication
Muscle loading	Descending pathways, peripheral nerve—afferent and efferent; myoneural junction muscle	Suspected hypertonicity, hypotonicity, dyskinetic patterning, low-back pain, myogenic and neurogenic atrophy
Fatigue studies	Descending pathways, peripheral nerve—afferent and efferent; myoneural junction muscle	Myesthenia gravis; low-back pain, dyskinetic patterning
Conduction velocity	Motor nerve integrity	Acute nerve injury, neuritis, compression neuropathy
H reflex	Afferent, efferent nerves; homologous neuronal pool	Excitability curves, suspected descending pathway lesions; potential use in subluxation undetermined
F reflex	Afferent nerve and motor neuron	Excitability curves, suspected descending pathway lesions; potential use in subluxation undetermined

EMG include muscular loading, fatigue studies, conduction velocity tests, F-wave responses, and H-wave responses, which all provide information relative to various different levels of the monosynaptic and multisynaptic control mechanisms of somatic muscle (Table 4).

Muscle loading and fatigue studies lend themselves well to the evaluation of muscular balance and coordination as the muscles act on the spinal structures. Chapman and Troup (1969) and Jaysinghe et al. (1978) have provided direct evidence of muscular force asymmetry and fatigue in low-back-pain patients. Simple testing of EMG activity during routine activities such as sitting, standing, and bending provides adequate load of postural muscles to record significant changes in as short a period as 6 minutes. Conduction velocity provides a measure of nerve trunk integrity and is used to evaluate significant compression.

H reflexes are a result of afferent stimulation of monosynaptic pathways with resultant homologous muscle response. The H reflex travels at a combined efferent and afferent av-erage conduction velocity of 46 m/sec following peripheral stimulation and may be utilized as an index of cord segment facilitation as well as another index of nerve compression. The electrode positioning and mechanisms of these measurements in man are shown schematically in Figure 14. Actual latencies will vary depending upon the nerve being tested and the site of the electrodes; standard texts carry tables of normals for clinically useful determinations.

F-wave responses are considered to be the antidromic excitation of anterior-horn cells following peripheral nerve stimulation. Of a similar latency as the H reflex but requiring stronger stimulation, the F wave may be indicative of the facilitated status of the motor neurons (Simpson 1973).

Monosynaptic reflexes in patients with L5-S1 nerve compression were studied by Deschuytere and Rosselle (1973). Using the extensor digitorum longus for S1 and triceps surae for L5 nerve roots, differences in latencies for the responses were seen. Up to 10 msec delay occurred in the affected limb as opposed to the

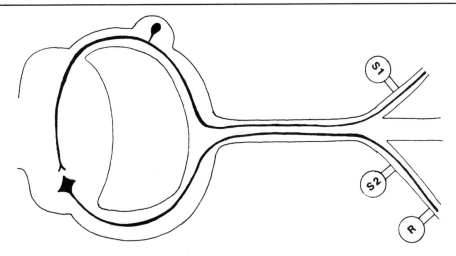

FIG. 14. **Schematic of nerves being tested by H and F reflexes. S1, stimulation transmitted through monosynaptic pathways to be recorded at R; S2, stimulation transmitted antidromically to motor neuron and returned to be recorded at R.**

normal limb. This led the investigators to conclude that a 2 msec difference in latency is evidence of chronic compression.

The facilitating or inhibiting effects of preconditioning stimuli, vibration, and slight volitional contraction of the muscle tested are variations which may also elicit clearer understanding of the excitability levels within the spinal cord. Exacting experimental research, however, requires diligence and experience to yield clinically useful data.

Traditional interpretation techniques are designed to elicit evidence of organic myopathy or neural degeneration. Both frequency and morphology of motor-unit action potentials recorded by needle electrodes may show alterations. Innervation ratio of muscle fibers may widen (Coers and Woolf 1959) and the action potential may become polyphasic (Fig. 15; Buchthal and Clemmesen 1941).

Additional phenomena associated with neurologic disorders include synchronization for motor unit potentials, fibrillation potentials, positive sharp waves, and fasciculation (Table 5). Myopathies, regardless of cause, have similar EMG abnormalities. The most characteristic is a diminished mean duration of action potentials. Other findings include all types of spontaneous activity, increased polyphasic potentials, and reduced motor unit field (Smorto and Basmajian 1977; Simpson 1973; Taylor 1962). There is no evidence to date that suggests that these types of findings are seen as a consequence of the subluxation lesion.

The majority of potential uses for EMG within the practice of chiropractic practice, however, are for kinesiologic evaluations dealing with the determination of hypertonicity, hypotonicity (Vennerson and Nimmo 1973; Walther 1976; Ny 1978; Triano and Davis 1976a, 1976b), dyskinetic movement patterning (Ortengren and Andersson 1977; Andersson and Ortengren 1974; Andersson et al. 1974; Andersson et al. 1976a, 1976b, 1976c; Jaysinghe et al. 1978), reduced conduction velocity (Eisen et al. 1977; Deschuytere and Roselle 1973), and potentially, altered sensitivity and refractoriness of the nerve trunk (Triano and Luttges 1978).

The findings of the authors listed above are far too extensive to discuss here. However, basic factors of muscular involvement in functional and structural disorders will be reviewed. Noninvasive differential diagnosis of spinal pain as well as radicular syndromes still remains difficult due to the poor reliability factors of all the methods thus far discussed. Although EMG interpretation is still in its infancy relative to this

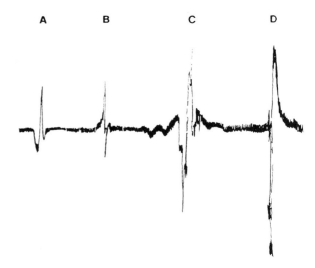

A   B   C   D

FIG. 15. **Action potentials from voluntary motor units. A), normal; B), myopathy; C), polyneuritis; D), motor neuron disease. (From Simpson 1973)**

TABLE 5. **Pathologic Electromyographic Findings of Nerve Degeneration**

Types of Activity	Peripheral Nerve	Anterior-Horn Cell	Descending Tracts
Spontaneous activity of short duration: 1) fibrillation potentials; 2) positive sharp waves	+	Spontaneous activity during sleep, infantile muscular atrophy	—
Fasciculations	Benign	Malignant	—
Pattern of maximal effort	Discrete activity; amplitude: acute stage—diminished < 1.5 mV (normal 2–4 mV); chronic stage—increased < 4 mV	Discrete activity; amplitude > 6mV	Possibly discrete activity; amplitude normal or decreased
Motor duration potentials (mean)	+30%	>30%	Normal (± 20%)
Incidence of poly-phasic potentials	Acute stage—normal (≤ 12%); chronic stage—> 12%	>12%	Normal (≤ 12%)
Maximum amplitude	Acute stage—normal (± 30%); chronic stage—increased (< 30%)	≥ + 500% giant waves	Normal (± 30%)

TABLE 6. **Conduction Times Between Knee and Ankle Measured by M and F Responses (msec—mean ± 2.5 SD)**

	Latency; stimulating at ankle	Latency; stimulating at knee	Difference: conduction time between knee and ankle
Posterior tibial nerve (n = 60)			
M response	5.85 ± 0.9	13.15 ± 1.5	7.3 ± 1.05
F response	47.4 ± 3.3	39.7 ± 2.95	7.6 ± 1.8
Peroneal nerve (n = 41)			
M response	5.2 ± 0.8	11.65 ± 1.2	6.4 ± 0.9
F response	44.6 ± 3.6	38.2 ± 3.1	6.3 ± 1.8

type of problem, some significant uses have been demonstrated. Recent studies by Eisen (1977) (Table 6) have provided a direct means of measuring the functional effect of compression by disc lesions through the evaluation of nerve conduction velocity. Animal studies in our laboratory suggest the possibility of future nerve trunk sensitivity studies by similar methods. Similarly, monosynaptic reflexes can be utilized to observe compression effects as previously described (Deschuytere and Rosselle 1973).

The work of Vannerson and Nimmo (1973), Goodheart (Walther 1976), Janda (1969, 1974, 1978), Janda and Stara (1971) and Stary et al. (1965) form a body of clinical and electromyographic evidence that describes the dependence of joint stability and integrity on the quality of movement patterns and the functional efficiency of cortical and spinal control systems. Poor movement pattern established by muscular weakness, spasm, or loss of normal coordination has been shown to exist in conjunction with joint dysfunction and may be responsible for its onset or persistence. Simultaneous recording of muscles suspected of contributing to joint dyskinesis can be quite fruitful by helping the clinician establish a rehabilitation program that will correct the disturbed joint movement and thus relieve the patient's discomfort. Obviously, this system of evaluation is too time consuming to be routinely used. However, in patients who have responded unsatis-

factorily to previous therapy, the EMG becomes an invaluable tool for the discrimination of deep-seated functional disturbances of the locomotor mechanisms. Through the use of H- and F-wave responses which give information as to the sensitivity of segmental neuronal pools, future work may expand the significance of functional evaluations even further. Gerren and Luttges (1978) have recently demonstrated a significant influence of peripheral nerve injuries on the facilitation of neuronal pools in mice. Vibrational inhibition (Wong 1977; Dindar et al. 1975; Barnes et al. 1970; Fra et al. 1968; Hagbarth 1973; Thomas and Lambert 1960; Sica et al. 1976; Hayes and Sullivan 1976; Ishikawa et al. 1966) of F- and H-wave responses also has not yet been turned to the evaluation of subluxation but appears to have the potential to further define its characteristics.

Kinesiologic evaluations and postural muscular loading studies are the most well defined and pertinent clinical areas available at this time. Although conflicting evidence exists and our knowledge is incomplete regarding electric and mechanical coupling, the evidence favors an interpretation where changes in electrical output parallel changes in force (Simpson 1973). Stary et al. (1965) and Grice (1974) have shown that a significant relationship exists between major EMG asymmetries and functional disorders of the spine. Triano and Davis (1976a, 1976b) have presented EMG evidence for loss of normal coordination between antagonistic muscle groups which logically would result in aberrant joint control and protection. Jaysinghe et al. (1978) found that patients with low-back pain demonstrate an imbalance in the force exerted by the postural muscles of the lumbar spine while standing.

The control subjects showed decreases in spinal muscle activity over the same time period. Chapman and Troup (1969) showed that muscle strength changes can readily occur over a small time period such as 5 days. Isometric contraction, as in muscle spasm, can result in increased activity of muscle fibers rather than an increase in muscle mass. Through this mechanism an acute low back can deteriorate into chronic instability. With the recent emphasis on normal biomechanics of various postures (Ortengren and Andersson 1977; Andersson and Ortengren 1976; Andersson et al. 1974; Andersson et al. 1976a, 1976b, 1976c), symmetry studies may prove useful in definitions of vertebrogenic disorders as well as in rehabilitation designs.

The evaluation by Johnson and Melvin (1971) of 314 patients with lumbar radiculopathy concluded that management and prognostic decisions may well be made based on the presence or absence of sharp waves within 7 to 10 days as well as disagreement between clinical and EMG findings at 19 to 21 days. If at 19 to 21 days pain persists but EMG findings show improvement, radical surgical approach can usually be avoided as the case is not likely to be an irreversible disc lesion.

Electrocardiography

The electrocardiogram (EKG) from its introduction in 1901 by Willem Einthoven has become the most significant diagnostic tool in cardiology. Extensive study of the electrical activity generated by the heart has been underway since that time. Today a significant degree of understanding of the meaning of various graphic patterns has been provided. The EKG is extremely useful in diagnosis of various heart diseases as well as differentiation of noncardiac disorders such as thyroid, renal, pulmonary, and electrolyte disorders (Table 7). Figure 16 illustrates the changes seen in the EKG pattern depending upon the net direction of the electrical activity, the *axis*, as it travels through the myocardium. These variations form the basis for the multilead EKG used in clinical diagnosis. The electrode positions and lead directions used in the standard electrocardiogram are shown in Figures 17 and 18.

Haldeman (1978) has listed the many sources where claims for efficiency of manipulative therapy in treatment of cardiovascular disease have been made. As he has noted, most of these claims are based on case study and noncontrolled evaluations. Specific disorders for which manipulative therapy has been advocated include congestive heart failure (Howell and Kappler 1973; Triano 1973, 1976) ischemic heart disease (Rogers and Rogers 1976; Tilley 1975) hypertension (Tran and Kirby 1977; Hodd 1974; Norris 1964; Fichera 1969), and certain arrhythmias (Egli 1962; Triano 1977). Several authors within the chiropractic profession over the years have attempted to identify specific vertebral levels of lesion that are found in association consistently with heart disease (Loban 1928; Janse 1947; Egli 1962; Triano 1977). Rogers and Rogers, and Triano have separately reported the findings of specific spinal patterns of lesions at multiple vertebral levels that seem to consistently be found in patients suffering from heart disorders. Statistical evaluation of these patterns by Triano suggest that the incidence of each lesion is significant to a p value of .05 and that the spinal pattern has a Pearson r coefficient of .99 and is likely to be better than a chance finding. Anecdotal and uncontrolled reports have been provided by many authors as to the occurrence of improvement within patients having both ischemic and arrhythmic disorders of the heart following correction of spinal lesions. The influence of the autonomic nervous system on the myocardium is well known; the effect of abnormal neurologic activity on the production of ar-

TABLE 7. **Classical EKG Pattern Changes Associated with Pathologic Conditions**

	Appearance	Interpretation
P wave	> .12 sec, > 3 mm high	Right atrial enlargement
	> .12 sec, > 3 mm high	Left atrial enlargement
QRS segment	> .12 sec	Bizarre complex of premature ventricular contraction
		Acute injury
	> .04 sec, > 1/3 of QRS height	Infarct
	M pattern in V_1 and V_2, > .12 sec	Right bundle branch block
	M pattern in V_5 and V_6, > .12 sec.	Left bundle branch block
T wave	Leads I, II, V_2–V_6	Ischemia
	Leads V_4–V_6	Left ventricular strain
	Leads V_1–V_4	Right ventricular strain

rhythmia is also well established, and it has been suspected to play a role in atherosclerotic (Thomas 1975; Gutstein et al. 1978) and congestive (Triano 1973) heart disease. However, no firm evidence is available at this time that would suggest the mechanism by which a spinal lesion would result in these cardiovascular abnormalities. Many authors (Phillips 1974; Sato 1975; Homewood 1963; Miller 1975; Tilley 1975; Bollier 1961) have presented a theoretical basis for somatic involvement with cardiac as well as other internal diseases and have provided laboratory evidence to support their ar-

guments. Referred pain, somatovisceral reflexes, nerve encroachment, altered proprioception, nerve root inflammation, and fibrosis are some of the supposed possibilities. Certainly combinations of these might also be possible. However, good correlation of these effects have not been found in man. Prinzmetal (1959) has written of his findings of a variant form of angina resulting in vasospastic activity within coronary circulation occurring both with and without atherosclerosis. This represents the most direct evidence to date that might implicate the nervous system during an ischemic at-

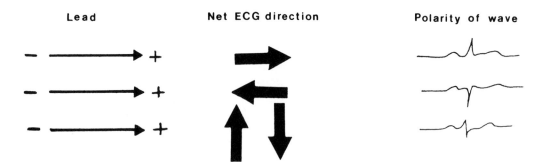

FIG. 16. Relationship of ECG lead direction and polarity of graphic deflection. Used to determine axis of electrical activity from which vector analysis may be derived.

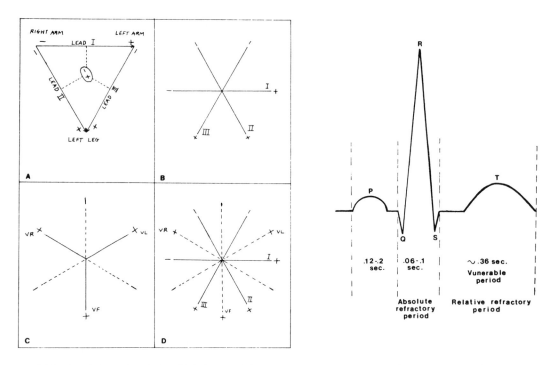

FIG. 17. Schematic of ECG limb lead position and polarity. The myocardium is visualized at the center of each. (A) Einthoven's triangular reference frame; (B) Transposition of legs of triangle to cross at center; (C) Orientation of unipolar leads; (D) Superimposition of bone to produce hexaxial reference frame. Normal deflection of lead II at right.

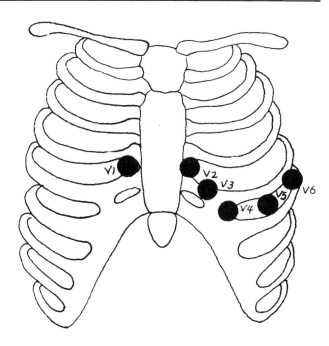

FIG. 18. **Position of unipolar chest leads for standard recording.**

tack (Yasue et al. 1974; Duhrandhar et al. 1972, Maseri et al. 1975; Levy 1971; Demany et al. 1968).

Norris (1964) and Tran and Kirby (1977) reported the influence of spinal manipulation on the "normalization" of blood pressure. Richman (1942) presented evidence indicating that manipulation of spinal lesions in patients with angina pectoris resulted in the lessening of the ST segment changes as well as absence in previously noted T-wave changes. The autonomic nervous system has been hypothesized in the development of arteriosclerosis. Gutstein et al. (1978) and Thomas (1975) have argued for this theory in experiments on animals. Atherosclerotic changes were produced by both direct and indirect stimulation of the autonomic nervous system. The findings of Gutstein et al. were particularly interesting because they were well controlled for diet and blood pressure changes. Tilley (1975) described a typical pattern of paravertebral abnormalities associated with ischemic coronary disease. This pattern included tension in the left upper thoracic pectoral areas with hyperesthesia over the shoulder

and supraspinatus and infraspinatus in the left pectoral areas. Treatment using manual methods, including manipulative therapy (Travell 1952), induced relief from this tension and discomfort but seldom has been noted to restore the EKG to a normal pattern. Triano (1977) has reported case studies of patients with congestive heart failure and arrhythmia that showed reduction in abnormal excitability of the myocardium immediately following manipulative therapy. Long-term studies are yet to be completed. Homewood (1963), Korr (1975, 1978), and Triano (1977) have speculated on the possible mechanisms involved. These findings tend to tantalize the practitioner. However, controlled studies are needed to establish the clinical impressions as being valid.

Clinical Laboratory Procedures

As might be expected, the utilization of the clinical laboratory by the chiropractor is primarily for the same purposes as those of others in the healing professions. For the present purposes, laboratory procedures will be arbitrarily sectioned into three hierarchial concerns: differential diagnosis of somatic lesions versus referred symptoms, contraindications for manipulative therapy, and nutritional evaluation and monitoring.

The literature is replete with references to referred pain and somatic changes where objective findings do not clearly rule out visceral involvement in somatic disorders nor somatic involvement with visceral disorders. In addition, the picture presented by the patient may be complicated by coexistence of separate entities, symptomatic or not. It is both legally and morally incumbent upon the clinician to identify the nature of the lesion from which a patient is suffering. The varying patterns of cardiac pain have been well documented and include the interscapular, precardial, sternal, submandibular, epigastric, brachial, and antebrachial regions. Other disorders with somatic reference of pain in the spinal region include peptic ulcer, aneurysm, pylorospasm, colitis, diverticulitis, abdominal carcinomas, prostatic carcinoma, obstructive uropathy, and others. These may all initiate back pain as their first symptom (Wintrobe et al. 1970). Laboratory procedures are helpful in making these differentiations and encompass the full gamut of standard tests and profiles included in hematology, serology, and urinalysis (Keiffer 1975).

Of special concern to the chiropractor is the identification of conditions specifically contraindicating manipulative therapy. Under certain pathologic circumstances the manipulative force may result in increased joint irritation, nerve compression, vertebral collapse, or hemorrhage. There exists a mild controversy over those conditions defined as being detrimentally affected by the manipulative approach. Stoddard (1969) and Jaquet (1976) attempted to rectify this discrepancy by defining classifications as "relative" or "absolute." It is doubtful that absolute contraindications would be disagreed upon by many. They include vertebral malignancy, tuberculosis, osteomyelitis, infectious arthritis, acute vertebral fracture, extreme osteoporosis, and extensive disc prolapse with evidence of severe nerve damage (Stoddard 1969; Jaquet 1976; Mennell 1960). Relative contraindications include osteoarthritis, disc prolapse, spondylolisthesis, hypermobility, severe scoliosis, and vertebrobasilar insufficiencies. Candidates for this category might also include hemangioma of the vertebral bodies, metabolic bone diseases, and diabetic neuropathy. Over these, there is likely to be disagreement. Stoddard's attempt to settle this dispute was to suggest that only "experienced" manipulative practitioners attempt to manage these patients.

More common tests used for these conditions include serum Ca and P, Ca/P ratio, alkaline phosphatase, acid phosphatase, complete blood count, erythrocyte sedimentation rate, urinalysis, protein electrophoresis, and immunoelectrophoresis (Schafer et al. 1977; Fisk 1977). Obviously, radiographic analysis should also be pursued where suspected diagnosis could be clarified by that procedure.

The chiropractic profession has, throughout the course of its history, been vitally interested in the clinical usefulness of nutrition and the rational approach of nutritional counseling as therapy for malnutrition, chronic undernutrition (Busse et al. 1978), overnutrition (Schneider et al. 1977) functional disease and some organic disorders. No specific claims are being made here; rather an attempt is made to represent the attitudes and approaches within the profession.

Nutritional science today is both young and controversial. Concepts of relative versus absolute deficiency, validity of the recommended daily allowance (RDA), type A lunch programs (Busse et al. 1978; Brin 1978; Albanese 1978; Head et al. 1973; Caliendo et al. 1977; Cichoke 1972; Frank et al. 1977; Kohrs 1978; Lowe 1970; Munro and Young 1978; Sims and Morris 1974; Thomas and Osner 1976; Ziegler et al. 1977), and variances of individual nutritional needs are hotly contested issues in which the profession has long immersed itself. The American society appears to be more susceptible to overnutrition and chronic undernutrition rather than frank malnutrition. Obvious segments of the population affected are low-income areas, children during rapid growth periods, and the elderly with psychosocial and chronic disease problems. Often in these patients, clinical symptoms as well as laboratory findings are nonspecific. Diagnosis, then, must rely on careful history and the absence of other conditions likely to be responsible for the patient's complaints. Periodic laboratory testing becomes extremely valuable as a means of monitoring patient response and affirming diagnosis.

Standard biochemical tests for specific nutritional deficiency are listed in Table 8. Tests for specific organ malfunction is often equally as important and informative.

Organic disorders often have their own characteristic laboratory findings which are available for review in any clinical laboratory or diagnosis text. In addition, however, there is a well-described systemic response that accompanies trauma, sepsis, or injury which is readily recognized via serum levels of sugar, urea nitrogen, ketones, and urinary urea nitrogen and ketones (Schneider et al. 1977). The "mobilizing" hormones, catecholamines and glucocorticoids, are released by central nervous system stimulus after significant injury or illness. Metabolic reserves are then released, including muscle protein. This response is quite different from the release of labile visceral protein of early starvation. Two phases, acute and adaptive, are supposed. During the acute phase, insulin release is inhibited by catecholamines which simultaneously stimulates hepatic gluconeogenesis. Meanwhile, glucocorticoids reduce peripheral sensitivity to the insulin remaining in circulation. Thus muscle mass will suffer in favor of maintaining a high circulatory level of nutrient substrates. The resulting effect on useful blood levels are an increased glucose, 17-ketosteroids, and blood urea nitrogen. After a short period of several days which is variable according to the degree of illness or injury, these levels fall and a state of ketosis introduces the onset of the adaptive phase. It is only after

TABLE 8. **Standard Tests Available for Direction Nutritional Evaluation**

Nutrient	Test
Vitamin A and carotene	Plasma vitamin A, plasma carotenoids, response to 200,000 IU vitamin A
Vitamin D	Serum Ca, serum P, serum alkaline phosphatase
Vitamin C	Whole blood, buffy coat
Protein	Plasma total protein, serum albumin, plasma essential amino acid/total amino acid
Riboflavin	Plasma flavin adenine dinucleotide, urinary riboflavin
Thiamine	Blood lactate, plasma pyruvate transketolase (TK) RBC, thiamine pyrophosphate effect on TK, urinary thiamine
Pyridoxine	Urinary xanthurenic acid after 10 gm D/L-tryptophane
Vitamin B$_{12}$	Plasma-B$_{12}$ level (*Euglena gracilis* in serum)
Pantothenic acid	Serum pantothenic acid
Iron	Serum iron, serum iron-binding capacity
Folic acid	Serum level (*L. casei*), forminimino glutamic acid after 20 gm 1-histidine HCl p.o.
Magnesium	Serum Mg
Zinc	Plasma Zn
Copper	Serum Copper
Vitamin K	Plasma prothrombine time
Sodium	Serum Na
Tocopherol	Plasma Tocopherol
Potassium	Serum K

this transition that nutritional supplementation is useful for tissue rehabilitation. Previous to this the hormonal mechanisms would only convert the nutrients to glucose.

Specific therapies are prescribed for certain

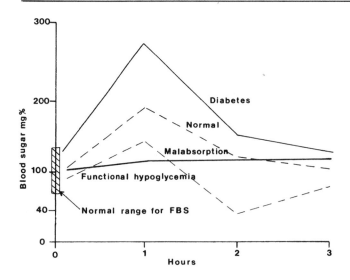

FIG. 19. **Typical responses seen with various conditions during 3-hour oral glucose tolerance test.**

conditions which are monitored by laboratory analysis. These include infection, cardiovascular disease, arterosclerosis, anemia, osteoporosis, renal disease, and diabetes (Schneider et al. 1977; Born 1972; Dudley 1972; Forshee 1971; Dold 1976; Goldman 1976; Hollen 1969; Palmeteer and Hollen 1971; Pressman 1971; Robinson 1965a, 1965b; Schroeder 1975; Wozny 1975; Jowsey 1976; Kritchevsky 1978).

Functional disorders are frequently misunderstood and misdiagnosed entities. A few of these have been found to have measurable biochemical alterations that allow easier diagnosis and monitoring but still remain poorly described. There remains a good deal of room for validation study and statistical analysis. Examples of the types of functional disorders for which laboratory evaluation is found to be useful include hypoglycemia, carbohydrate malabsorption, hypothyroid, and functional hypoadrenia (Hollen 1969; Jessen 1967; Walther 1976; Buehler 1971; Sisson 1976).

The only reliable means of determining the presence of functional hypoglycemia or malabsorption of carbohydrates is through the use of an oral glucose tolerance test. A typical 3-hour response to glucose loading is shown in Figure 19. As the clinical differentiation of hypo-

glycemia can be perplexing and easily confused with anxiety, thyroid disorders, hypoadrenia, anemia, undernutrition, chronic inflammatory disease, Addison's disease, insomnia, and others, all of which may cause chronic fatigue, the suspicion of the alert clinician often can be clarified by testing. It is Walther's opinion that a drop in blood glucose levels can still occur at a later time in a patient with a normal 3-hour glucose tolerance test. For this reason he strongly advocates use of the 6-hour test which he feels is most accurate and representative of a reliable response to sugar loading.

Functional hypoadrenia is an incompletely defined condition, suspected and responsive clinically, but also without substantial laboratory or pathologic characterization. Symptoms similar to those of hypoglycemic states with an associated postural hypotension (Sewall 1918; Crampton 1915; Goodheart 1965) and failure to maintain direct pupillary light response was described by Goodheart (1965). Considered to be a response to chronic emotional, physical, or dietary "stress," the syndrome is purported to be a minimally underactive response of the adrenal glands. Laboratory evaluation includes a marginally high serum sodium–osmalality ratio (Lobdell 1970) at a value of 0.51 or more while 24-hour urinary 17-KS, 17-KGS, and free cortisol (Smilo and Forsham 1969) would be low to low normal. Some unpublished evidence exists that there may be an early phase which demonstrates a marked elevation up to twice normal levels of urinary steroid followed in the chronic phase by a decline.

The primary importance of laboratory techniques is directly related to the clinician's need dictated by the frequency of somatic pain which is associated with nonsomatic disease. The convenience of the laboratory as a source of patient monitoring makes the laboratory even more desirable.

Hair Analysis

The evaluation of the constituents of hair has been developed within the decade as a more widely available technique of analysis of mineral and protein concentrations. A sample is taken, usually from the nape of the neck, where relatively new growth can be expected. It is washed with acetone for removal of lacquers, dried, treated with nitric acid, incubated, and diluted with deionized water. Final analysis is achieved by use of atomic absorption spectroscopy and flame emission spectroscopy (Harrison et al. 1968). The degree of "tampering" with hair, inherent to today's society, introduces variables that must be communicated to the technician if any meaningful result is to be expected. Record of natural hair color, shampoos, and hair tints or dyes must be made as these can markedly alter mineral concentrations (Schroeder et al. 1966, 1969; Tipton 1963). For these reasons, a pubic hair sample is often desirable.

In addition to contaminants, it has also been noted that there are mineral concentration changes occurring between sexes, within differing age groups, and in different hair colors. Schroeder demonstrated wide variations in eight trace minerals studied. For example, more magnesium, copper, and cobalt were found in female patients. Gray hair showed more accumulation of magnesium and less cadmium while other hair colors also show

further variance in concentrations. Petering and co-workers (1971) demonstrated a linear logarithmic increase in mineral concentration during childhood and decrease after "maturity." All of these factors make the use of hair analysis in the clinical practice a highly involved process. Supposing a careful charting of these variables in the early stages of patient evaluation would be the only means by which any succeeding change could be meaningful.

Of greater significance for clinical use were conclusions (Petering et al.) that single-hair analysis and blood evaluation bore no relationship to each other. However, hair analysis holds a direct relationship to the level of ingestion of minerals over time. Even so, it is inferred that this time necessary to follow the patient is several months.

Based on known mineral-mineral and mineral-vitamin interactions, interpretation of the results of these test procedures have been carried beyond pure-mineral recommendations (Parmae Labs 1976). Evaluations of these results are presented as "tendencies toward" and indications of potential health problems. To quote a simple example, "High calcium and magnesium with relatively low sodium and potassium is a classic pattern for hypoglycemia; a 6 hour glucose tolerance test should be run to confirm it." It would be interesting to see the results of correlative studies based on such observations.

Other Instruments

Several other types of examining instruments have been or are still being used within the profession. As none of these are widespread, only the fundamentals of their use will be described.

Phonocardiography

First introduced by Einthoven in 1894 these recordings are of greatest use in the determination of the timing of cardiac sounds and for the documentation of physical findings (Hurst 1974; Wintrobe 1970). A microphone transducer is used with a filtration system that will alter the sensitivity of the recording ranging anywhere from 0 to 400 Hz. With the microphone placed at the base of the heart, precise timing of the aortic and pulmonary components of the second sound as well as respiratory vibrations may be made. Obviously any murmurs located in this area would also be picked up. The filtration setting for sounds in this region should be between 200 and 300 Hz as the usual loud sounds in this area have a frequency range of 100 to 400 Hz. The second microphone is used over the lower sternal area. Filtration systems setting here should range between 30 and 40 Hz wherein lies the recording for low-frequency sounds such as mitral or ventricular gallups, and diastolic murmurs.

Cameron Heartometer

The Cameron heartometer was a pulse pressure recording device said to be sensitive to very small variations (Cameron 1963). A clutch operated graphic disc with mechanical ink writing channels was used to record both pulse pressures and standard readings of systolic and diastolic pressures. It is well known that many inferences may be made from pulse pressure alterations.

Obviously alterations of pulse wave due to reduced stroke volume, increased stroke volume, irregular rhythms, abnormal rhythms, as well as abnormal pulse shapes, anocrotic, dicrotic, and bisferrens may all be detected (Hurst 1974; Wintrobe 1970).

With the advent of electronic recording systems and heat sensitive paper, more reliable means are available for confirmation of pulse pressure diagnosis.

Plethysmography

The plethysmograph is an instrument that records the changes in size of a body part resulting from alterations in vascular flow. Blood volume can be measured directly as a result of pressure-volume changes accompanying constriction or dilation of the blood vessels.

This method has been successfully used by Figar and Krausova (1965) and Figar, Krausova and Lewit (1967) to portray improvement following manipulation in 32 of 44 previously determined abnormal finger plethysmograms of patients with radicular syndromes involving the sixth to eighth cervical segments.

Further use of this instrument should be encouraged particularly in specific neurocirculatory disturbances and may also prove useful in radicular syndromes involving the extremities.

Spirometry

The detrimental influence of scoliosis and restricted chest expansion on cardiopulmonary function is well documented (Beglu 1959; Bergofsky et al. 1965; Bjure et al. 1970; Davis 1950; O'Donovan 1951; Weber et al. 1975). These sources have reported asthematic patients whose symptoms were relieved after treatment of thoracic scoliosis or radiculitis of the spine. Goldman (1972) further listed a high incidence of spinal lesions involving third to fifth thoracic vertebrae in such patients, but no statistical significance was given nor effect of treatment described. Wilson (1946) concurred with the location of spinal lesion but also listed the need of "freeing" the fourth and fifth ribs bilaterally during the therapeutic process. He additionally stressed the value of patient's responsibilities for rest, diet, breathing exercise, and avoidance of allergies. Purse (1966) reported a study of 4600 cases of respiratory infection. Treatment of these cases was through spinal manipulation alone. He concluded that patients so treated not only recovered from the primary infection but also showed an apparent reduction in the frequency of complications compared to those treated by other means.

The types of spirometric findings associated with these conditions are divided into two main categories: obstructive findings and restrictive findings (Wintrobe et al. 1970; Ayres 1972). The air trapping mechanisms of inflamed bronchi result in characteristic obstructive signs which are summarized by reduction in forced expiratory flow and forced midexpiratory flow rate with evidence of "stair stepping" of maximal voluntary ventilation. Disorders causing reduced expansion, such as scoliosis, are considered restrictive diseases and are characterized by reduced vital capacity, increased forced expiratory volume, and normal flow rates. Reports providing description of changes in these more objective parameters have not been found in the literature.

Good controlled studies are needed to evaluate the nature of manipulative therapy for these conditions.

Summary

The use of instrumentation and laboratory techniques by the chiropractor have increased the ease and accuracy of his diagnosis and therapy. Much continued research is necessary to accomplish optimal utilization of the instruments available as they are applied to the spine. However, there is adequate current knowledge to markedly improve the practitioner's reliability. Postural evaluation has been standardized and made more reliable by Moiré topography where axial rotation of the torso may be quantified, by the anatometer which can measure pelvic asymmetry and leg length discrepancies, and by computer-aided x-ray analysis which can mathematically reduce radiographic distortion to being insignificant and allow exact identification of vertebral position and attitude.

One of the most rapid and exciting areas of growth in our knowledge lies in the measure of functional changes resulting from the spinal lesion. Thermography, plethysmography, and electromyography rank as the most useful of these techniques. Thermography provides a direct measure of vascular and muscular reaction in the area of the lesion. Patterns observed have been adequately studied to allow significant differentiation of spasm, disc rupture, and spondylitis. Plethysmography gives direct vascular measurement of changes associated with radiculopathies. Finally, electromyographic patterns can identify many neuromusculoskeletal lesions. However, its greatest potential lies in the identification of dyskinetic patterns that cause the persistence of more difficult cases.

The laboratory examination is a vital and integral part of the doctor's practice. Used as a means to diagnose the patient's status and to follow his progress, laboratory results allow the constant assurety of appropriate care.

REFERENCES

Adelman G: Infrared photography, and infrared thermography. Dig Chiropr Econ 1963

Agar Wol L, Dovey T: Dermography of the spine and sacroiliac joints in spondylitis. Rheumatol Phys Med 10:342, 1970

Ayres S: Pulmonary function studies. In Holman CW, Muschenheim C (eds): Bronchopulmonary Diseases and Related Disorders. Hagerstown, MD, Harper & Row, 1972

Albanese AA: Calcium nutrition in the elderly: maintaining bone health to minimize fracture risk. Med 63:167, 1978

Andersson BJG, Örtengren R: Myoelectric back muscle activity during sitting. Scand J Rehabil Med [Suppl] 3:73, 1974

Andersson BJG, Jonsson B, Örtengren R: Myoelectric activity in individual lumbar erector spinae muscles in sitting. Scand J Rehabil Med [Suppl] 3:91, 1974

Andersson BJG, Herberts P, Örtengren R: Myoelectric back muscle activity in standardized lifting postures. In Komi PV (ed): Biomechanics 5-A. Baltimore, University Park Press, 1976a

Andersson BJG, Örtengren R, Nachemson A, Elfstrom G: Lumbar disc pressure and myoelectric back muscle activity during sitting: I. studies on an experimental chair. Scand J. Rehabil Med [Suppl] 3:104, 1976b

Andersson BJG, Örtengren R, Nachemson A: Quantitative studies of back loads in lifting. Spine 1:178, 1976c

Atkins A, Wyndham C: A study of temperature regulation in the human body with the aid of an analog computer. Pfluegers Arch Ges Physiol 307:104, 1969

Bailey HW, Beckwith DO: Short leg and spinal anomalies. J Am Osteopath Assoc 134, 1937

Bailey HW: Theoretical significance of postural imbalance especially the "short leg." J Am Osteopath Assoc 77:452, 1978

Barnes CD, Pompeiano O: Presynaptic and postsynaptic effects in the monosynaptic reflex pathway to extensor motorneurons following vibration of synergic muscles. Arch Ital Bio 108:259, 1970

Basmajian JV: Muscles Alive: Their Function Revealed by Electromyography. Baltimore, Williams & Wilkins, 1974

Bergofsky EH, Turnio GM, Fishman AP: Cardiorespiratory failure in kyphoscoliosis. Medicine 38:263, 1959

Beyeler W: Experiences in the management of asthma. Swiss Ann 3:111, 1965

Bjure J, Grimby G, Gasalicky J, Lindh M, Nachemson A: Respiratory impairment and airway closure in patients with untreated idiopathic scoliosis. Thorax 25:451, 1970

Bollier W: Spine and internal disease. Ann Swiss Chiropr Assoc 5:167, 1961

Born B A: Nutritional aspects in the prevention and treatment of arteriosclerosis. ACA J Chiropr 9:VI, S53, 1972

Brin M, Bauernfiend S: Vitamin needs of the elderly: maintaining bone health to minimize fracture risk. Postgrad Med 63:167, 1978

Buchthal F, Clemmesen S: The electromyogram of atrophic muscles in cases of intramedullar affections. Acta Psychol Neurol 18:337, 1943

Buehler MT: The hypoglycemic state. ACA J Chiropr 8, 51: V, S33 1971

Busse EW: How mind, body, and environment influence nutrition in the elderly. Postgrad Med 63:118, 1978

Caliendo MA, Sanjur D, Wright J, Cummings G: Nutritional status of preschool children. J. Am Diet Assoc 71:20, 1977

Cameron: Cameron Heartometer: Cardiovascular and Related Facts Graphically Depicted. Chicago, Cameron Heartometer Corp., 1963

Champan AE, Troup JDG: The effect of increased maximal strength on the integrated electrical activity of lumbar erectores spinae. Electromyography 9:263, 1969

Changes in vasomotor reflexes in painful vertebrogenic syndromes. Rev Czech Med 10(4):238, 1964

Chung EK: Electrocardiography. New York, Harper & Row, 1977

Cichoke AJ: Protein malnutrition and introduction of low-cost protein-rich supplements. ACA J Chiropr 9, 2:S11, 1972

Coërs C, Woolf AL: The Innervation of Muscle. Oxford, Blackwell, 1959

Coggins WN: Basic Techniques and Systems of Body Mechanics. Florrissant, MO, Elco, 1975

Connel JF, Morgan E, Rouselout LM: Thermography and herniated disc. Am J Roent 102:790, 1968

Cooper P, Randall WC, Hurtzman AB: Vascular convection of heat from active muscle to overlying skin. J Appl Physiol 14:207, 1959

Cramptom CW: The blood ptosis test and its experimental work in hygiene. Proc Soc Exp Biol Med 12:119, 1914–1915

Daniels L, Worthingham C: Therapeutic Exercise for Body Alignment and Function. Philadelphia, W. B. Saunders, 1977

Davis D: Respiratory manifestations of dorsal spine radiculitis simulating cardiac asthma. Ann Int Med 32:954, 1950

Davison C: Res Publ Assoc Res Nerv Ment Dis 20:774, 1940

DeBois EF: The Mechanism of Heat Loss and Temperature Regulation. Stanford, Stanford University Press, 1937

Demany MA, Tambe A, Zimmerman HA: Coronary arterial spasm. Dis Chest 53(6):714, 1968

Deschuytere J, Roselle N: Diagnostic use of monosynaptic reflexes in L5 and S1 root compression. In Desmedt JE (ed): New Developments in Electromyography and Clinical Neurophysiology. Basel, Karger, 1973

Dhurandhar RW, Watt DL, Silver MD, Trimble AS, Adelman SG: Prinzmetal's variant form of angina with arteriographic evidence of coronary arterial spasm. Am J Cardiol 30:902, 1972

Dindar F, Verrier M: Studies on the receptor responsible for vibration induced inhibition of monosynaptic reflexes in man. J Neurol Neurosurg Psychiatr 38:155, 1975

Dold WR: Anemia investigation and classification. ACA J Chiropr 13, 4:X, S35, 1976

Dudley WN: Preliminary findings in thermography of the back. ACA J Chiropr 15:S83, 1978

Dudley WN: Triglycerides and sucrose. ACA J Chiropr 9(11):VI, S79, 1972

Duensing F, Becker P, Rittmeyer K: Thermographic findings in lumbar disc protrusions. Arch Psychiatr Nervenkr 217:53, 1973

Eason RG: Electromyographic study of local and generalized muscular impairment. J Appl Physiol 15:479, 1960

Edeiken J, Wallace JD, Curley RF et al.: Thermography and herniated lumbar disc. Am J Roent Radiol Therapeu Nuclear Med 102:790, 1968

Edrich J, Toftness IN: Spine thermography at millimeter wave length. Dig Chiropr Econ 19:17, 1976

Egli A: Spine and heart vertebrogenic cardiac syndromes. Ann Swiss Chiropr Assoc 6:95, 1962

Einthoven W, Geluj M: Dieregistrierung der herztone. Pfluegers Arch Ges Physiol 57:617, 1894

Eisen A, Schomer D, Melmed C: An electrophysiological method for examining lumbosacral root compression. J Can Sci Neurol, May 1977, p 117

Electronic Development Laboratories: Instructions for Using Nervo-Scopes. Plainview, NY, EDL, no date

Evans FG, Lissner HR: Biomechanical studies of the lumbar spine and pelvis. J Bone Joint Surg 21A:278, 1959

Fichera AO, Celander DR: Effect of osteopathic manipulative therapy on autonomic tone as evidenced by blood pressure changes and activity of the fibinolytic system. J Am Osteopath Assoc 23:1036, 1969

Figar S, Krausova L: A plethysmographic study of the effects of chiropractic treatment in vertebrogenic syndromes. Acta Univ Carol, Med, Suppl 21:84, 1965

Figar S, Krausova L, Levit K: Plethysomographic examination following treatment of vertebrogenic disorders by manipulation (German). Acta Neuroveg 29:618, 1967

Fipps G: A simple method of measuring and graphically plotting spinal curvature and other asymmetries by means of a new direct reading scoliometer. Am Psych Ed Rev 11:18, 1906

Fisk JW: The Painful Neck and Back. Springfield, IL, Charles C. Thomas, 1977, p 10

Forshee GK: Arterio and atherosclerosis with relation to vitamin D. ACA J Chiropr 8, 11:V, S81, 1971

Fra L, Brignolio F: F-and H-responses elicited from muscles of the lower limb in normal subjects. J Neurol Sci 7:251, 1968

Fradd NW: A new method of recording posture. J Bone Joint Surg 2:757, 1923

Frank GC, Voors AW, Schilling PE, Berenson GS: Dietary studies of rural school children in a cardiovascular survey. J Am Diet Assoc 71:31, 1977

Free RV: Spinal analysis utilizing moiré topography. Dig. Chiropr Econ 17(4):26, 1975

Fuhrer M: Effects of stimulus site on the pattern of skin conductance responses evoked from spinal man. J Neurol Neurosurg Psychiatr 38:749, 1975

Fuhrer M: Electrodermal study of patients with spinal-cord injuries. Arch Phys Med Rehabil 34:728, 1978

Gerren R, Luttges M: Proceedings of the 9th Annual Biomechanic Conference. Boulder, University of Colorado, 1978

Goldberg HI, Heines ER, Taveras JM: Thermography in neurologic patients: preliminary experiences. Acta Radiol 5:786, 1966

Goldman SR: Pathogenesis of the diabetic syndrome. ACA J Chiropr 4(3):S22, 1967

Goldman SR: A structural approach to bronchial asthma. Bull Eur Chiropr Union 21(3):66, 1972

Goodheart GJ: Postural hypotension and functional hypoadrenia. Dig Chiropr Econ 7, 6:43, 1955

Green D, Joynt RJ: Vascular accidents to the brain stem associated with neck manipulation. J Am Med Assoc 522, 1959

Gregory R, Seeman DC: Subluxations: short leg and pelvic distortions. The Upper Cervical Monograph 2:1, 1978

Gregory R: Personal communication, 1978

Grice AC: Posture and postural mechanics. J Can Chiropr Assoc 13:85, 1970

Grice AC: Muscle tonus changes following manipulation. J Can Chiropr Assoc 19:29, 1974

Gutstein WH, Harrison J, Parl F, Kiu G, Avitable M: Neural factors contribute to atherogenesis. Science 199:46, 1978

Hagbarth KE: The effect of muscle vibration in normal man and in patients with motor disorders. In Desmedt JE (ed): New Developments in Electromyography and Clinical Neurophysiology. Basel, Karger, 1973

Halberg F: Temporal coordination of physiologic function. Cold Springs Harbor Symp Quant Biol 25:289, 1960

Halberg F: Chronobiology. Ann Rev Physiol 31:675, 1969

Haldeman S: Observations made under test conditions with the synchro-therme. J Can Chiropr Assoc 9, 1970b

Haldeman, S: First impressions of the synchro-therme as a skin temperature gauge. J Can Chiropr Assoc 1970b

Haldeman S: Clinical basis for discussion of mechanisms of manipulative therapy. In Korr I (ed): Neurobiologic Mechanisms of Manipulative Therapy. New York, Plenum Press, 1978

Harrison WW, Yurachej, JP, Benson C: The determination of trace elements in human hair by atomic absorbtion spectroscopy. Clin Chim Acta 33:83, 1968

Hartman K, Knebel A, Semel CJ, Cougar J: Clinical

studies in thermography: application of thermography in evaluating musculoligamentis injuries of the spine: a preliminary report. Arch Environ Health 20:412, 1970

Hayes KC, Sullivan J: Tonic neck reflex influence on tendon and hoffman reflexes in man. Electromyogr Clin Neurophysiol 16:251, 1976

Head MK, Weeks RJ, Gibbs E: Major nutrients in the type of A lunch. J Am Diet Assoc 63:31, 1973

Heines R, Goldberg H, Taveras J: Experiences with thermography and neurologic patients. Ann NY Acad Sci 121:171, 1964

Hildebrandt RW: Chiropractic Spinography. Des Plains, IA, Hilmark Publication, 1977

Hoag JM: Musculoskeletal involvement in chronic lung disease. J Am Osteop Assoc 71:698, 1972

Hollen WV: Clinical carbohydrate evaluation. ACA J Chiropr 6:ii, S73, 1969

Homewood AE: The Neurodynamics of the Vertebral Subluxation. Willowdale, ONT, Chiropractic Publishers, 1963

Hood RP: Blood pressure. Dig Chiropr Econ 16:36, 1974

Hoppenfield S: Scoliosis: A Manual of Concept and Treatment. Philadelphia, Lippincott, 1969

Houdas Y, Guier JD: Environmental factors affecting skin temperature. Thermography Proceedings of the 1st European Conference (Amsterdam) held in 1974. Bibl Radiol 6:1, 1974

Howell RK, Kappler RE: The influence of osteopathic manipulative therapy on a patient with advanced cardiopulmonary disease. J Am Osteop Assoc 73:322, 1975

Huskisson EC, Berry H, Browett J, Wykeham Balme H: Measurement of inflammation. Ann Rheum Dis 32:99, 1973

Hurst JW et al.: The Heart. New York, McGraw-Hill, 1974

Illi FW: The phylogenesis and clinical import of the sacroiliac mechanism. J Can Chiropr Assoc 1965

Ishikawa T: Viscero-cutaneo-vascular reflex and its clinical significance. Ann Rep Res Inst Tuberc 18:1, 1960

Ishikawa K, Ott K, Porter R, Stewart D: Low frequency depression of H-wave in normal and spinal man. Exp Neurol 15:140, 1966

Janda V: Postural and phasic muscles in the pathogenesis of low back pain. Proceedings of the 11th Congress of the International Society of Rehabilitation of the Disabled. Dublin, 1969

Janda V: Muscle and joint correlation. Proceedings of the 4th Congress of the International Federation of Manipulative Medicine. Prague, 1974

Janda V: Muscles, central nervous motor regulation and back problems. In Korr I (ed): The Neurobiologic Mechanisms in Manipulative Therapy. New York, Plenum Press, 1978

Janda V, Stara B: Comparison of movement in healthy and spastic children. Proceedings of 2nd International Symposium—Cerebral Palsy. Prague, 1971

Janse J, Wells FF, House RH: Chiropractic Principles and Technique. Chicago, National College, 1947

Jaquet P: An Introduction to Clinical Chiropractic. Geneva, Jaquet and Grinard, 1976

Jayasinghe WJ, Harding RH, Anderson JAD, Sweetman MR: An electromyographic investigation of postural fatigue in low back pain. Electromyogr Clin Neurophysiol 18:191, 1978

Jenness M: The role of thermography and postural measurement in structural diagnosis. In Goldstein M (ed): Research Status of Spinal Manipulative Therapy, NINDCS Monograph No. 15. Washington, U.S. DHEW, 1975

Jenness M, Speijers F, Silverstein H: Use of the conformateur and line of gravity apparatus in the new technique for assessing posture. Dig Chiropr Econ 14, 1974

Jessen AR: Diagnosis of thyroid dysfunction. ACA J Chiropr 4:S49, 1967

Johnson EW, Melvin JL: Value of electromyography in lumbar radiculopathy. Arch Phys Med Rehabil 27:239, 1971

Jones C: Physical aspects of thermography in relation to clinical techniques. Bibl Radiol 6:157, 1974

Jowsey J: Osteoporosis. Postgrad Med 60:75, 1976

Judovick B, Bates W: Pain Syndromes: Treatment by Paravertebral Nerve Block. Philadelphia, F. A. Davis, 1949

Keiffer JD: Laboratory procedures in the low back syndrome. ACA J Chiropr 2:17, 1975

Kimmel E: Electro-analytical instrumentation. ACA J Chiropr, May 1966, p 9

Kimmel E: Electro-analytical instrumentation. ACA J Chiropr, June 1966, p 9

Kimmel E: Electro-analytical instrumentation. ACA J Chiropr, July 1966, p 13

Kimmel E: The dermathermograph. J Clin Chiropr 2:78, 1971

Kohrs MB, O'Neil R, Preston A, Eklund D, Abrahams O: Nutritional status of elderly residents in Missouri, Am J Clin Nutri 31:2186, 1978

Korr I: Proprioceptors and the behavior of lesioned segments. In Osteopathic Medicine. Action, MA, Sciences Group, 1975

Korr I: Sustained sympathicotonia as a factor in disease. In Korr I (ed): The Neurologic Mechanisms in Manipulative Disease. New York, Plenum Press, 1978

Kouvalchouk JF: Les scolioses. Conc Med 16:2941, 1971

Kritchevsky D: How aging affects cholesterol metabolism. Postgrad Med 63(3): 133, 1978

Lebkowski J, Polocki B, Borucki Z, Dudek H, Szepakovicz P, Tomcqyk KH: Determination of the level of prolapsed intervertebral disc ischalgia by means of an electric thermometer. Pol. Tgy Lek 28(24):907, 1973

Levy MN: Sympathetic-parasympathetic interactions in the heart. Circ Res 29(5):437, 1971

Loban J: Technic and Practice of Chiropractic. Bunn-Loban, 1928

Lobdell DH: Freezing point osmometry—simple and valuable procedure. Lab Med 433, 1970

Lowe CU et al.: Reflections of dietary studies with children in the ten-state nutrition survey of 1968-1970. Nutrition Program Center for Disease Control, Washington, DHEW

Mac Rae JE: Roentgenometrics in Chiropractic. Toronto, Canadian Memorial College, 1974

Maseri A, Mimmo R, Chierchia S, Marchesi C, Pesola A, L' Abbate A: Coronary artery spasm as a cause of acute myocardial ischemia in man. Chest 68:625, 1975

Meadows DM, Johnson WO, Allen JB: Generation of surface contours by moiré patterns. Appl Optics 9:942, 1970

Mennell J: Back Pain. Boston, Little, Brown 1960

Miller WD: Treatment of visceral disorders by manipulative therapy. The Research Status of Spinal Manipulative Therapy, NINCDS, Monograph No. 15. Bethesda, MD, U.S. DHEW, 1975

Missiuro W, Kirchner H, Kozolowski S: Electromyographic manifestations of fatigue during work of different intensity. Acta Physiol Pol 13:11, 1962

Mitchell FL, Pruzzo NL: Investigation of voluntary and primary respiratory mechanisms. Am Osteopath Assoc J 70:120, 1971

Moe J et al.: Scoliosis and Other Body Deformities. Philadelphia, Saunders, 1978

Munroe HN, Young VR: Protein metabolism in the elderly: observations relating to dietary needs. Postgrad Med 63:143, 1978

Naito R, Morisue S: Screening of transfusion hepatitis by means of electrodermatography. Proceedings of the 8th Congress International Society of Blood Transfusion, Tokyo, 1960

Nichols P: The accuracy of measuring leg length differences. Br Med J 29:1247, 1955

Nichols P: The short leg syndrome. Br Med J 1:1863, 1960

Norris T: The study of the effect of manipulation on blood pressure. Acad Appl Osteop Yearb 1964

Ny YJ: Hypertonic psoas syndrome. J Am Chiropr Assoc 15, 9:1978

O'Donovan D: The possible significance of scoliosis of the spine in the causation of asthma and applied allergic conditions. Ann Allergy 16:184, 1951

Örtengren R, Andersson GBJ: Electromyography studies of trunk muscles with special reference to the functional anatomy of the lumbar spine. Spine J 2:44, 1977

Owen E, Holt GA: Thermographic patterns in sacroilitis and ankylosing spondylitis. Presented to the Annual Meeting of the American Thermographic Society, New York, 1973

Palmateer DC, Hollen SV: Urinary tract calculi diagnosis and treatment. ACA J Chiropr 8:V, S25, 1971

Parmae Laboratories: Trace Minerals and Hair Analysis. Dallas, Parmae Laboratories, 1976

Petering HG, Yeager DW, Witherup SO: Trace metals content of hair. Arch Environ Health 23:202, 1971

Pettibon BR, Loomis WP: Bio-mechanical research by Pettibon and associates. Today's Chiropr 1:22, 1973

Pfeiffer J, Bauer J, Berkova L, Sussova J: Electromyography of the abdominal and dorsal muscles in initial disorders of spinal dynamics. Acta Univ Carol, Med. Suppl 21:33, 1965

Phillips RB: The irritable reflex mechanism. J Can Chiropr Assoc 22, 1974

Poole D: Thermography proceedings of the first European conference (Amsterdam). Bibl Radiol 6:19, 1974

Pressman R: Calcium and neglected minerals. ACA J Chiropr 8, 6:v, S45, 1971

Prinzmetal M, Kennamer R, Merliss R, Wada T, Bor N: Angina pectoria, I: a variant form of angina pectoris. Am J Med 7:375, 1959

Pry J: Personal communication, 1947

Pulella S et al.: Correlative study of various instruments and procedures in chiropractic. ACA J Chiropr 11(2):S42, 1976

Purse FM: Manipulative therapy of upper respiratory infections in children. J Am Osteop Assoc 65:964, 1966

Raskin M: Thermography in low back diseases. Medical Thermography: Theory and Clinical Applications. Los Angeles, Brentwood, 1976

Raskin M, Martinez L, Sheldon J: Lumbar thermography and discogenic disease (in preparation)

Reinberg A: Circadian changes in the temperature of human beings. Bibl Radiol 6:126, 1974

Remond A: Handbook of EEG and Clinical Neurophysiology. Amsterdam, Elsevier, 1973

Reynolds E, Levitt R: A method of determining the

position of the center of gravity in its relation to certain boney landmarks in the erect position. Am J Physiol 24:286, 1909

Richman WG: Influence of somatic manipulation in coronary artery disease—evaluated by controlled method. J Am Osteopath Assoc 41:217, 1942

Robinson R: Calcium and vitamins C and D in nutrition on bone, muscle, and nerve. ACA J Chiropr 2, 6:14, 1965a

Robinson R: Calcium and vitamins B and C in nutrition of bone, muscle, and nerve. ACA J Chiropr 2, 7:17, 1965b

Rogers JT, Rogers JC: The role of osteopathic manipulative therapy in the treatment of coronary artery disease. J Am Osteopath Assoc 76:71, 1976

Rozeboom D, Davis B: Personal communication, 1977

Ruch WA, Steiner HA: A study of lower extremity leg inequality. Am J Roent 56:616, 1946

Ruch TC, Patton HD, Woodbury JW, Towe AL: Neurophysiology. Philadelphia, Saunders, 1965

Sato A: The somatosympathetic reflexes: their physiological and clinical significance. In The Research Status of Spinal Manipulative Therapy, NINCDS Monograph No. 15. Washington, DHEW, 1975

Schafer RC (ed): Basic Chiropractic Procedural Manual. Des Moines, American Chiropractic Association, 1977

Schneider H, Anderson C, Coursin D: Nutritional Support of Medical Practice. Hagerstown, MD, Harper & Row, 1977

Schroeder, HA, Nason AP: Trace metals in human hair. J. Invest Dermatol 53:71, 1969

Schroeder HA, Nason AP, Tipton IH, Balassa JJ: Essential trace metal in man. J Chronic Dis 19:1007, 1966

Schroeder RM: Diseases related to the pathologic biochemistry of calcium, phosphorus, and alkaline phosphatase metabolism. ACA J Chiropr 12, 1:IX, S13, 1975

See DH, Kraft GH: Electromyography in paraspinal muscles following surgery for root compression. Arch Phys Med Rehabil 56:80, 1975

Sewall H: Clinical significance of postural changes in blood pressure. Am J Med Sci 158:786, 1918

Sica R, Sanz OP, Columbi A: Potentiation of the F-wave by remote voluntary muscle contraction in man. Electromyogr Clin Neurophysiol 16:623 1976

Simpson JA: Neuromuscular diseases. In Remond A (ed): Handbook of Electroenciphalography and Clinical Neurophysiology. Amsterdam, Elsevier, 1973

Sims LS, Morris PM: Nutritional status of preschoolers. J Am Diet Assoc 64:492, 1974

Sisson JA: Handbook of Clinical Pathology. Philadelphia, Lippincott, 1976

Speijers F, Jenness M, Blackmon C, Perdew W, Solomon A: The use of moiré topography in a 3-dimensional assessment of spinal conformation. Presented to 6th Annual Biomechanics Conference on the Spine, University of Colorado, Boulder, 1975

Smilo RP, Forsham PH: Diagnostic approach to hypofunction and hyperfunction of the adrenal cortex. Postgrad Med 56:146, 1969

Smorto MP, Basmajian JV: Electrodiagnosis: A Handbook for Neurologists. New York, Harper & Row, 1977

Stary, O, O'Brda K, Pfeiffer J, Barankova M: Polyelectromyographic studies of proprioceptive analysis disorders during the initial phases of vertebrogenic disorders in children. Acta Univ Carol Med [Suppl.] 21:21, 1965

Stoddard A: Manual of Osteopathic Practice. New York, Harper & Row, 1969

Stoddard A: The short leg and low back ache syndrome. Proceedings of the International Congress of Physical Medicine, London, 1952

Stolwijk J: Heat exchanges between body and environment. Bibl Radiol 6:144, 1974

Stolwijk J, Hardy J: Temperature regulation in man: theoretical study. Pfluegers Arch 291:129, 1966

Suh C, West H: Biomechanics of the spine. Part 1. J Am Chiropr Assoc 8:S1, 1974

Tachio I: Viscero-cutaneous-vascular reflex and its clinical significance. Res. Inst. Tuberc 18(1): 1960, Kanazawa University, Japan.

Taylor A: The significance of grouping of motor unit activity. J Physiol (London) 162:259, 1962

Terada H, Kamazawa E: The position of euryon on the human skull analyzed 3-dimensionally by moiré contourography. J Anthro Soc Nippon 82:10, 1974

Thomas JE, Lambert EH: Ulnar nerve conduction velocity and H-reflex in infants and children. J Appl Physiol 15(1):1, 1960

Thomas PE: The role of the autonomic nervous system on arterosclerosis. In Clinical Review Series-Osteopathic Medicine. Action, MA, Publishing Sciences Group, 1975

Thomas PE, Korr IM: Relationship between sweat gland activity and electrical resistance of the skin. J Appl Physiol 10:505, 1957

Thomas S: Patterns of muscle activity in the leg, hip, and torso associated with anomalous 5th lumbar conditions. J Am Chiropr Assoc 67:1039, 1958

Tilley RM: The somatic component in heart disease.

In Clinical Review Series-Osteopathic Medicine. Action, MA, Publishing Sciences Group, 1975

Tipton DH, Cook MJ: Trace elements in human tissue. Part 2, adult subjects in the United States. Health Phys 9:103, 1963

Tran TA, Kirby JD: The effect of upper cervical adjustment upon the normal physiology of the heart. ACA J Chiropr 11:S58, 1977

Travell J: The myofascial genesis of pain. Postgrad Med 11:425, 1952

Triano J: The pathophysiology of congestive heart failure. Chiropr Econ 1973

Triano J: Typical spinal distortion of 19 cardiopulmonary patients treated chiropractically. Proceedings of Winter Meeting, International College of Applied Kinesiology, San Diego, 1977

Triano J, Davis BP: Experimental characterization of the reactive muscle phenomenon. Chiropr Econ 1976a

Triano J, Davis BP: Reactive muscles: reciprocal and crossed reciprocal innervation phenomenon. Proceedings of 7th Annual Biomechanic Conference on the Spine. Boulder, University of Colorado, 1976b

Triano J, Luttges M: Effects of intermittent mechanical irritation on sciatic nerves of mice. Proceedings of the 9th Annual Biomechanics Conference on the Spine. Boulder, University of Colorado, 1978

Trott PH, Maitland GD, Gerrard B: The neurocalometer: a survey to assess its value as a diagnostic instrument. Med J Aust 1:464, 1972

Van den Burg JW: Thermal conductivity and heat transfer of the skin. Bibl Radiol 6:166, 1974

Vannerson JF, Nimmo RL: Specificity and the law of facilitation in the nervous system. ACA J Chiropr 10, 3:VII, S78, 1973

Walshe P: Diseases of the Nervous System. London, Churchill Livingston

Walther DS: Applied Kinesiology. Pueblo, Systems D.D., 1976

Weber B, Smith JP, Briscoe, WA, Friedman SA, King TK: Pulmonary function in asymptomatic adolescents with idiopathic scoliosis. Am Rev Respir Dis 111:389, 1975

Weiant CW, Adelman G: Photography through the skin proves chiropractic as science. J Nat Chiropr Assoc 21, 1952

Wilson PT: The osteopathic treatment of asthma. J Am Osteop Assoc 35:491, 1946

Wintrobe MM et al. (eds): Harrison's Principles of Internal Medicine. New York, McGraw-Hill, 1970

Wong P, Verrier M, Ashby P: The effect of vibration on the F-wave in normal man. Electromyogr Clin Neurophysiol 17:319 1977

Wozny PJ: Iron and Anemias. ACA J Chiropr 12, 11:IX, 21, 1975

Yasue H, Touyama M, Shimamoto M, Kato H, Tanaka S, Akiyama F: Role of autonomic nervous system in the pathogenesis of prinzmetal's variant form of angina. Circulation 50:534, 1974

Ziegler EE, O'Connell AM, Stearns G, Nelson SE, Burmeister LF, Fomon SJ: Nitrogen balance studies with normal children. Am J Clin Nutr 30:939, 1977

Zimmerman HM: Res Publ Assoc Nerv Ment Dis 20:824, 1940

CHAPTER THIRTEEN
Physical and Spinal Examination Procedures Utilized in the Practice of Chiropractic
HENRY G. WEST, JR.

Chiropractors have been accepted as health care providers and their patients are eligible for first- and third-party reimbursement. The chiropractor, therefore, has a professional, ethical, and moral obligation to make an adequate physical examination.

There are four primary reasons for an adequate physical examination:

1. To identify the patient's health problem and to correlate the subjective symptoms with the objective clinical findings;
2. To determine if the patient is a candidate for manipulative therapy or whether the patient's health problem could best be treated by another health provider;
3. To identify any unrecognized health problems;
4. To determine where and how the patient is to be treated and whether there are any contraindications for manipulative therapy.

In order to arrive at a correct diagnosis a systematic examination of the patient is necessary. The procedure begins with the initial interview when the patient consults the chiropractor for a health problem which has produced unpleasant symptoms that interfere with his comfort or productivity.

Patient History Taking

An accurate history is often worth many hours and may save money which would otherwise be spent on unnecessary supplemental procedures. The objective of the clinician is to obtain an organized, logical history and to perform a systematic examination to properly assess the patient's health problem.

Initially, the examiner observes the patient as he enters the office and continues this observation while the history is being obtained. Although this observation is commonly thought of as part of the physical examination, it is an inseparable and important part of the history taking.

In order to derive the maximum information from the history, the clinician must become skilled in eliciting the patient's story. The examiner should not be hurried or interrupted. By listening carefully to the patient's story the examiner can obtain factual information regarding the patient's health problem. The clinician's desire to understand and help will become evident to the patient. Realization that the examiner cares about him will remind the patient of aspects of his problem and may lead to the disclosure of additional information which may be of significant diagnostic importance to the clinician. The clinician who can combine sensitive insight and understanding with a sensible objective approach to the patient's problem usually will establish an excellent professional rapport with the patient.

Chief Complaint

The chief complaint should constitute, in a few simple words, the main reason why the patient has consulted the chiropractor. The chief complaint or complaints should be stated as nearly as possible in the patient's own words. It should be simply a notation of the thing or things that are troubling the patient. The chief complaint should not include diagnostic terms.

The examiner should not accept the patient's own diagnosis and, similarly, he should not accept the unqualified diagnosis of any other chiropractor or physician the patient may have previously consulted. It is the responsibility of the chiropractor to arrive at the diagnosis and this can only be done accurately after all of the available information has been obtained. Failure to obtain an accurate chief complaint may ultimately result in an incorrect diagnosis.

Patient's History

The patient's health history should be a well-organized sequentially developed elaboration of the chief complaint or complaints. The patient is asked to describe his symptoms in terms of their nature, location, mode of onset, duration, and what activities accentuate or relieve them. In addition, each symptom is qualified as to its characteristics, i.e., ache, burning, numbness, or tingling.

Since the chiropractor's major mode of therapy is spinal manipulation, the most important aspect of the patient history is the anatomical location of the symptoms and the mode of onset. The examiner should insist on specific localization of pain or discomfort by asking the patient to point to the site of his discomfort.

Taking this portion of the history requires the meticulous development of each symptom from its inception until the patient consults the chiropractor. It cannot be too strongly emphasized that a careful, detailed history is of great importance to the clinician in trying to evaluate the patient's health problem.

Since back pain is the most common symptom afflicting mankind (Wiles 1959; Shands 1967; Calliet 1968; McNabb 1977) a chiropractor must, from necessity, differentiate the etiology of back pain, whether it be viscerogenic, neurogenic, vascular, psychogenic, or vertebrogenic. Viscerogenic back pain is not aggravated by activity, nor is it relieved by rest. The patient displaying symptoms that are visceral in origin,

such as from the kidney or gallbladder may writhe around to get relief, whereas the patient suffering from vertebrogenic back pain may have comparative symptomatic relief in a recumbent position. Neurogenic back pain may be caused from a spinal cord tumor or from nerve root compression from a protruded or herniated intervertebral disc. Frequently the patient gives a history of having to get out of bed at night to walk around in order to obtain relief from back or leg pain. Back pain from peripheral vascular disease may give rise to symptoms resembling sciatica. Characteristically, the pain is not precipitated or aggravated by activities such as bending, stooping, and lifting. The symptoms of vascular back pain are aggravated by walking and relieved by standing still. Psychogenic or psychosomatic back pain is not common. The examining clinician must be prepared to accept the responsibility of eliminating all the possibilities of underlying pathology before considering this classification.

Vertebrogenic back pain may be defined as pain coming from the spinal column and its associated structures. The pain may be aggravated by general and specific activities and relieved, to some extent, by recumbency. Spondylogenic lesions constitute the most common source of back pain seen in clinical practice (McNabb 1977) and represent the greatest area of interest to the chiropractor.

Many patients will have already applied some home remedy on their own. Such measures may vary from proprietary medications to the physical application of heat, cold, or various appliances. The effect of such treatment, either beneficial or harmful, may be of importance and should be recorded as a part of the history. In addition, the patient may have previously consulted a physician who prescribed various medications. The patient's response to these measures is equally important and constitutes a pertinent segment of his history.

The clinician should know what medication the patient is presently taking such as diuretics, urocosuric agents, steroids, antidepressants, and anticoagulants to name a few. This information is important to determine whether or not the medication has any relationship to the present problem or constitutes a contraindication to spinal manipulation. On occasion the patient's symptoms may be a reaction to the medication he is taking.

When the history is completed, it should give the examiner, in chronologic sequence, a clear picture of the date and mode of onset of each symptom, its course and duration, precise location, character, exacerbations and remissions, what relieves or makes it worse, and any relationship to other symptoms, activities, or medications.

History of Past Health Problems

The past history should include a review of all past illnesses and surgical procedures. All statements made by the patient regarding his previous illnesses should be thoroughly evaluated and clarified.

History of Accidents and Spinal Hygiene

It is an important part of the case history and the overall evaluation of the patient's health problem to record information relative to past injuries whether they be major or trivial. A patient may fail to mention minor injuries unless closely questioned. Patients will often admit that they had a previous car accident but that there was no apparent injury at the time. They seem to equate a fracture or the appearance of blood as the criterion for being injured.

It is important to obtain the patient's evaluation of any previous treatment for a spinal complaint especially if it is a recurrence, and his comprehension of the condition for which he was being treated.

Occupational History and Activities of Daily Living

Spinal hygiene is integrally related to occupational history and activities of daily living (ADL). The chiropractic examiner is interested in the patient's physical comfort in the performance of his occupational duties. It is necessary to know what kind of work the patient does and

what influence this has upon the musculoskeletal system. The occupational history should include a record of all past and present types of work. It should also include a history of any work time loss as a result of an industrial accident or workman's compensation claim. The chiropractic examiner should likewise be aware of occupational exposures to dust, fumes, and chemicals. It may be necessary in certain circumstances to recommend a change of occupation.

It is important to evaluate the influence of the patient's activities of daily living upon the patient's musculoskeletal system. Some activities of daily living such as lifting furniture, making beds, and gardening may be more injurious or place the patient in greater jeopardy than his occupational duties.

In addition, a history of the patient's recreational pursuits such as breaking horses, athletics, snowmobiling, or motorcycle racing should be included.

Family History

Heredity and constitutional factors play an important role in the etiology of certain disease processes, such as diabetes mellitus, cancer, hypertension, arteriosclerosis, gout, and coronary artery disease. The chiropractor is particularly interested in the history of musculoskeletal disorders in blood relatives, such as degenerative disc disease, arthritis, and anomalies of the spine. The hereditary nature of the present illness or spinal pain may be revealed by asking, "Are there any other members of your family who have had a similar problem?" Frequently this question will uncover evidence of a familial factor that can not be found in any other way.

Social and Marital History

The course of organic disease and spinal pain is influenced by the patient's emotional reaction to his health problem and his environment. Questioning is directed, therefore, into the patient's personal habits, his emotional adjustments, sexual habits, business life, personality factors, and recreation habits.

Supplemental History by Questionnaire

Many chiropractic physicians utilize health questionnaires such as the Cornell Medical Index (CMI) or its equivalent. The pain drawing and self-questionnaire by Mooney et al. (1976) is a very useful history-taking aid (Fig. 1). Such questionnaires help to obtain a maximum amount of information in a minimum amount of time. The disadvantage is overreliance on questionnaires with a loss of the doctor's personal attention.

General Physical Examination

Assessment of the patient's health condition is predicated upon an adequate physical examination. The examination begins with a general inspection of the patient's posture, body movements, gait, speech, state of nutrition, and stature.

Vital Signs

The height and weight should be vocalized. If the patient challenges the height, it may be a clue to a spinal distortion such as a lateral curvature, an increase in the thoracic curve, or progressive disc degeneration. If the patient remarks about a weight change the examiner should investigate the cause for the change. An involuntary weight loss may be a sign of significant systemic disease.

Systolic arterial blood pressure in persons under 40 years of age is usually 110 to 140 mm Hg and the diastolic pressure is 60 to 90 mm Hg (Prior 1959). Comparison of the blood pressure of both upper extremities should not vary more than 10 percent. Variance of more than 10 percent may be due to a neurovascular compression syndrome or an aneurysm. If the patient complains of undue fatigue or light headedness the blood pressure should be taken in a recumbent as well as in the upright position. The systolic blood pressure should increase 4 to 10 mm

Hg from recumbency to weight bearing (Sewell 1919; Raglund 1920). In postural hypotension there is a significant drop in the systolic pressure on standing which may account for fatigue or light-headedness.

Pulse rate varies with age, sex, physical activity, and emotional status, with 72 beats per minute being the average. Increased pulse rate may be due to fever, tachycardia, or hyperthyroidism. Decreased pulse rate may be seen in intracranial pressure, syncope, and complete heart block. The radial pulse in both upper extremities and the pedal pulse of both lower extremities should be palpated and evaluated for circulatory sufficiency.

The examiner should observe the type, rate, and depth of quiet breathing. In the adult at rest, the normal respiratory rate is 16 to 20 beats per minute and is regular in depth and rhythm. The normal ratio of respiratory to pulse rate is 1:4. There is a definite increase in the respiratory rate with fever, usually at the rate of four additional respiratory cycles per minute for each degree of fever (Prior 1959).

Body temperature is measured with an oral thermometer and normally does not exceed 37 C. Subnormal temperatures are important and may occur during shock, congestive heart failure, excessive exposure to cold, or hypothyroidism. Hyperthermia is primarily the result of tissue injury and occurs in many conditions, i.e., infections, malignancies, injuries, cerebral vascular accident, and hemmorrhage into various body cavities.

Systems Review

After recording the vital signs one should examine the body in a systematic manner from head to feet. A systems review includes examination of the head, cardiovascular system, respiratory system, gastrointestinal system, and genitourinary system.

The examiner should develop a fairly standard routine so that he can examine a patient smoothly and efficiently without forgetting important steps. Failure to follow a systematic procedure may result in the omission of important signs or symptoms. If only positive signs are recorded, the physician may be in doubt when reviewing the case history with regard to those signs and tests which are not listed. The absence as well as the presence of symptoms and signs should be recorded.

Head. With the patient seated, the clinician should examine the head, hair, scalp, skull, and face of the patient. Of particular interest is the sensitivity of the frontal and paranasal sinuses to palpation. A postnasal discharge along with a pain response to palpation over the sinus cavities may be due to sinusitis.

Eyes. The examiner should check the visual acuity with a Snellen eye chart and the visual fields by confrontation. In addition, he should check the alignment of the eyes, the eyebrows, eyelids, lacrimal apparatus, conjunctiva and sclera, cornea, iris, pupils, and extraoccular movements. An opthalmoscopic examination should be performed at all initial examinations. Opthalmologic disorders are important etiological factors in headache.

Ears. The examiner should inspect the ear canal and eardrum with an otoscope and check auditory acuity with the ticking of a watch. If acuity is diminished the examiner should check for lateralization and compare bone conduction with air conduction using a tuning fork. Impacted cerumen, otitus externa, or otitus media may result in hearing loss, pain, or dizziness.

Nose. The clinician should examine the external nose and by means of nasal speculum inspect the nares, the mucosa, the septum, and the terminates.

Mouth and Pharynx. The clinician should inspect the lips, buccomucosa, gums and teeth, roof of the mouth, tongue, tonsils, and pharynx. Bad teeth are a well-known health hazard, and the patient should be referred for proper dental care. Palpation of the temporomandibular joint is of particular importance to the chiropractor. This is performed by opening and closing the mouth. Symmetry of occlusion should be noted. Gelb (1977) states

that malrelationship of the jaws may have a consequent effect upon the entire neuromuscular system involved in the various static and active functions of the structures in the head, neck, and shoulders. A temporomandibular joint syndrome may respond to specialized manipulative therapy. In certain cases the patient should be referred to a dentist specializing in oral orthopedics.

Neck. The clinician should inspect and palpate the cervical nodes, trachea, and thyroid. Deviation of the larynx on deglutition may be indicative of a space occupying lesion or adhesions. If lymphadenopathy is present the examiner should look for an infectious source of the lymphatic drainage.

Cardiovascular System. The heart is assessed chiefly by examination through the anterior chest wall by means of inspection, palpation, percussion, and auscultation. The palmar surface of the hand at the base of the fingers is sensitive to vibrations and therefore is useful in detecting thrills associated with murmurs. Percussion is used in evaluating the size of the heart. The first heart sound (S1) and the second heart sound (S2) are identified by listening at the following locations:

1. Aortic area (second right interspace close to the sternum);
2. Pulmonic area (second left interspace close to the sternum);
3. Third interspace close to the sternum where murmurs of both aortic and pulmonic orginin may often be heard;
4. Tricuspid area (fifth left interspace close to the sternum);
5. Mitral area (fifth left interspace just medial to the mid clavical line).

The carotid arteries are examined one at a time with the index or middle finger around the medial edge of the sternocleidomastoid muscle. Decreased or absent carotid pulse suggests arterial narrowing or occlusion. Auscultation of the carotid should be performed. Upper cervical manipulation may be contrain-

Name _____

Date _____

Mark the areas on your body where you feel the described sensations. Use the appropriate symbol. Mark the areas of radiation. Include all affected areas.

Numbness = = =   Pins and needles 000   Burning xxxxx   Stabbing ///

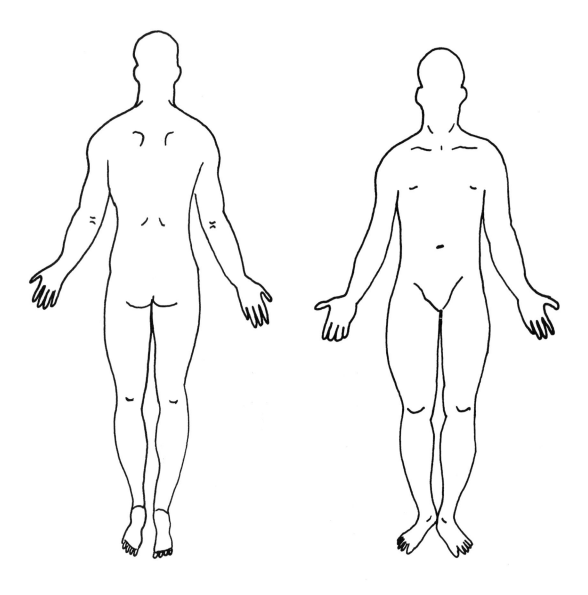

1. How long have you had the present pain? _____ Weeks _____ Mos _____ Years

2. How long have you had any trouble with your
   back, legs, or neck? _____ Weeks _____ Mos _____ Years

3. How long have you been off work or unable
   to do normal housework? _____ Weeks _____ Mos _____ Years

4. Did your pain begin: [] Gradually [] Suddenly [] From an injury [] At work

5. Is your pain: [] Continuous [] Off & on [] Neither

6. My pain is:

	Better	Worse	Unchanged
A. With cough or sneeze	[]	[]	[]
B. Sitting down at a table	[]	[]	[]
C. Sitting in an automobile	[]	[]	[]
D. Bending forward to brush teeth	[]	[]	[]
E. Walking short distance	[]	[]	[]
F. Lying flat on back	[]	[]	[]
G. Lying flat on stomach	[]	[]	[]
H. Lying on side with knees bent	[]	[]	[]
I When I awake in the morning	[]	[]	[]
J. Mid-morning	[]	[]	[]
K. Middle of night	[]	[]	[]

7. My back sometimes gets "stuck" when I bend forward. [] Yes [] No
   My back feels it is likely to give way when I bend forward. [] Yes [] No
   My pain stops me after I walk a certain distance. [] Yes [] No
   After walking, bending forward improves my pain. [] Yes [] No

8. How many times have you been in a hospital for back, leg, or neck problems? _____

9. Have you had previous back injuries? [] Yes [] No Type _____

10. Have you had other types of surgery? [] Yes [] No Type _____

11. Have any treatments made your pain better? [] Yes [] No What treatments _____
    _____

12. Have any treatments made your pain worse [] Yes [] No What treatments _____

13. What is the most aggravating thing about your pain? _____
    _____

Occupation _____
Date _____ Age _____

FIG. 1. **Pain drawing (facing page) and self-questionnaire (above). (Adapted from Mooney V, Douglas C, Robertson R: A system for evaluation and treating chronic back disability. West J Med 124:370, 1976)**

dicated in the presence of carotid insufficiency (see Chapter 16, this volume).

Respiratory System. The respiratory tract is assessed by examination through the anterior and posterior chest wall by means of inspection, palpation, percussion, and ascultation.

1. Examination of the posterior thorax and lungs is made with the patient seated.
   a. Palpatation of the chest is useful in identifying areas of tenderness, assessing observed abnormalities such as masses, assessing respiratory excursion from inspiration to expiration, and evaluating vocal or tactile fremitus. Fremitus is decreased or absent when the bronchus is obstructed or the pleural space is occupied by fluid, air, or solid tissue.
   b. Auscultation of the lungs is useful in assessing the amount of airflow through the trachial bronchial tree and in evaluating the presence of fluid or a friction rub in the pleura.
2. Examination of the anterior chest, using the procedure of inspection, palpation, percussion, and auscultation is made with the patient supine. The examiner assesses the quality of air flowing through the bronchial tree and lungs for the presence of crepitus, mucus, or fluid. This should be done in a systematic manner covering each lobe of both lungs.

While examining the anterior thorax a breast examination of the female patient is performed, both in the sitting and supine positions. With the patient seated, properly disrobed and arms at the side, the examiner inspects the breast, noting size, symmetry and contour with special reference to masses, dimpling or flattening. The patient is asked to raise her arms over her head and then to press her arms against her hips as the examiner looks for any change in contour of the breast. The breast should be palpated for lumps and masses. Nipple retraction and a discharge from the breast needs further consultation. With the arms extended over the head, the examiner palpates the axillary lymph nodes. Lymphadenopathy may result from infection or other diseases of the breast or neck. Enlargement of the lymph nodes may also come from habitual use of certain deodorants.

Gastrointestinal System. The abdomen is examined with the patient supine. Inspection of the skin is carried out to determine the presence of scars, dilated veins, the contour and symmetry of the abdomen, and the contour and location of the umbilicus. The abdomen is palpated for any masses of focal tenderness. The examiner should make a habit of visualizing each organ in the region that he is examining. The abdomen should be examined with superficial and deep palpation. Percussion is useful for general orientation of the abdomen, for measurement of the liver and sometimes of the spleen, and for identification of air in the stomach and bowel. The examiner should auscultate all four quadrants of the abdomen, noting the frequency and character of the sounds of peristaltic movement. A friction rub may be audible with enlargement of the liver or spleen. The examiner can identify the aortic pulsation by deep palpation slightly to the left of the midline. A prominent pulsation with lateral expansion suggests an aortic aneurysm for which heavy dorsal spinal manipulative therapy which increases intraabdominal pressure would be contraindicated.

Genitourinary System. With the patient supine, each kidney is examined by deep bimanual palpation. With the patient prone, Murphy's percussion test is made by placing the palm of the hand over the costovertebral angle. The examiner strikes the posterior surface of the hand with the opposite hand. Normally the patient should receive a painless jar or thud; pain suggests kidney infection. A genitourinary examination may include a pelvic examination of the female especially in patients who complain of menstrual cycle related low-back pain. The external genitalia are examined followed by a bimanual examination, noting the size, shape, consistency, mobility, and tenderness of the uterus, fallopian tubes and ovaries.

Both sexes are examined for inguinal and femoral hernia. On the male, examination of the penis and palpation of the testes and scrotum is performed noting any abnormalities.

No examination of the genitourinary tract is complete without a urinalysis. Since viscerogenic reflexes can cause spinal pain, the chiropractic examiner uses the urinalysis to eliminate urinary tract infection as a cause of referred back pain.

A physical examination may require a rectal examination in order to be complete. While this examination is technically a part of the gastrointestinal system, the examination is more easily performed with the genitourinary system. With a gloved hand, and properly lubricated index finger, examine the anus, the sphincter, and the rectal wall for lumps, masses, and hemorrhoids. In the male, palpate the prostate for size, tenderness, and nodules. While making a rectal examination the examiner palpates the internal contours of the coccyx and the sacrococcygeal junction by lifting posterior on the coccyx. A pain response may be indicative of coccydenia.

While approximately 80 percent of all lowback pain is vertebrogenic (Shands 1967; Calliet 1968; McNabb 1977) the chiropractic examiner must be cognizant that the remaining percentage comes from a variety of causes, some of which are referred pain from a prostatic disorder, urinary tract infection, rectal pathology, pelvic inflammatory disease, or malposition of the uterus. Spinal manipulative therapy will not produce satisfactory results without special attention to the possibility of referred pain.

Spinal Examination

Since the primary therapeutic tool of the chiropractor is manipulation, the spinal and extremity examination becomes the focal point of patient evaluation. It is of paramount importance to have a keen working knowledge of anatomy, physiology, biomechanics, and kinesiology of the spinal column and extremities before an adequate determination of normal and abnormal function can be made.

When dysfunction is determined, treatment is instituted to return the affected tissues to as near normal a physiological state as possible.

Posture is defined as the relative arrangement of bodily parts. Good posture is a state of muscular and skeletal balance. Poor posture is an abnormal relationship of bodily parts which produces stress on the musculoskeletal system and in some cases may impair visceral function.

Posture Examination

A simple tool to aid the clinician in the evaluation of posture is a double string plumbline with a T board placed on the floor to separate the feet by approximately 3 inches so that the knees do not touch each other. Hypothetically, the halves of the skeletal structure are essentially symmetrical and the two halves of the body are exactly counterbalanced. Therefore, the center of the plumbline should bisect the skull and be superimposed upon the spine and the gluteal crease in viewing a normal subject from the rear (Fig. 2). The patient is placed in front of the double string plumbline with his feet straddling the T square on the floor as the examiner evaluates the patient's posture. The examiner should look for head tilt, rotation of the head, comparative shoulder levels, obvious lateral distortion or curvature of the spine, the level of the iliac crests, and vertical alignment of the gluteal crease.

Head tilt and/or rotation of the head can easily be evaluated by having the examiner place his index fingers in the ear canals of the patient. Through clinical experience head tilt can be determined by noting unequal levels of the examiner's fingers. In the absence of rotation this is thought to be due to a lateral occipital condyle sideslip upon the lateral masses of the atlas.

Superior head tilt accompanied by posterior rotation of the occiput on the same side is usually due to laterality of the atlas. DeJarnette (1961) feels that the lateral wedge shape of the lateral masses of the atlas causes any lateral shifting of the atlas to produce elevation of the occiput.

Inferior head tilt, attended by posterior rotation of the head is felt to be due to a rotational malposition of the axis with the spinous process of the axis rotating away from the midline of the spine.

Any alteration of structure may produce an alteration of function which, in turn, may increase the strain on the supporting structures resulting in a compromise in the efficient balance of the body. Occipital-atlantal-axial distortion may produce hypertonicity of the suboccipital muscles and alter the range of motion. Studies by Wolff (MacBride 1970) reveal that sustained contraction of neck muscles is associated with neck pain, shoulder pain, and headaches. Suboccipital tension resulting from structural disrelationship of the upper cervical spine is a frequent finding in patients complaining of headaches.

Unilateral elevation of a shoulder may be associated with a structural problem, the most frequent of which is a lateral curvature of the spine or scoliosis. A lateral curvature of the spine is defined here as a functional muscular distortion, whereas scoliosis is defined as a structural distortion associated with a lateral wedging and torsion of the vertebral body which is usually attended by prominence and winging of the scapula (Keim 1972). Bilateral elevation of the shoulders is a sign of hyperinflation of the lungs (Brewis 1975).

Distortion from the normal vertical alignment of the gluteal crease may be due to rotation of the pelvis, paraspinal muscle spasm, sacroiliac distortion, or an inequality of leg length. If the pelvis is level with the gluteal crease, aligned with the plumbline, and there is a lateral tilt of the lumbar spine superior to L4-5, there may be unilateral spasm of the erector spinae. Acute strain is characterized by sharp angular deviation due to unilateral muscle spasm of the erector spinae. Chronic strain, on the other hand, is characterized by a "C" type distortion.

A body list is significant when radicular symptoms are present. A body list toward the side of sciatic radiculopathy is probably due to an angular protrusion or a nuclear herniation of the intervertebral disc on the medial side of the nerve root (Fig. 3). A body list away from the side of a lumbar radiculopathy is probably

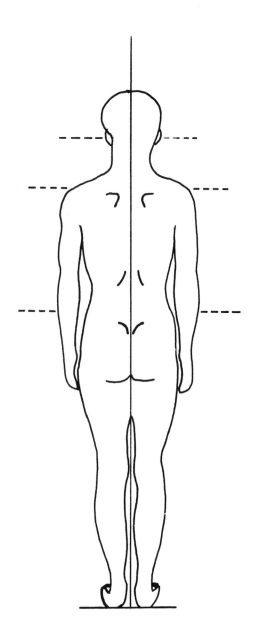

FIG. 2. **Standard posture—posterior view. Using a double string plumbline to evaluate spinal distortion, head tilt, head rotation, shoulder level, iliac crest level, and rotation of the pelvis.**

due to a disc lesion on the lateral side of the nerve root (Fig. 4) (Finneson 1973).

Observation of the hip joint in a weight-bearing position in front of the plumbline is difficult since it is the most deeply seated of any joint. The position of the hip is the key to body posture because it determines the angle of the pelvis, and the pelvis is the foundation upon which the spine is erected (Wiles 1959). Hip joint pathology is characterized by a flexion of the knee together with abduction and external rotation of the leg on the affected side in the weight-bearing position. This is particularly noticeable on walking. Patrick's FABER (*flex*ion, *ab*duction, *e*xternal *r*otation) test and x-ray examination are an essential part of any evaluation of the hip joint.

While the patient is still in front of the plumbline the clinician examines the posture of the knees and feet since they also are part of the complex foundation for the spine.

In the side view, a vertical line of reference represents the plane which hypothetically di-

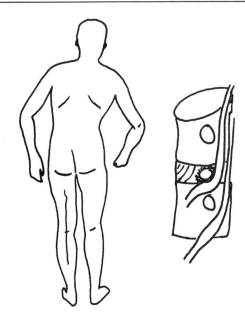

FIG. 4. **Body list away from the side of radicular symptoms is usually attended by a protrusion of the intervertebral disc on the lateral side of the nerve root.**

vides the body into front and back sections of equal body weight. These sections are not symmetrical and therefore there is no obvious line of division on the basis of anatomical structure. The plumbline should pass through the mastoid, midway between the back and abdomen, the great trochanter, and the lateral malleolus (Fig. 5) (Kendall 1955). As the chiropractic examiner views the patient from the side, he is interested in the anatomical balance of the head in relationship to the body and should note the anterior lordotic curve of the cervical spine, the thoracic curve, and the lumbar lordosis.

Hypolordosis, or cervical kyphosis, has been considered an etiologic factor in neck pain and in vertebrogenic suboccipital-frontal cephalalgia. A decrease in the thoracic curve is frequently associated with vertebrogenic chest pain. An increase in the thoracic curve is found in poor posture, anterior wedge deformity of a thoracic vertebral body, shoulder sag, and emphysema.

A flat lumbar spine may be due to hyper-

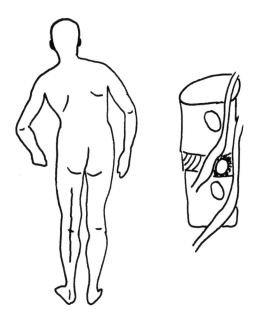

FIG. 3. **Body list toward the side of radicular symptoms (left) is usually attended by a protrusion of the intervertebral disc on the medial side of the nerve root (right).**

tonicity of the paraspinal musculature. Hypolordosis in turn, increases the shearing stress at the lumbosacral joint (Lipe 1963).

Circumference Measurement of the Chest

The circumference of the chest should expand 1.5 to 2.5 inches for the male and 1 to 1.5 inches for the female from expiration to inspiration. Limited chest expansion may be due to restrictive pulmonary function, such as emphysema or ankylosing spondylitis.

Spinal Palpation

Spinal palpation has two components: static and motion. While static palpation is performed easily in both recumbent and weight-bearing positions, motion palpation is best performed in the sitting or standing position.

The findings on palpation may be expressed as a sense of resistance on one side to a sense of yield on the other side (Johnston 1975). A trained, skillful examiner can feel fine differences in tissue texture and muscle tone. Both superficial and deep palpation should be employed, keeping in mind that undue painful pressure is not necessary.

Normally there is no pain response to palpation and no tenderness on palpation of connective tissue. In patients with symptomatic structural or functional distortion a skilled examiner should be able to locate areas of hypertonicity which are tender to palpation. In symptomatic lesions of the upper cervical spine, palpation may reveal painful fibrotic cordlike strings, or pulpy, soft edematous connective tissue. In a patient with a lateral shift of the atlas there may be a palpable fullness on the side of laterality. To the experienced palpator the muscle mass overlaying the lamina of the axis will have a fullness on the side of posterior rotation, whereas the spinous process will deviate to the opposite side.

The remainder of the cervical spine is palpated from the spinous processes laterally across the lamina which are covered by six muscle layers (Bateman 1972) toward the articular

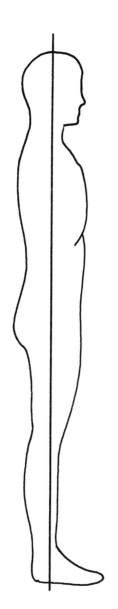

FIG. 5. **Standard lateral posture using the double strength plumbline for the evaluation of the primary curves of the spine and anteroposterior weight distribution.**

pillar. Localized muscle contraction is definable and will elicit a pain response upon palpation. Motion palpation will confirm the plane of restricted motion which may be used as a guide in the application of the manipulative thrust. Localized palpatory tenderness at the posterolateral margin of C-5, 6 will frequently give rise to referred pain in the middorsal spine and across the vertebral border of the homolateral scapula, following the origin and course of the dorsal scapular nerve (Lipe 1963).

Palpation of the first rib head is accentuated by having the patient flex the head and neck toward the chest. In the normal subject there is no undue tenderness. If palpable tenderness is present it may be due to costovertebral disrelationship. In addition, it has been suggested that this condition is associated with a homolateral sacroiliac slip (DeJarnette 1961).

Static palpation of the spinous processes with the thumb is normally painless (Maigne 1972). If painful, the spinous process should be percussed with the spine in a flexed position. Exquisite pain is frequently correlated with a fracture, disc herniation, or bony pathology.

In a normal subject in the prone position, the spinous processes are spread equidistant. An abnormal palpatory finding is a "flat" spot in the thoracic curve. The spinous process of the offending vertebra tips inferiorly, causing a disproportionate interspinous spacing. This is commonly referred to as "an anterior dorsal vertebra" and is invariably tender to axial pressure on the spinous process. It is frequently associated with referred pain into the anterior chest wall. A viscerotropic reflex from the lung may produce a difference in pigmentation in the interscapular space with wasting of the subcutaneous tissue and loss of elastic tone, characterized by a saucerlike depression of the dorsal spine (Pottinger 1925). This is commonly referred to as a "Pottinger saucer."

Based on this author's clinical experience, a long-standing chronic gastric, peptic, or duodenal ulcer may produce a viscerotrophic reflex, resulting in a saucerlike depression in the midthoracic spine. In patients complaining of dorsalgia, it is not infrequent to find a localized circumscribed area of redness which can be produced by the weight of the palpating fingers. It has been postulated by DeJarnette (1961, 1963) that these areas of hyperemia are produced by a vasomotor reaction for which there is no adequate explanation at the present time. These areas of hyperemia consistently respond to specific manipulative therapy with an immediate significant change or complete disappearance of the hyperemia.

In addition to palpation of the spinous processes, the examiner should also palpate the tissues over the costovertebral articulations. Relative position of vertebral rotation and tippage can be determined by a skillful examiner. This becomes meaningful if it is attended by a pain response or a vasomotor change.

Palpation of the lumbar spine is most readily performed by using the thumbs in axial pressure over the spinous processes, the mammillary processes, and the interspinous spaces. Additional information can be obtained if the examiner places his thumb against the side of the spinous process and applies pressure not only in a forward direction but in a lateral direction as well, thereby applying a rotatory strain to the segment. If there is reproduction of the symptomatic pain by this maneuver, it is of diagnostic significance in helping to differentiate a rotational strain from a flexion-extension strain.

Digital pressure with the thumbs in the iliolumbar angle will elicit a pain response on the side of hypertonicity of the sacrospinalis (erector spinae). The examiner should compare the level of the posterior superior iliac spines with his thumbs as he grasps the ilium with the thenar surface of the index finger. A comparative inferiority of the posterior iliac spine on one side may be indicative of a posterior inferior rotation of the innominate.

With spondylolisthesis of L5 there may be a pronounced spinous process of L5 and a depression at the L4 level because of the anterior displacement of the lumbar spine superior to L5.

The examiner should palpate the sacroiliac joints with the thumbs. A pain response will be elicited when a sacroiliac disrelationship exists with either an anterior or posterior rotation of the innominate or in the presence of sacral crest rotation.

Skin Rolling

This examination is made by grasping a large fold of skin between the thumb and index finger and rolling the skin as one rolls a cigarette (Maigne 1972). This maneuver is normally barely perceivable by the patient. The examiner looks for tender nodules or large folds in the skin which are sensitive to the least amount of pressure. Over the spine the skin appears thickened and has a nodular consistency at involved levels, while vertebral levels above and below appear to be normal. These cutaneous tender infiltrations often show a distribution following the posterior branch of the spinal nerve (Bateman 1972; Maigne 1972). Skin rolling is used for diagnosis and treatment of subcutaneous lesions and connective tissue lesions over the spine, abdomen, and chest. (Mennell 1960, Zohn 1976)

Motion Palpation

No matter what is revealed with static palpation, consideration must be made for the presence of joint fixation. This is defined as failure of motion in a particular plane of joint motion as a function of dynamic motoricity (Stonebrink 1969). Motion palpation in contrast to static palpation evaluates the dynamics of regional body movement (Johnson 1973).

The examiner evaluates segmental movement to determine whether the segment contributes to the gross movement pattern. An accurate history may be the only help to determine if a lesion is a response to a biomechanical lesion or if the position is due to some neuromusculoskeletal reflex from deeper underlying pathology.

With the patient seated each cervical segment should be tested in flexion, extension, lateral bending, and rotation. For the most part, motion palpation is made with passive movement controlled by the examiner's nonpalpating hand.

Occipital-Atlas. This motion palpation is carried out with the examiner's palpating fingers halfway between the occipital notch and the mastoid process on either side and immediately beneath the occiput. The other hand, controlling the head, moves the head forward and backward, not up and down. Normally, motion is present. The second contact point is the space between the transverse process of the atlas and the ramus of the jaw. This space should open and close on anterior and posterior movement of the occiput.

Atlas-Axis. With the palpating fingers over the atlas-axis articulation the examiner moves the head posterior and anterior. The second contact point is made with the palpating forearm held horizontally, the palm forward with the index finger on the occipital notch, the middle finger on the posterior tubercle of the atlas, and the ring finger on the spinous process of the axis. The examiner rotates the patient's head with the opposite hand. The spinous process of the axis in a normal subject should not follow the occiput in its early movement. If it does follow the occiput, there is fixation between the atlas and the axis.

Occiput-Atlas-Axis. With normal flexion of the head upon the neck the occipitoatlantal and the atlantoaxial interspaces should increase. Likewise, these spaces should decrease in extension of the head.

Motion Palpation of C3 Through C7. With the palm of the examining hand resting on the upper dorsal spine and the tip of the index and middle fingers lateral to the spinous process of C3, the examiner rotates the head from side to side. This is followed by bending the head laterally from side to side, then flexing and extending the head and neck. Normally, segmental motion is present in all planes. Each cervical vertebra is tested in descending order.

The interspinous spaces and the ligamentum nuchae are examined during flexion and extension of the neck. Degenerative changes associated with spondylosis may have a characteristic palpable click which is often associated with decreased intervertebral disc space, telescoping of the facets, and laxity of the ligaments.

Thoracic Spine.   There are three areas to be evaluated with motion palpation in the thoracic spine: intervertebral motion, costovertebral motion, and intercostal motion.

With the patient seated, there are two ways to evaluate intersegmental movement:

1. With the examiner seated behind the patient the examiner uses the dorsal surfaces of the fingers over the spinous processes. The free arm is anchored across the front of both shoulders of the patient. The examiner holds the patient in the erect position with the free arm and pushes forward with the examining fingers in a short pistonlike manner to evaluate the resistance to motion.
2. With the patient and the examiner in the same position as above, the examiner uses the tip of the index, middle, and ring fingers over the spinous processes. The patient is guided in motion with the examiner's other arm into flexion and then extension. Range of motion or resistance of the segments is evaluated. This is repeated in lateral bending to each side followed by rotation to each side. The costovertebral joints and the rib heads are palpated for intercostal motion in lateral bending only, using the three fingers with one finger above and one finger below the segment being tested.

Lumbar Spine.   With the patient seated and the examiner seated behind the patient on one side, the examiner palpates the spinous processes and guides the patient in flexion and extension with the nonpalpating hand. In flexion the spinous processes should separate in a flaring fashion. In extension the spinous processes normally approximate each other. In lateral bending it should be possible to feel compression of the lateral vertebral elements on the side of concavity with separation the side of convexity. To evaluate the lumbar spine in rotation,

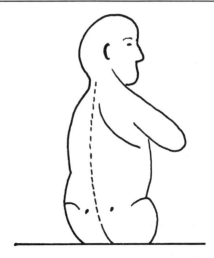

FIG. 6.   **The spinous processus in lumbar rotation should slant in an unbroken manner. Intersegmental fixation will restrict the slant from the involved vertebral segment downward.**

the examiner places the index and middle finger paraspinally, and with the free arm, rotates the patient without flexion (Fig. 6). The palpating fingers follow the line of the spinous processes from the first lumbar to the sacrum. This line should curve in an unbroken manner. Intersegmental fixation will restrict the curve from the involved vertebral segment downward.

Sacroiliac.   With the patient standing, the examiner grasps the ilium with the index finger along the crest of the ilium and the thumb over the posterior superior iliac spine. The patient is asked to lift his leg to a right angle with the knee bent at 90 degrees and the foot pointing toward the floor. The palpating thumb on the side of the lifted knee should move posteriorly and inferiorly on a normal subject. Another check point is made inferiorly as close as possible to the ischium and with the patient elevating the leg in a similar manner. The palpating thumb should move anteriorly (Gillet 1963).

Motion palpation requires practice and skill for correct interpretation. The chiropractor must be able to determine partial fixation, complete fixations, erratic motion, hypermobility, and other qualities of motor unit disharmony. As the examiner develops the skill of kinetic palpation, he will have a greater appreciation of spinal biomechanics and kinesiology which is necessary for the correct application of manipulative therapy.

Percussion

Percussion of each spinous process is done with a pleximeter striking the examiner's thumb which has been placed over the spinous process. The spinous processes become accentuated in flexion which is the more desirable position for this examination. When percussion produces acute pain which immediately subsides, it is likely due to traumatic joint pathology (Arnold 1978). Dull pain which slowly disappears suggests fracture, neoplasm, or other bone disease. If the pain persists for an extended period of time it is a sign of bone pathology.

Percussion of the interspace of the lumbar spine which produces a radiating pain into the lower extremity usually signifies a disc lesion. Patients with a low-pain threshold or who may suffer from hysteria or functional overlay will often say that " . . . all joints are painful."

Range of Motion

Use of the goniometer allows for quantification in the measurement of range of motion. Specific instructions are necessary to insure accuracy. For measuring flexion and extension of the cervical spine a long-handled goniometer is placed on the shoulder adjacent to the neck with the center of the goniometer at the level of C-6 with the long arm of the goniometer extending vertical between the mastoid and external auditory canal. From the neutral position, the patient is asked to bend his head down and touch his chin to his chest (flexion). For extension the patient is asked to bend his head backwards as far as he can. The second arm of the goniometer measures the exact range of motion (Fig. 7).

Lateral bending of the spine is measured with

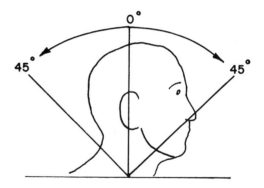

FIG. 7. **Measurement of flexion and extension of the cervical spine using a long-handled goniometer.**

the goniometer resting on the spinous process of T1. The patient is asked to bend his head to the side in an attempt to touch the ear to the shoulder (Fig. 8). On measuring cervical rotation the patient begins in a neutral position, looking straight ahead, with the examiner standing above the patient and the goniometer above the head. The patient is asked to turn his head to the right and look over his shoulder. The examiner uses the long arm of the goniometer to measure the arc of motion, using the patient's nose as a reference point (Fig. 9). The maneuver is repeated to the opposite side. The American Academy of Orthopedic Surgeons (1965) lists the following normal ranges of mobility:

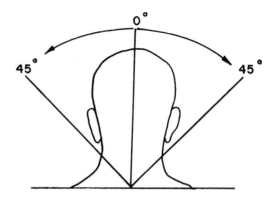

FIG. 8. **Lateral bending of the spine.**

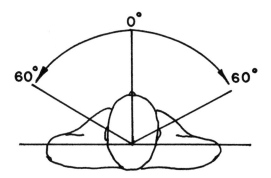

FIG. 9. **Rotation of the cervical spine.**

Flexion	45°
Extension	45°
Lateral bending, right	45°
Lateral bending, left	45°
Rotation, right	60°
Rotation left	60°

Dorsolumbar ranges of motion can likewise be measured with the goniometer. The following values are obtained with the goniometer placed over the sacrum for lateral bending and over the hip for flexion and extension. Rotation is best estimated with the patient's hand grasping the hips and measuring the rotation of the elbow from an imaginary horizontal line.

Flexion	80°
Extension	30°
Lateral bending, right	35°
Lateral bending, left	35°
Rotation, right	45°
Rotation, left	45°

An estimate of flexion can be obtained by recording the distance of the fingertips from the floor when the patient is asked to bend forward. Extension is measured with the goniometer when the patient is asked to bend backward as far as he can. Lateral bending is measured with a goniometer resting on the base of the sacrum. An estimate of lateral flexion can be obtained by noting where the extended arm touches the homolateral leg in lateral bending. Rotation is measured with the examiner stabilizing the patient and asking the patient to twist

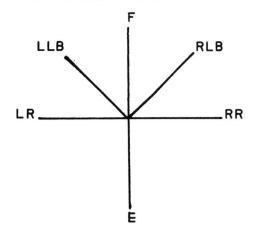

FIG. 10. **"Star diagram." Adapted from Maigne (1972), using a shorthand method for the evaluation of range of motion of the cervical spine, thoracic spine, and the lumbar spine.**

the upper half of the body as far as he can.

Limitation of range of motion becomes significant if there is an unequal measurement of one side compared to the other, particularly if there is pain or muscle spasm. A shorthand method of recording spinal range of motion has been developed by Maigne (1972) and is presented in Figures 10 and 11.

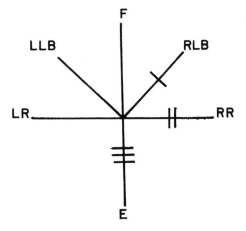

FIG. 11. **Example of limited motion using the star diagram with / = 25%, // = 50%, /// = 75%, //// = complete loss of motion.**

Range of motion may vary considerably with difference in body build, i.e., a long willowy neck versus the short bull neck. The important factor is the comparative range of motion of one side versus the other.

Soto-Hall. The examiner places one hand on the sternum of the patient, who is supine and without a pillow, exerting light pressure so that no flexion can take place at either the lumbar or thoracic regions of the spine. With the other hand under the occiput, the head is flexed upon the neck and the sternum. Flexion of the head and neck upon the sternum progressively produces a pull on the posterior spinous ligaments from above downward. A noticeable localized pain will be experienced at the level of a lesion such as a fracture of the spinous tip or vertebral body. There will also be localized pain at the level of a sprain or strain.

If, during the performance of the Soto-Hall maneuver the patient develops a sudden, transient electriclike shock spreading down the body and into the upper and lower extremities, the patient has Lhermitte's sign which is seen in multiple sclerosis, cord degeneration, and cervical cord injuries (Dorland 1965).

Flexion of the head and neck on the chest that causes flexion of the knees is due to meningeal irritation (Brudzenski's sign). If neck and head flexion produces low-back symptoms (Lindner's sign) there may be a localized vertebrogenic lesion of the low back.

Iliopsoas-Quadrantus Lumborum Test. Michelle (1962) lists six different ways to test for tension of the iliopsoas muscles. DeJarnette (1940) uses a bilateral arm stretch overhead. With the patient supine the examiner grasps the wrists of the patient and extends the arms overhead with the fingers extended. In this position the comparative length of the arms is measured. The arm length will be shorter on the side of contraction of the iliopsoas and quadratus lumborum muscles. This is followed by palpatory verification of the psoas muscles through the abdominal wall. With the patient's knee flexed, the foot flat on the table, and the abdominal wall relaxed, the examiner palpates

through the abdominal wall with the dorsal surface of the first and second phalanges of the four fingers, thus pressing the contents of the abdomen into the psoas muscle. An uncomfortable palpable tension over the muscle is considered a positive test.

Leg Length. The causes of leg length discrepancy are numerous and varied (Shands 1967; Wiles 1959). Clinical estimation of leg length discrepancy by palpating the iliac crests in the weight-bearing position or by tape measurements from the anterior superior iliac spine to the tip of the medial malleolus with the patient supine are unreliable (Clark 1972; Fish 1978). Opinions vary regarding the importance of leg length difference in the pathogenesis of back pain (Fisk 1978). However, Giles (1966) states that leg length disparity is a significant etiological factor in scoliosis. Travell (Gelb 1977) reported that if one leg is only a quarter of an inch shorter, the entire body can be tilted enough to cause pain throughout the skeletal system. So slight a difference can distort the entire skeleton, causing a "seesaw" condition that pulls one shoulder down a full inch. This may never be recognized until, for example, the person is hurt in a fall or an accident. According to Stoddard (1959), inequality of leg length leads first to sacroiliac strain and secondly to lumbosacral or lower lumbar strain. Therefore, to the chiropractic examiner, leg length evaluation is a very important aspect of the spinal examination. Observation of the paired internal malleoli in both supine and prone positions, when the patient is lowered into either position from a high-low table, is probably as accurate as any other clinical examination.

Thompson (1973) has claimed to provide a system of clinical examination to differentiate anatomical leg length deficiency from that due to functional muscular contraction. The Derefield-Thompson Leg Check begins with the patient prone on the lowered table. The relative leg length in the extended position is checked using the internal malleoli or the bottom of the heel as a reference point. The second phase of the examination is done by grasping the ankles of the patient and flexing the patient's leg at the knee to a point just beyond 90 degrees. In the flexed position, the comparative leg length, using the same reference point, is noted. If one leg is short in the extended position and remains short in the flexed position, an anatomical difference probably exists. If the short leg in the extended position equalizes in the flexed position, the leg length difference is due to a functional muscular deficiency due to a posterior rotation of the innominate at the sacroiliac joint on the involved side (Thompson 1973). In order to differentiate an innominate rotation from a rotation of the sacrum, the examiner places the heel of one hand on the base of the sacrum with the fingers pointing toward the patient's feet. Sufficient pressure is applied at the sacral base to prevent the patient from raising the pelvis off the table during the test. The patient is requested to raise one leg at a time as high as possible without flexing the knee and without raising the pelvis from the table. Normally, the legs should rise to approximately the same level. According to Thompson (1973), a positive finding is noted when there is a marked difference in the ability of the patient to raise the extended leg.

Thompson claims to differentiate a functional short leg caused by pelvic distortion from a functional short leg caused by a cervical lesion. With the patient prone, the comparative lengths of the extended legs are noted. The patient is then asked to rotate the head fully to the left while the legs remain in the extended position and then to turn the head to the right. Thompson states that if there is any change in the comparative leg length, palpation of the upper cervical spine will reveal a painful nodular mass over the posterior arch of the lamina of the cervical segment involved.

Upper Extremity Examination

Even though symptoms in the upper extremities are due more often to a lesion of the cervical spine than to any other cause (Wiles 1959), the chiropractic examiner must also con-

sider visceral referred pain, such as angina pectoris, as well as regional disorders of the shoulder, elbow, wrist, and hand. The following tests are helpful.

Cervical Compression Test

With the patient sitting and the head bent obliquely backward, the examiner applies compression force to the head. If pain is exaggerated down the course of a specific nerve root, this is a positive test and indicates nerve root compression which may come from a subluxation, edema, degenerative joint disease, or disc herniation. Local pain in the neck without radiating pain along the nerve root is not a positive test. If moderate traction relieves the pain, it is particularly indicative of nerve root compression (Shaffer 1977).

Cervical Distraction Test

The physician should check visual acuity one eye at a time using a Snellen eye chart, then recheck visual acuity while manually tractioning the cervical spine with one hand under the occiput and one hand under the mandible. If there is improvement in visual perception, there may be an impairment in vertebrobasilar circulation for which cervical manipulative therapy is contraindicated without further evaluation (DeRusha 1977).

Shoulder Depression Test

The patient laterally bends the head which is stabilized by the examiner's hand while the other hand manually depresses the shoulder. If this maneuver causes reproduction or aggravation of radicular pain, it is believed to be indicative of adhesions about the dural sleeve of the nerve root and the adjacent capsular structures (Shaffer 1977).

Neurovascular Compression Tests for Thoracic Outlet Syndrome

Compression of the subclavian or axillary vessels and/or the brachial plexus will produce certain typical signs and symptoms in the upper extremity which may include pain, paresthesias, numbness, weakness, discoloration, swelling, ulceration, gangrene, and in some cases Raynaud's phenomenon (Lord 1958). The neurovascular bundle traverses the following structures where abnormal structural variation may compress the nerves and vessels:

1. Intervertebral foramina (brachial plexus roots only);
2. Interscalene triangle;
3. Costoclavical space;
4. The axilla beneath the coracoid process and the pectoralis minor tendon.

Foramina Compression Test

Axial pressure is applied by the examiner to the cervical spine in lateral bending, thereby causing compression of the contents of the intervertebral foramen. The test is positive if there is a localized pain response in the neck or referred pain into the arm and shoulder (Lipe 1963).

Adson's Maneuver

The test is performed by having the patient take and hold a deep breath, extend his neck fully, and turn his chin toward the side being examined. The test is repeated by turning the head to the opposite side. The examiner should grasp both wrists and check the radial pulses during the maneuver. A decreased or absent pulse represents a positive finding indicating compression by the scalenus anticus muscle on the neurovascular bundle. A cervical rib may produce compression on the neurovascular bundle at the same anatomical location and will also cause a diminution in the radial pulse during this maneuver. The cervical rib can be confirmed by x-ray examination.

Costoclavicular Test (Eden's Test)

The patient is asked to take a deep breath and hold it. He is then asked to assume an exagger-

ated military posture with the shoulders drawn downward and backward with the neck in flexion. This maneuver narrows the costoclavicular space by approximating the clavicle to the first rib, thus tending to compress the neurovascular structures within the costoclavicular space. Modification or obliteration of the radial pulse by this maneuver indicates arterial compression and is a positive test. The radial pulse of both arms is checked at the same time.

Hyperabduction Test (Wright's Test)

As the arm is abducted from the side of the body to a position overhead, the radial pulse is palpated through an arc of 180 degrees. The components of the brachial plexus and axillary vessels are bent to form a 90-degree angle around the coracoid process beneath the pectoralis minor tendon. A decrease or obliteration of the radial pulse is a positive finding.

Examination for Combined Neurovascular Compression Syndrome

This is a combination of two or more of the above disorders, such as, hyperabduction syndrome and costoclavicular syndrome.

Shoulder Examination. The shoulder possesses the largest range of motion of any joint in the body. It has less stability and less mechanical protection than any other large joint of the body. The shoulder joint is examined by inspection, palpation, and measurement of range of motion. Ranges of motion of the shoulder are:

Abduction	180°
Anterior flexion	180°
Posterior flexion or extension	45°
Circumduction	360°

Rotation of the arm at the side:

Internal rotation	80°
External rotation	60°

Rotation of the arm at the shoulder level:

External rotation	90°
Internal rotation	70°

Adduction is measured by reaching across and touching the other shoulder. Posterior internal rotation is measured by reaching backward and medially to touch the opposite scapula.

Drop Arm Test. The examiner passively abducts the patient's extended arm. If the patient cannot maintain the extended arm in the abducted position it is a positive "drop arm sign." It is indicative of a partial or complete tear of the musculotendinous rotator cuff.

Bicipital Tendon Test. The patient flexes the forearm at the elbow with the elbow against his side. The examiner stabilizes the patient's elbow as the patient resists the examiner's efforts to extend the arm. The patient also resists external rotation of the flexed arm at the elbow. The test is positive if pain over the intertubercular groove develops or is aggravated. This is suggestive of bicipital tendinitis at the transverse humeral ligament.

Elbow. The examiner inspects, palpates, and measures range of motion of the elbow. The normal ranges are: flexion, 150 degrees; extension, 0 to 10 degrees; pronation, 80 degrees; and supination, 80 degrees. Weakness of grip in a twisting motion accompanied by a pain response on deep palpation is a positive sign for lateral epicondylitis.

Wrist and Hand. Since traumatic lesions and infections are the most common afflictions of the wrist and hand (Shands 1967) and can lead to disabling sequelae if not recognized and treated properly, the chiropractic examiner's chief interest is to differentiate local lesions from spinal referred pain.

The wrist and hand are inspected for deformities, palpated for swelling and hypertrophy of the connective tissue, and palpated for cre-

pitus. The range of motion of the wrist is: flexion, 90°; extension, 70°; ulnar deviation, 50°; radial deviation, 20°.

If flexion of the wrist produces paresthesia of the fingers (Phalen's sign) and if percussion of the volar surface of the wrist over the median nerve at the transcarpal ligament produces tingling into the fingers (Tinnel's sign) a carpal tunnel syndrome probably exists.

The hand is examined by asking the patient to actively flex and extend the fingers. This is followed by flexing the fingers against resistance.

Neurological Examination

The neurological examination and its related special sensory and performance tests are the most important parts of the premanipulation physical examination. A screening examination for sensory changes, motor changes, autonomic disturbances, mental, psychological, and cerebellar disturbances will help the chiropractic examiner determine whether or not a patient is a candidate for manipulative therapy.

Cranial Nerve Examination

The physiologic and anatomic implications of disturbed function of the cranial nerves is extremely important in the premanipulation clinical evaluation of the patient. The cranial nerves should be evaluated in the following manner.

1. Olfactory nerve (I). Using a familiar odor, such as menthol on a cotton ball, the patient, with eyes shut and one nostril held closed, is asked to identify the test substance. The test is repeated with the other nostril held closed.
2. Optic nerve (II):
   a. Visual acuity: Test each eye, one at a time with a Snellen eye chart.
   b. Fundus: Examine the fundi with an opthalmoscope. The normal disc is yellow-

ish-red, flat with clearly defined margins. If papilledema is present the optic disc is swollen, the margins are blurred, and the physiologic cup is not visible. The disc will be pink due to venous statis and engorgement secondary to increased intracranial pressure from a space occupying lesion or concussion. If papilledema is present, manipulative therapy is contraindicated and an emergency neurological referral is required.

c. Visual fields: The visual fields should be tested by confrontation.

d. Color blindness: The patient is asked to identify colored wool or the numbers in Ishihara plates.

3. Occulomotor, trochlear, and abducen nerves (III, IV, VI): The occulomotor, trochlear, and abducens nerves are checked when the patient is asked to follow an object or light with their eyes vertically, horizontally, and obliquely to the extremes. The following shorthand formula identifies the muscles with the direction of movement: $ER_6 (SO_4) 3$. External rotation is cranial nerve VI, superior oblique cranial nerve IV, and all other eye movements are supplied by cranial nerve III. The III nerve is also tested by looking for pupillary constriction when light is shined in the eye.

4. Trigeminal nerve (V):

a. A blink reflex or corneal stimulation is elicited by touching the cornea from the side with a strand of cotton while the patient is looking upward. The examiner should then stroke the patient's face with a camel hair brush in the opthalmic, maxillary, mandibular distributions of the trigeminal nerve testing for disturbances of sensation.

b. Motor function of the trigeminal nerve is tested by palpating the contraction of the masseter and temporalis muscles with the jaws clinched.

5. Facial nerve (VII): Muscles of the face are checked by asking the patient to smile and frown while observing the face for symmetrical movements.

6. Cochlear nerve (VIII):

a. Hearing acuity: The examiner can compare the acuity of hearing in each ear with a ticking watch. The examiner places a vibrating tuning fork on the vertex of the head and asks the patient if he senses the vibration equally in both ears. When unilateral hearing loss is due to middle ear disease, the patient reports louder vibration on the diseased side. When there is nerve deafness on one side the sound will be louder in the normal ear (Weber's test). Next the examiner should check bone conduction in both ears by using a vibrating tuning fork placed on the mastoid until the patient can no longer detect the vibration. The vibrating tuning fork is then held in front of the ear in this way testing air conduction. In a normal subject the patient should be able to detect vibration by air conduction after bone conduction ceases.

b. The caloric test for vestibular function is performed by irrigating ice water into the ear. Nystagmus shows that the vestibular portion of the VIIIth nerve is intact.

7. Glossopharyngeal nerve (IX): This is tested by the identification of taste over the posterior one-third of the tongue and the presence of a gag reflex on stimulation of the tonsillar pillars.

8. Vagus nerve (X): Hoarseness and loss of strength in coughing suggests paralytic involvement of the vagus nerve. The examiner should touch the posterior pharyngeal wall with a tongue depressor to elicit a gag reflex. The examiner should then palpate the larynx for muscle strength on deglutition.

9. Spinal accessory nerve (XI): The patient is asked to turn his head and shrug his shoulders, to test the strength of the sternocleidomastoid and trapezius muscles.

10. Hypoglossal nerve (XII): The patient is asked to stick out his tongue. The tongue should be in the mid-line. If it deviates laterally, the test is positive.

Muscle Testing. Muscular weakness is a cardinal sign of dysfunction in many parts of the nervous system. The ability of the patient to move a joint against gravity as well as against resistance should be observed and recorded. One method of quantification of muscle strength is based on an index of 0 to 5 (Van Allen 1969) where:

5	normal strength
4	full normal movements possible but strength of contraction can be overcome by examiner
3	normal range or movement against gravity but not against added resistance
2	movement when gravity does not act in opposition
1	flicker of movement only
0	no movement

Comparison of muscle functions will indicate whether the patient is improving or worsening.

Grip Test with Hand Dynamometer. Quantification of strength of grip is easily measured with a hand dynamometer such as the Jaymar or equivalent. Normally the dominant hand is stronger.

Deep Tendon Reflexes. Reflexes are inborn stimulus-response mechanisms involving a reflex arc which includes both a sensory and a motor neuron. The presence or absence of the reflex has localizing value in reference to peripheral pathways and to vertical cord levels. The loss of a reflex in a painful extremity may well mean that nerves or roots innervating the painful area are being compressed. Exaggeration of the deep tendon reflex is found in lesions involving the pyramidal track (upper motor neuron lesions) including diseases of the cord, brain stem, and the cerebral hemispheres.

The following system is used for estimating the degree of reflex muscular contraction (Van Allen 1969):

4+	very brisk response-evidence of disease and associated with clonus
3+	a brisk response, possibly indicative of disease
2+	a normal, average response
1+	a response in low normal range
0	no response and possible evidence of disease, depending on the circumstances. If a reflex response is elicited by reinforcement, then the arc is intact although possibly inhibited. The reinforcement may be recorded 1+ (R)

Reflex testing is done with the patient sitting. The examiner, using a reflex hammer taps the triceps tendon at the posterior aspect of the elbow. Next, the examiner locates the biceps tendon in the antecubital fossa with his thumb, then strikes the thumb with the reflex hammer. The distal radius is located at the wrist with the examiner's thumb and tapped in the same manner with the reflex hammer looking for contraction of the brachioradialis muscle. The patellar tendon is tapped while the patient is seated; the Achilles reflex is easily examined with the patient prone.

Deep-tendon reflexes on one side are always compared with the other side. A loss or a diminished reflex is seen in nerve root compression and other peripheral nerve lesions.

Deep-Sensory-Reflex Examination. The somatic sensory examination is the most difficult and least reliable part of the neurological investigation. Consistency of findings of several sensory examinations gives some assurance of their validity. The sensory examination is performed with a Wartenberg pinwheel or sharp instrument along the dermatomal patterns of the upper and lower extremities. Any area of sensory disturbance is noted.

Use of a vibrating tuning fork over bony prominences tests the integrity of the posterior columns of the cord. Diminished vibratory sense is found in posterior column diseases, peripheral neuropathies, and lesions of the midbrain and cerebrum.

Test for Cerebellar Function. Tandem walking is a much better test of balance and is more sensitive than Romberg's test (Van Allen

1969). The patient is asked to walk heel to toe down a line on the floor. Another coordination test is to have the patient close his eyes and alternately touch his nose with the index finger of each hand. Patients with disease of the cerebellum will have difficulty with these tests.

Heel Walk. Walking on the heels tests the strength of the tibialis anterior (L4, 5 nerve distribution). Weakness of the tibialis anterior may be produced by compression of the peroneal nerve, an L4–L5 radiculopathy or an upper motor neuron lesion such as a cerebral vascular accident. The major criteria of differentiation would be the increased reflexes and spasticity in the upper motor neuron lesion.

Toe walk. The patient is asked to walk on his tiptoes to test the strength of the calf muscles (L5, S1 distribution). Unilateral weakness may be indicative of nerve root compression.

Straight-Leg Raise (SLR). With the patient supine, the examiner grasps the foot with one hand and maintains the knee in a fully extended position with the other hand raising the leg slowly toward a 90-degree angle. During straight-leg raising the first 15 to 30 degrees of elevation cause no movement of the nerve roots at the foraminal level. When the leg has reached an angle of 30 degrees there is traction on the sciatic nerve followed by a downward movement of the roots in their foramina (Calliet 1968). It is important to record the range through which the leg must be raised before the pain is experienced. Reproduction or aggravation of the sciatic pain by a forced dorsiflexion of the ankle at the limit of straight-leg raising (Braggard's test) is highly suggestive of root tension and this impression is confirmed if the patient admits relief on bending of the knee (McNabb 1977). If the straight-leg raise is positive the examiner should lower the leg slightly and internally rotate the femur. If this maneuver reproduces the sciatic pain it is due to increased tension of the piriformis muscle on the sciatic nerve and is not a sign of root tension. This is a positive piriformis sign. A non-neurogenic pain may be elicited with tight ham-

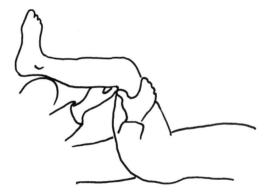

FIG. 12. **Bow string examination. Resting the semiflexed knee upon the examiner's shoulder and pressing on the sciatic nerve in the popliteal fossa. Tenderness will be elicited from the patient with nerve root compression. (After McNabb 1977)**

string muscles, a sacroiliac lesion, or hip joint pathology. When pain is exacerbated in the affected extremity by straight-leg raising of the opposite leg it is strongly suggestive of a disc herniation, usually lying medial to the root (Fajerstajn's well-leg raising sign).

Bowstring Sign. According to McNabb (1977) this is the most reliable test of root tension. In this test, straight-leg raising is carried out until pain is reproduced. At this level, the knee is slightly flexed until the pain abates. The examiner rests the limb on his shoulder and places his thumb in the popliteal fossa over the sciatic nerve. If sudden firm pressure on the nerve gives rise to pain in the back or down the leg (Fig. 12), the patient is almost certainly suffering from significant root tension.

Specific muscle tenderness has been considered a sign of root irritation. With first sacral root irritation the calf muscles may become tender to deep palpation. With fifth lumbar root irritation the anterior tibial muscles may be tender to palpation in addition to being weak on heel walking. With fourth lumbar root irritation the quadriceps may be tender to deep palpation.

Circumference Measurements. The examiner measures the circumference of the upper and lower extremities with a steel tape for the detection of muscle atrophy. The measurements are taken at the same comparative level: midpoint of the biceps, the largest circumference of the forearm, midthigh, and the greatest circumference of the calf.

Pathological Reflexes. While there are many pathological reflexes that can be tested, the single most important sign is dorsiflexion of the big toe when the bottom of the foot is stroked with a sharp instrument (Babinski's sign). This indicates dysfunction of the corticospinal system.

Lower Extremity Examination

The following regional orthopedic tests will allow for the determination of abnormal function:

Lumbosacral Spine, Sacroiliac, and Hips

Bilateral Leg Raise. Bilateral, active straight-leg raising in the supine position causes the pelvis to rotate posteriorly by the weight of the legs and thereby hyperextends the spine. Instability of the lumbosacral joint or disc thinning at L5, S1, may cause pain in this region.

Belt Test. With the use of a belt as a trochanteric cinch around the pelvis, the patient is instructed to bend forward (as an alternative the physician can stabilize the patient with his arms around the pelvis). If bending forward with support is more painful than without support, the problem is more likely to be a lumbosacral lesion. Conversely, if bending over with the support is less painful than without support, a sacroiliac lesion should be suspected (Shaffer 1977).

Gaenslen's Test. There are two ways to perform this test:

1. The supine patient flexes one knee and holds the flexed knee against his chest as the opposite leg is dropped over the side of the table, producing a hyperextension strain on the spine and torsion on the sacroiliac joint of the extended leg. With sacroiliac lesions, this maneuver is painful.

2. With the patient lying on his side the lower leg is flexed and held against the chest while the upper leg is extended and rotated posterior, thus applying a rotary strain. The maneuver is painful with a sacroiliac lesion.

Abduction Test of the Extended Leg. With the patient lying on his side the superior leg is abducted against resistance. When the gluteus medius contracts to abduct the hip, it pulls the ilium away from the sacrum. With sacroiliac joint lesions, abduction against resistance is painful (McNabb 1977).

Ely's Heel-to-Buttock Test. This is performed with the patient prone as the knee is flexed and approximated to the opposite buttock. Pain or restricted movement may come from contraction of the psoas muscle, contracture of the tensor fascia lata, or a sacroiliac or lumbosacral lesion.

Hibb's Test. With the patient prone the knee is flexed to a right angle and the ankle and foot are rotated laterally toward the floor, causing an inward rotation of the hip. A positive test indicates a sacroiliac lesion.

Patrick's FABER Test. With the patient supine, flex the knee and place the foot on the opposite knee and externally rotate the thigh. The hip joint is now flexed, abducted, and externally rotated. Limited range of motion or pain is indicative of hip joint pathology. This is an important test to differentiate hip joint pathology from a sacroiliac or lumbosacral lesion.

Tensor Fascia Lata Syndrome (Tensor Fascia Femoris Contracture). With the patient lying on his side the superior leg is passively abducted by the examiner. A normal tensor fascia lata will permit the leg to drop in adduction to the table.

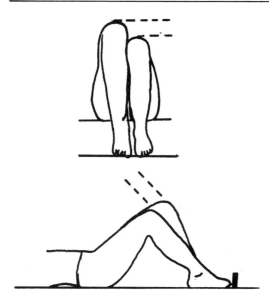

FIG. 13. **Allis sign. Disparity of the height of the knees in the anteroposterior plane is due to the shortness of the tibia. Disparity in leg length in the lateral view is due to a shortness of the femur or acetabular dysplasia. (From Hoppenfield 1976)**

Contracture of the tensor fascia lata will produce symptoms in the hip and thigh and the patient will hold the leg in abduction. This test helps to differentiate symptoms of nerve root compression, lumbosacral lesions, or hip joint pathology from a contracture of the tensor fascia lata.

Allis Test. With the patient supine, both knees are flexed to 90 degrees and the patient's feet are flat on the table. If one knee appears higher than the other the tibia of that extremity is longer. If one knee projects further anteriorly than the other, the femur of that extremity is longer (Fig. 13) (Hoppenfield 1976). This differentiates anatomical shortness of the femur from anatomical shortness of the tibia. Hip joint pathology may also cause an apparent shortness of the femur.

Trendelenberg Test. With the patient standing, one leg is raised to 90 degrees with the knee flexed at right angles. If the gluteus medius muscle is functioning properly, there will be an elevation of the hip on the side of the raised leg. If the pelvis on the unsupported side descends, the gluteus medius muscle on the supported side is either weak or nonfunctioning. This is a positive Trendelenberg sign. There are a number of conditions that weaken the gluteus medius muscle including coxa vera, slipped femoral capital epiphysis, poliomyelitis, and root lesions within the spinal canal.

Examination of the Knee

The knee is the largest joint in the body and is susceptible to traumatic injury and degenerative joint disease. The examiner should inspect and palpate the osseous and soft-tissue structures of the knee. In addition the examiner should grasp the patella and move it superiorly and inferiorly then laterally from side to side. Normally there is movement of the patella in all planes without crepitus.

The range of motion of the knee in flexion is measured and recorded with the normal being 135 degrees.

Genuvalgus or genuvarum may have an adverse effect on posture, particularly if one leg is more involved than the other. Medial knee pain in the absence of a local lesion of the knee is frequently referred from the hip (Lipe 1963).

To test the stability of the medial collateral ligament apply valgus stress to the open knee by applying force with one hand at the knee joint on the lateral side, with the other hand on the lower leg to counterbrace the valgus stress. Excessive motion is indicative of a sprain or tear of the medial collateral ligament.

To test for stability of the lateral collateral ligament, apply varus stress to the open knee joint. Abnormal motion may be due to a sprain or tear of this ligament.

Drawer Sign. With the patient supine, the knee flexed, the foot on the table and the patient stabilized with the knee of the examiner, the examiner grasps the leg below the knee and applies a push-pull motion of the lower leg on the femur. A positive anterior draw sign is indicative of a torn anterior cruciate ligament.

A positive posterior draw sign is indicative of a torn posterior cruciate ligament. Either condition requires immediate surgical consultation.

McMurray's Click Test. During knee flexion and extension, a torn meniscus may produce a palpable or audible "clicking" in the region of the joint line. With the patient supine and the legs flat in a neutral position, the examiner grasps the heel and flexes the leg fully. The examiner's free hand is then placed on the knee joint with the fingers touching the medial joint line and the thumb against the lateral joint line. Valgus stress is applied while rotating the leg externally and extending the leg. If this maneuver causes a palpable or audible "click" within the joint, there is a probable tear of the medial meniscus.

Ankle and Foot Examination. The ankle and foot provide the foundation for the musculoskeletal system and are the focal points to which total body weight is transmitted in ambulation. Because of this concentrated stress, the foot and ankle are involved in static deformities which may affect posture which, in turn, may cause spinal distress. The chiropractic examiner should evaluate the foot for pes planus, pes cavus, ankle pronation, hammer toes, and claw toes.

Palpation of the metatarsal arch will reveal tenderness over the metatarsal heads if there is an inferior disrelationship of one of the metatarsal heads. This may be attended by a tyloma as a result of a pressure point. A tyloma or a hemoloma durum may cause the patient to favor that foot, resulting in a limp which may cause a postural distortion eventually resulting in biomechanical stress of the back.

Conclusion

The purpose of the physical examination is to assess the patient's health problem and to arrive at a diagnosis. It is then determined whether the patient is a candidate for manipulative therapy or whether the patient's health prob-

lem could be best treated by a practitioner in another discipline.

Before any manipulative therapy is administered the chiropractor must conscientiously consider the reason why the patient is seeking his advice, why the patient is complaining of symptoms, and what reasonable course of manipulative therapy would benefit the patient.

REFERENCES

Arnold LE: Chiropractic Procedure Examination. Seminole, FL, Seminole Printing, 1978

Bateman JE: The Shoulder and Neck. Philadelphia, Saunders, 1972

Bates B: A Guide to Physical Examination. Philadelphia, Lippincott, 1974

Beckerstaff ER: Neurological Examination in Clinical Practice, 3rd ed. London, Blackwell, 1975

Brewis RAL: Lecture Notes on Respiratory Disease. London, Blackwell, 1975

Calliet R: Low Back Pain Syndrome, 2nd ed. Philadelphia, Davis, 1968

Chusid JG, McDonald JJ: Correlative Neuroanatomy and Functional Neurology, Los Altos, CA, Lange, 1964

Clark GR: Unequal leg length: an accurate method of detection and some clinical results. Rheumatol Phys Med 11:385, 1972

DeJarnette MB: Spinal Distortions. Nebraska City, 1935

DeJarnette MB: Sacro-Occipital Technique of Spinal Therapy. Nebraska City, 1940

DeJarnette MB: Unpublished notes, 1961

DeRusha JL: Personal correspondence

Dorland's Illustrated Medical Dictionary. 24th ed. Philadelphia, Saunders, 1965

Drum DC: Posterior gravity syndrome. Dig Chiropr Econ, May–June, 1968, p 36

Finneson BE: Low Back Pain, Philadelphia, Lippincott, 1973

Fisk JW, Baigent ML: Clinical and radiological assessment of leg length: N Z Med J 81:477, 1978

Gelb HG: Clinical Management of Head, Neck and TMJ Pain and Dysfunction. Philadelphia, Saunders, 1977

Giles LGF: Leg length inequalities associated with low back pain. J Can Chiropr Assoc, March 1966, p 25

Gillet H: The Anatomy and Physiology of Spinal Fixations. Brussels, 1963

Gray H: Anatomy of the Human Body, Philadelphia, Lea & Febiger, 1956

Grice AS: Harmony of joint and muscle function in the prevention of lower back syndrome. J Can Chiropr Assoc 1976

Hoppenfield S: Scoliosis, A Manual of Concept and Treatment. Philadelphia, Lippincott, 1967

Hoppenfield S: Physical Examination of the Spine and Extremities. New York, Appleton-Century-Crofts, 1976

Jackson RB: Atherosclerosis: Precursor to arterial insufficiencies and occlusive vascular disease processes. ACA J Chiropr 10:137, 1976

Janse J, Houser RH, Wells BF: Chiropractic Principles and Technique. 2nd ed. National College of Chiropractic, Lombard, IL, 1947

Johnston LC: The Theory and Practice of Postural Measurements, Toronto, Canadian Memorial Chiropractic College, 1961

Johnston WL: The role of static and motion palpation in structural diagnosis. In Goldstein M (ed): The Research Status of Spinal Manipulative Therapy. NINCDS, Monograph 15, U.S. DHEW, NIH, Bethesda, MD, 1975

Keim HA: Scoliosis. Clin Symp 24:18, 1972

Kendall HO, Kendall FP, Boynton DD: Posture and Pain. Baltimore, Williams & Williams, 1955

Lewit K: Meniere's Disease and the Cervical Spine. Rev Czech Med 7:129, 1961

Lewit K: Pain arising in the posterior arch of the atlas. Eur Neurol 16:263 1977

Lipe FM: Unpublished notes. Los Angeles College of Chiropractic, 1963–65

Lord JW Jr, Rosalie LM: Neurovascular Compression Syndromes of the Upper Extremity. Clin Symp 23, 2:3, 1971

MacBryde CM, Blacklow RS: Signs and Symptoms. 5th ed. Philadelphia, Lippincott, 1970

McNabb I: Backache. Baltimore, Williams & Wilkins, 1977

McRae RK: Clinical Orthopedic Examination. London, Churchill Livingston, 1976

Maigne R: Orthopedic Medicine. Springfield, IL, Charles C Thomas, 1972

Mennell JM: Back Pain. Boston, Little, Brown 1960

Michele AA: Iliopsoas. Springfield IL, Thomas, 1962

Mooney V, Douglas C, Robertson R: A system for evaluating and treating chronic back disability. West J Med 124:370, 1976

Pottinger FM: Symptoms of Visceral Disease. 3rd ed. St. Louis, Mosby, 1925

Prior JA, Silberstein JS: Physical Diagnosis. St. Louis, Mosby, 1959

Ragland DC: Postural blood pressure method of evaluating adrenal hypofunction. In Ragland DC (ed): Essays on Internal Secretions. Harrower, 1920

Raus R, Raus M: Manual of History Taking, Physical Examination and Record Keeping. Philadelphia, Lippincott, 1974

Schafer RC: Basic Chiropractic Procedural Manual. 2nd ed. Des Moines, American Chiropractic Association, 1977

Sewall H: Clinical Significance of Postural Changes in Blood Pressure and the Secondary Waves of Atrial Blood Pressure. Philadelphia, Lea & Febiger, 1919

Shands AR, Raney RB: Handbook of Orthopedic Surgery. St. Louis, Mosby, 1967

Stoddard A: Manual of Osteopathic Technique, London, Hutchinson, 1959

Stonebrink RD: Common Orthopedic Tests and Signs. Physician's General Reference, Portland, OR, Association of Chiropractic Physicians, 1967

Stonebrink RD: Palpation for vertebral motoricity. ACA J Chiropr 3:11, 1969

Thompson JC: Derefield-Thompson Leg Check. Davenport, IA, Palmer College of Chiropractic 1973

Van Allen MW: Pictoral Manual of Neurological Tests. Chicago, Year Book, 1969

Wiles P: Essentials of Orthopedics. 3rd ed. Boston, Little, Brown, 1959

Winterstein JR: The Short Leg Syndrome. Dig Chiropr Econ March–April 1974 p 78

Zohn DA, McM Mennel J: Diagnosis and Physical Treatment of Musculoskeletal Pain, Boston, Little, Brown, 1976

CHAPTER FOURTEEN
A Chiropractic Approach to Biomechanical Disorders of the Lumbar Spine and Pelvis
RONALD GITELMAN

A review of the clinical trials on the effectiveness of spinal manipulation on patients suffering from low-back pain (Tables 1 [page 298] and 2 [pages 300–5]) demonstrates the difficulties which face a clinician making a definitive diagnosis. A common problem in all of these studies is the failure to recognize the fact that a practitioner of spinal manipulative therapy must make two diagnoses rather than one. He must vary his therapeutic approach to the requirements of the individual patient rather than use a single uniform approach or technique in all patients with low-back pain.

The integrated approach must be to first diagnose the lesion or discrete locus of pathomechanical behavior with its local tissue responses. Secondly, an assessment of the spatial ecology or broader status of the statics and dynamics of the locomotor system of the patient must be made. Only after reaching these two decisions can the practitioner identify the syndrome which he will treat. He must, at the same time, be cognizant of the temporal factors involved in any disease process and look at a patient as being in the midst of an ongoing process. Developmental factors leading to a spinal lesion and the adaptive mechanisms which the body has adopted in response to the symptomatic lesion must all be considered in selecting an approach to treatment and rehabilitation.

While it is usually pain which motivates the patient to seek help, this pain should be considered the end result of a long process (except in the case of acute trauma). In order to understand the application or mode of action of spinal manipulation there must be an appreciation of the normal and abnormal dynamics of movement as well as the functional reflexes which may be disturbed. Many of these reflexes, under normal circumstances, enable the patient to adapt to internal and external environment stresses (Gitelman 1975).

In the discussion of the various techniques of adjusting, the following workable diagnostic methods of classification of low-back pain syndromes will be used.

1. *Pain Patterns*
   a. Low-back pain
   b. Low-back and leg pain
   c. Leg pain
2. *The Lesion*
   a. Sacroiliac syndrome
   b. Posterior facet syndrome
   c. Posterior facet and sacroiliac syndrome
   d. Intervertebral disc syndrome
   e. Lateral nerve root entrapment syndrome
   f. Central spinal stenosis
3. *Structural*
   a. The dynamic and static configurations of the spine and pelvis
   b. Major muscle length and strength
   c. Individual subluxation

TABLE 1. **Review of Literature on the Effectiveness of Manipulative Therapy in Low-Back Pain: Demographics**

Source	Male	Female	Total	Ages
Riches (1930)	28	47	75	37.5 avg
Henderson (1952)	314	186	500	30–50
Mensor (1955)	104	31	205	16–65 39.8 avg
Coyer and Curwen (1955)	84	52	136	30–59
Parsons and Cumming (1958)			2000	
Chrisman et al. (1964)	28	11	39	19–62 40 avg
	17	5	22	22–69 39 avg
Hutton (1967)			100	
Mathews and Yates (1969)			10	
Edwards (1969)			184	
Fisk (1971)			328	
Siehl et al. (1971)			47	
Warr et al. (1972)	273	227	500	15–75
Kane et al. (1974)			232	
Glover (1974)	73	11	84	16–64
Doran and Newell (1975)	245	211	456	20–50
Breen (1977)			1598	47 avg
Potter (1977)			528	
Evans (1977)			32	
Bergquist-Ullman and Larsson (1977)	189	28	217	17–64 34.5 avg
Heyse-Moore (1978)	71	49	120	17–72
Sims-Williams et al. (1978)	65	29	94	20–65

The pain pattern in a particular patient is established on the basis of the case history and may serve as part of the classification. The pain pattern may also serve to establish the significance of the lesion. In order to identify the active lesion it is important to understand the pathomechanical process leading to advanced spondylosis. A review of these processes is included in this chapter followed by a description of the significant examination findings which are used to establish not only the presence of a spinal lesion but also to give a better appreciation of the overall structural diagnosis. Each

syndrome associated with the various spinal lesions will be discussed. The specific manipulation techniques which are felt to be of greatest value in correcting these problems will be described.

The Sacroiliac Syndrome

The question of whether the sacroiliac joints move should be settled once and for all (Illi 1940; Weisl 1950; Colachis 1963; Coventry

1972; Fick 1911; Meyer 1878; Sashin 1930; Frigerio et al. 1974; Egund et al. 1978). The major question is, "How does it move?" The most logical hypothesis to explain sacroiliac motion is that proposed by Illi (1940). He states that the sacrum is the keystone of the pelvis and that the sacroiliac joint moves about three separate axes of motion: one in flexion, one in extension, and a third movement which occurs as the sacrum flexes and extends about a central axis at approximately the level of S2. Janse (1978) and Illi (1971) have expanded this concept by suggesting that a gyroscopic figure 8 type of motion takes place at the sacroiliac joint on one side during normal walking with a mirror action taking place at the opposite sacroiliac joint. The acceptance of this proposed mechanism of sacroiliac motion makes it much easier to understand and appreciate individual distortions of the pelvis, including the existence of an oblique axis of motion as described by Mitchell (1965).

Clinical Picture

Patients with sacroiliac syndrome often report a recent fall on the buttock, a twist, or a sprain. Hormonal changes which occur during pregnancy and produce relaxation of the pelvic ligaments may have an effect on the sacroiliac joint for up to 12 weeks after delivery (Hagen 1974; Cox 1972; Colachis et al. 1963). Therefore, recent pregnancy should be noted in taking the case history. The pain in sacroiliac syndrome is unilateral, dull in character, and located over the buttock. It may radiate to the groin, to the anterior thigh, or even down the leg, presenting a pain pattern similar to sciatica (Hacket 1956). A patient with this problem often complains of tenderness over the posterior superior iliac spine (PSIS) and may describe a sense of heaviness or fatigability of the lower limb on the involved side. The pain is aggravated by standing on the affected side, sitting and arising from a chair, twisting or going upstairs, and it is often present at night when the patient lies on his or her back or turns. The gait in these patients may show less deviation of the pelvis on the involved side and the stride is usually shorter on that side. On visual exam-

ination in front of the plumbline, torsion and laterality of the pelvis will usually be found. Inequality in the height of the PSIS, the anterior superior iliac spine (ASIS), and the iliac crests may be noted in front of the plumbline. Asymmetry of the gluteal crease may be present, and the contour of the buttock usually appears flatter on the side of the fixation (the side of limitation of normal movement of the sacroiliac joint). In lateral bending away from the involved side, the pelvic shift is usually limited, although not necessarily painful. Rotation to the side opposite the lesion is often painful. Forward flexion may be limited and disruption of the lumbopelvic rhythm may be seen with trunk deviation occurring to the side of the lesion.

Movement Palpation Tests for the Sacroiliac Joints

Specific techniques for motion palpation of the sacroiliac joint and pelvis have been developed by Gillet and Liekens (1969) and modified by the Department of Biomechanics and Kinesiology at the Canadian Memorial Chiropractic College under the direction of A.S. Grice (Fig. 1, p. 306).

Test No. 1. Place the index finger on the PSIS, on one side pushing up the skin slack. Place the thumb of the same hand on the sacral apex. Instruct the patient to forward flex. With normal lumbopelvic rhythm and functioning sacroiliac joints, separation of up to a half inch occurs between the thumb and index finger at the end of this movement. This test should be repeated on the other side. Normally, the extensors of the spine (multifidus and sacrospinalis muscles) relax in full flexion. Failure to do so may compromise movement of the sacroiliac joint. On the other hand, contraction of the gluteus maximus, the hamstring, or the lateral rotator muscles, especially the piriformis, may compromise the sacroiliac joint from below and prevent normal movement from occurring.

Test No. 2. Place the thumbs on the PSIS bilaterally and grip the ilia with the fingers. Instruct the patient to bend laterally to the right

TABLE 2. **Review of Literature on the Effectiveness of Manipulative Therapy in Low-Back Pain: Sample, Treatment, and Success**

Source	Sampling	Exclusions	Inclusions
Riches (1930)	Retrospective orthopedic hospital records	None	Chronic low-back traumatic strain
Henderson (1952)	Unselected orthopedic hospital patients	Evidence of lumbar root or neurologic involvement	Backache
Mensor (1955)	Unselected patients: 72 private, 133 industry	None	92.2% injured; 71% leg signs; 34% leg atrophy; 26% sensory disturbances; 6.8% motor weakness; 53% reflex change
Coyer and Curwen (1955)	Unselected orthopedic hospital patients	Pain referral past buttock; neurological signs	Low-back pain
Parsons and Cumming (1958)		Bilateral sciatica; coccydynia; sacral paresthesia; bowel/bladder signs; impotence	Low-back pain
Chrisman et al. (1964)	Private orthopedic patients Controls	None	Low-back pain with sciatic radiation
Hutton (1967)	Private practice 5 treated, 5 controls	None	Backache and/or sciatica
Mathews and Yates (1969)		Neurological signs	Low-back pain
Edwards (1969)	Selected, uncontrolled	Hip or sacroiliac pain; psychiatric disturbances	Neurological signs
Fisk (1971)	Retrospective, unselected, private practice	None	Low-back pain

Diagnosis	Treatment	Reassessed	Success (%) and Comments
1. Chronic strain 2. Sacroiliac strain 3. Lumbosacral strain 4. Arthritis only 5. Arthritis + sciatica 6. Neurotic spine	Bilateral, rotatory manipulations under anesthesia	Reexamination and questionnaire	1. 86.7% 2. 92.0% 3. 33.3% 4. 40.0% 5. 50.0% 6. 0%
Lumbar IVD protrusion	1. Bed rest 2. Plaster jacket 3. Lumbosacral support 4. Manipulation 5. Extension exercises	Period of 18+ months	1. 21.1% 2. 46.5% 3. 9.6% 4. 33.8% 5. 19.4%
Lumbar IVD syndrome	Bilateral, rotatory manipulations under anesthesia	6 months–10 years 22.8 month avg	64% private, 45% industry Higher % relief from manip. than from surgery with less permanent disability
Low-back pain	1. Manipulations (Cyriax 1950) 2. Rest, pillow, analgesics	1. 1 week 2. 6 weeks	1. 50% after manip. 2. 27% of controls 1. 88% after manip. 2. 72% of controls
Disc syndrome in 90% of cases	Manipulation in hyperextension, rotation, and distraction	Daily for a maximum of 4 manipulations	75% of simple backache (annular); 40% or less with nerve root irritation
Lumbar IVD syndrome	Modified Pitkin rotatory manipulations under anesthesia Conservative therapy alone (controls)	2–4 days, 6–8 weeks, 5–12 months, after 3 years	51%; myelograms showed no changes after manipulation but those without a defect did better
Lumbar disc syndrome	Manipulation		85% improved symptomatically
Lumbar disc prolapse with epidurography	Rotational manipulations (Cyriax 1965)		Manipulation relieved lumbago symptoms and repeat epidurography showed prolapses reduced in size
1. Central back 2. Buttock radiation 3. Posterior: thigh to knee 4. Posterior: leg or foot	a. Heat, massage, and exercises b. Maitland's manipulation and mobilization techniques	At each treatment	1a. 82.5% in 9.7 tr. 1b. 82.5% in 4.8 tr. 2a. 69.5% in 10.2 tr. 2b. 78.1% in 4.3 tr. 3a. 65.2% in 8.5 tr 3b. 95.7% in 6.2 tr. 4a. 51.7% in 13.3 tr. 4b. 78.5% in 6.4 tr.
Regional spinal disturbances	Manipulation	After 1 year	90%

(continued)

TABLE 2 *(continued)*

Source	Sampling	Exclusions	Inclusions
Siehl et al. (1971)	Randomized hospital in-patients	Malignancy; TB; osteoporosis; fracture/dislocation	Fibrillation potentials and EMG observed neuropathic motor units
Warr et al. (1972)	Selected hospital patients: unresponsive to conservative therapies	Cauda equina; sepsis; neurological disease; hemorrhagic diatheses	Low-back pain
Kane et al. (1974)	Retrospective: patients seeking chiropractic or medical care	None	Workmen's compensation
Glover (1974)	Randomized, controlled trial on individual patients	Bilateral pain and hyperesthesia, other treatment at same time, neurological signs	Back pain, skin hyperesthesia, tenderness and limited trunkal movements
Doran and Newell (1975)	Randomized, stratified—7 hospitals	Psychological disturbances; pregnancy, root pain, scoliosis, SLR below 30°, paresthesia, corset, bladder signs, neurological signs, OA hip, previous manipulations, osteoporosis, sacroilitis	Low-back pain
Breen (1977)	Retrospective, questionnaire records	None	Pain for longer than 3 months
Potter (1977)	Preselected referrals	None	Low-back pain
Evans (1977)	Blind assessment	Root compression, more than 3 weeks of pain, steroid therapy, chronic disease, psychological disturbances, spondylitis, polyarthritis	Root pain

Diagnosis	Treatment	Reassessed	Success (%) and Comments
Nerve root compression	1. Manipulation under anesthesia 2. Conservative (bed rest, leg traction, muscle relaxants) 3. Laminectomy and diskectomy	6 months, 12 months	1. 14% improved 43% unchanged 43% worse 2. 0% improved 71% unchanged 29% worse 3. 47% improved 42% unchanged 11% worse
Chronic lumbosciatic syndrome	Epidural injection plus rotation of the spine and bilateral sciatic nerve stretch	2 weeks, 6 months	63% relieved 7% surgical 30% failed
Claimable neck and back injuries	Unspecified		Chiropractor as effective as M.D. in patients' assessment of function and satisfaction
1. 1st attack 2. 2+ attacks 3. under 7 days 4. over 7 days	15 min. placebo (detuned SWD); placebo plus one rotational manipulation, side of pain up	15 min, 3 and 7 days, 1 month	Manipulation more effective within 15 min in group 3 only; 75% improved in all groups after 1 week; population size too small for number of group
Low-back pain	Manipulation, physiotherapy, corset, analgesics	3 weeks, 6 weeks, 3 months, 1 year	80/98 relieved in 1 week after manipulation 74/104 after physiotherapy 64/93 with corset 69/100 on analgesics After 6 weeks, all groups were equal; after 3 mo and 1 yr, no treatment superior
Low-back pain	Manipulations	After 7 visits	Within about 7 visits chiropractic achieved 43% success
1. acute no leg 2. acute + leg pain 3. Acute + neurolog. 4. chronic no leg 5. chronic + surgery 6. chronic + leg pain 7. chronic + leg + surg. 8. chronic + leg + neurol. 9. chronic + leg + neurol. + surg.	Manipulations	Over 1 year	1. 93.8% 2. 76.4% 3. 48.2% 4. 64.0% 5. 66.7% 6. 59.0% 7. 58.8% 8. 36.1% 9. 37.5%
Chronic low-back pain	Manipulation plus analgesics; analgesics only	1 week, 3 weeks, repeated in crossover	Manipulation and analgesics provided improved spinal flexion and decreased pain scores

(continued)

TABLE 2 (*continued*)

Source	Sampling	Exclusions	Inclusions
Bergquist-Ullman and Larsson (1977)	Randomized, stratified (psychologic and vocation), controlled: light industry & clerical	Chronic pain; rhizopathy; tumor; pregnancy; senile osteoporosis; back surgery; infection; spondylolisthesis; structural scoliosis; fractures; ankylosing spondylitis	Acute or subacute lumbosacral pain ± radiation to thigh; less than 3-months duration
Heyse-Moore (1978)	Retrospective, unselected	None	Mechanical low-back pain and sciatica
Sims-Williams et al. (1978)	Randomized, general practitioner referrals	Psychological disturbances, spinal surgery; pregnancy; bowel/bladder signs; inflammatory or other spinal disorders; muscle wasting; other medical contraindications and the physiotherapists' judgement that patient unlikely to benefit from mobilization	Sensory changes; lost reflexes; muscle weakness without wasting

Compiled by D.J. Brunarski.

and then to the left. Normally, the sacrum rotates within the two ilia with one ilium abducting and the other adducting simultaneously while the PSIS remain level.

When the PSIS on one side moves higher it suggests that either the lateral stabilizers of the spine (the quadratus lumborum and iliopsoas muscles) or the sacrospinalis and multifidus are preventing normal lumbar rotation. Alternately, the abductors of the hip (gluteus medius and minimus) and/or the tensor fascia lata muscles are hypertonic and preventing normal movement and in this way contributing to the sacroiliac fixation.

Test No. 3. The contact is the same as in Test No. 2. The patient is instructed to elevate the flexed knee as high as possible (Trendelen-

burg-like maneuver). Normally, the PSIS on the flexed-leg side moves lower than its mate. This indicates the ability of one ilium to rotate posterior relative to the other. When fixation is present, the whole pelvis tends to move as a unit.

Test No. 4. Place one thumb on the PSIS and the other thumb on the 2nd sacral tubercle. Instruct the patient to raise his/her leg as in Test No. 3. Normally the sacrum can be felt to move to the anterior and inferior while the ilium moves to the posterior and inferior. An excursion of 1/4 to 1/2 inch should be perceived. This tests the movement at the upper part of the sacroiliac joint. The test is repeated on the other side. If the sacroiliac joint is fixed, the sacrum and ilium will move as a unit. This is the most

Diagnosis	Treatment	Reassessed	Success (%) and Comments
Acute and subacute low-back pain	1. Back school (ergonomic advice) 2. Manual and combined physiotherapy 3. Placebo (low-intensity SWD)	10 days, 3 weeks, 6 weeks, 3 months, 6 months, 1 year	1. 20.5 days; 14.8 days pain 2. 26.5 days sick-leave; 15.8 days duration of pain 3. 26.5 days sick-leave; 28.7 days pain
Acute first episode less than 6 months; chronic more than 6 months and failed other treatments	Methylprednisolone injection; hyalase and cortisone acetate (H+CA); manipulation under anesthesia (MUA) and straight-leg stretch (SLS)	After 1 year	H+CA 63% Injection alone 60% MUA+SLS 50% Injection alone 67% Apparent worsening of acute cases with MSU+SLS Overall success with injection in 81–87% acute and 44% chronic
Nonspecific lumbar pain	Maitland style of mobilization and manipulation; and placebo (low-intensity microwave radiation)	1 month	Both groups were improved but more significantly in the treated group
		3 months	Most still improved but differences in groups near 0
		After 1 year	66% better in both groups but no significant difference between groups was observed

common sacroiliac fixation and is thought to be caused by any weight-bearing muscular imbalance.

Test No. 5. One thumb is placed on the ischium as close to the inferior aspect of the joint as possible while the thumb of the other hand is placed on the sacral apex. The patient is instructed to elevate his or her knee as in tests No. 3 and No. 4. Normally, an excursion of 1/4 to 1/2 inch should be perceived with the ischial contact moving anterior, superior, and laterally. If the sacral apex and ischium move together, the lower aspect of the sacroiliac joint is fixated. This is usually seen in so-called "extension subluxations" and often appears in combination with flexion subluxations or fixation of the upper sacroiliac joint on the opposite side. The most common muscles involved in this fixation

are iliopsoas, piriformis, and gluteus medius and maximus. This fixation is commonly seen in conjunction with the piriformis syndrome (Maxwell 1978; Yeoman 1928; Robinson 1947; Edwards 1962; Janse 1947).

Further evaluation of the sacroiliac joint can be carried out in the prone position where the difference in the height of the iliac crests is noted. The depth and tenderness of the sacral sulcus and any fullness or tenderness of the inferior angle can be determined in this position. Springing the sacroiliac joint obliquely and rocking the apex of the sacrum may be painful. Heel to buttock testing and internal and external rotation of the hip will often not be equal on the two sides. In the sitting position, the difference between the two PSIS should decrease approximately 1/4 inch (Gillet 1969; Mennell

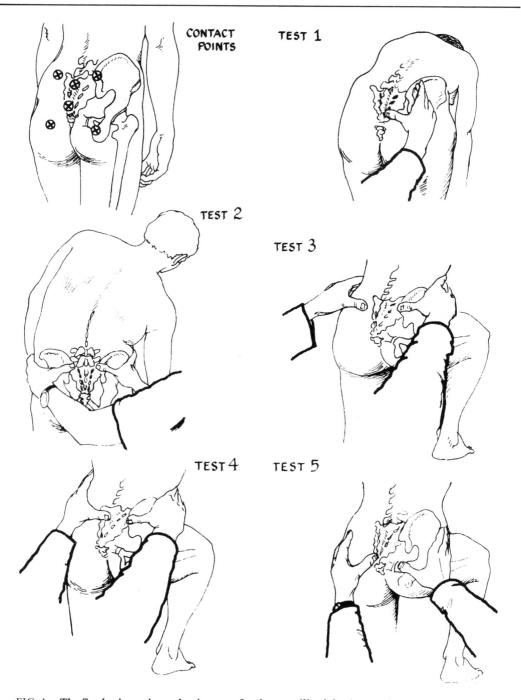

FIG. 1. The five basic motion palpation tests for the sacroiliac joint (see text).

1960). Failure to do so indicates fixation at the sacroiliac joint. As the patient sits, the height of the iliac crests and the configuration of the lumbar curve should be noted. If the curvature decreases, a leg deficiency or psoas spasm should be suspected.

In the supine position a sacroiliac fixation will often cause inequality in the height of the iliac crests and ASIS and perhaps even of the pubic ramus. In the case of a sacroiliac joint which is fixated in flexion, the pubic ramus will often palpate superior on that side. Classically the leg appears short on the same side. Tenderness of the tensor fascia lata may be present on the opposite side as can tenderness at the anterior acetabular region and the insertion of the hip adductor muscles. This may result in limited range of movement during Patrick's FABER test. Straight-leg raising is often limited in sacroiliac fixations but to a much lesser degree than in nerve root syndromes. With fixation of the sacroiliac joint, the straightened leg can be coaxed up higher, whereas in the root syndromes it is impossible to elevate the leg beyond the point of pain. During straight-leg raising it is important to note any flexion of the opposite leg. This is a positive Thomas test and indicates increased tonicity of either the iliopsoas and/or the rectus femoris muscle. Bragard's sign and the Bowstring sign are both negative in sacroiliac fixations. The Goldthwaite test allows one to evaluate movement at both the sacroiliac and lumbosacral joints in the non-weight-bearing position. In addition, by carrying the knee across to the opposite shoulder, it is possible to determine the relative length of the gluteus maximus which often shows hypertonicity during sacroiliac fixation. The contralateral sign in straight-leg raising is not usually present. However, in acute sacroiliac syndromes the transference of torsion stresses across one sacroiliac joint to the other on straight-leg raising may, on occasion, result in pain on the opposite side.

Inequality of internal and external rotation of the hip when tested at 90° flexion with the knee flexed to 90° is usually present in lesions of the sacroiliac joint. This test, along with the comparison of internal and external rotation of the hip during the prone examination, allows for further differentiation between the various muscle hypertonicities at the hip joint. To complete the picture, adduction and abduction movement must be assessed. If inequality is noted in any of these movements, the individual groups of muscles must be tested for both length and strength. The tendon reflexes are usually intact in sacroiliac fixations. However, a slightly diminished Achilles reflex has, on occasion, been noted on the side of the lesion. Sacroiliac separation and compression tests are usually not painful except in severe cases of sacroiliac sprain, ankylosing spondylitis, spondylitis associated with psoriasis, Reiter's syndrome, or infectious arthritis. At the conclusion of this examination the biomechanical relationships of the pelvis should be clearly appreciated. The muscles which surround the sacroiliac joint, none of which are intrinsic to it, should have been assessed and the major muscular components of the sacroiliac fixation should be evident.

Sacroiliac fixation combinations are fairly common. These include bilateral upper-joint fixation in the presence of increased lumbar lordosis and anterior tipping of the sacrum. Upper joint fixations on one side with lower joint fixations on the other side can occur when there is fixation on the oblique axis of motion of the sacrum. This is often seen in the presence of a leg deficiency. In the presence of complete fixation of one sacroiliac joint where both the upper and lower aspect of the joint are fixed, hypermotoricity of the opposite sacroiliac joint can occur. The side of hypermotoricity may be the symptomatic side. Therefore the choice of which sacroiliac to manipulate should be based on the palpation findings rather than on symptoms. The spine and pelvis should be viewed as a single organ rather than as a group of individual segments. For example, the sacrospinalis muscle may react to distortional factors in the dorsal spine or even higher. This may compromise movement at the sacroiliac joint and in this way make the manipulation of choice one which is directed at the dorsal spine.

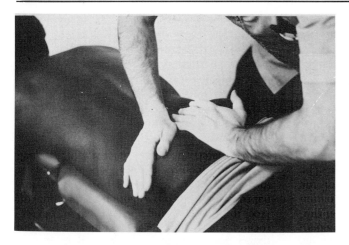

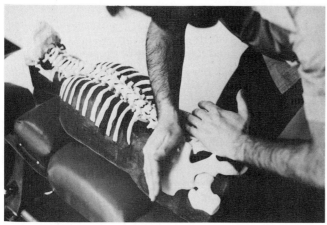

FIG. 2. **(Top) A technique for mobilizing an upper joint or flexion fixation of the sacroiliac joint. (Bottom) Illustration of the contact points for this mobilization technique on a skeleton model.**

Mobilization Techniques

Mobilization of a typical upper joint or flexion fixation (demonstrated most dramatically in Test No. 4) may be accomplished in the prone position. Contact is taken at the superior aspect of the PSIS and the force is directed laterally and caudally. The other hand is used to take contact on the inferior aspect of the sacrum on the same side with its force directed rostrally and anteriorly (Fig. 2). A springing action is used to produce a shearing stress between the two osseous contacts. If desired, a shallow thrust may be delivered equally with each hand. Increased leverage may be gained by utilizing the so-called "Dutchman's roll" or pelvic wedges

(DeJarnette 1966; Gravel 1966). If more force is required, the lower limb may be used in extension as a long lever in the prone or side posture position. Care must be taken when using the last two techniques as they both produce hyperextension of the lumbar spine.

Mobilizing techniques (Fig. 3) can be utilized in a similar manner for lower joint or extension fixations (demonstrated most dramatically in Test No. 5). Stoddard (1959) has described a leg tug method of sacroiliac mobilization where the leg on the side of flexion is tractioned at an angle of approximately 45° (short-leg side) and the leg on the side of extension (long-leg side) is tractioned at approximately 10° (Fig. 4). These maneuvers are carried out separately. An-

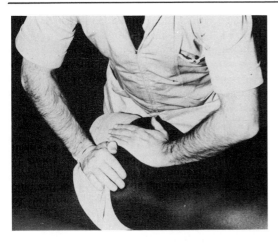
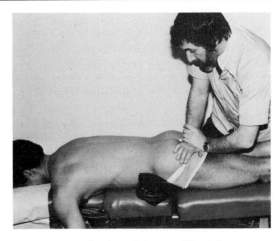

FIG. 3. **Two techniques for mobilizing a lower joint or extension fixation of the sacroiliac joint.**

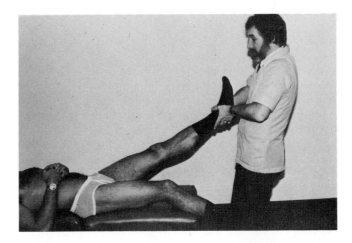

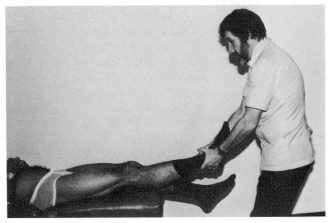

FIG. 4. **The leg tug method of sacroiliac joint mobilization. (Top) The leg on the side of sacroiliac flexion is tractioned at 45°. (Bottom) The leg on the side of the sacroiliac extension is tractioned at 10°.**

other mobilizing maneuver (Fig. 5) is carried out by elevating the knee on the flexed side toward the chest and externally rotating the hip while straightening the leg (Fig. 5A). This should be done on the side of the short leg. To compliment this maneuver the muscles of the hip on the long-leg side may be passively stretched by internally rotating the femur on the side of thigh flexion as the leg is extended (Fig. 5B). Passive mobilization can also be achieved by utilizing the block techniques as described by DeJarnette. Gillet has demonstrated a mobilizing technique which can be utilized in the sitting position (Fig. 6). Figure 7 illustrates some of the many alternate techniques for mobilizing the sacroiliac joint.

Adjustment Techniques for the Sacroiliac Joint

Perhaps the most frequently used and, in most cases, the manipulation of choice for the typical upper joint or flexion fixation is performed in a side posture position with the fixed innominate upward (Fig. 8). The patient is asked to hold the side of the table with the superior hand. The lower arm is tractioned beneath the patient in a rostal direction toward the clinician. This prevents undue lumbar torsion. The patient is then asked to release his hold on the side of the table. The patient's inferior leg is flexed slightly to bring the lumbar lordosis to a neutral position. The patient's superior leg is flexed to approximately 75° and the foot placed comfortably in the popliteal space of the inferior leg. The pelvis should now be perpendicular to the table. The contacts made by the clinician are on the deltoid with one hand and on the superior aspect of the PSIS with a pisiform eminence of the other hand. Traction is applied to the leg through the thigh, and a rostral force is exerted on the deltoid. As the patient relaxes by taking a deep breath and exhaling, traction is taken up. Two or three breaths can be utilized and increased traction applied with each breath until the limit of the paraphysiological range of motion of the joint is reached. A shallow impulse is then delivered in

the direction of the superior femur through the inferior contact hand, while the upper hand stabilizes the trunk of the body. It should not be necessary to place the weight of the clinician on the femur as this may introduce an unnecessarily traumatic force to the hip.

Manipulation of a flexion fixation of the sacroiliac joint where the sacrum has moved inferiorly can be achieved by taking a contact on the inferior aspect of the sacrum with the pisiform (Fig. 9). The corrective thrust is given in a straight rostral direction along the long axis of the body (see Fig. 9A). The same sacral contact can be used with the fixed sacroiliac side down. This may be necessary in the presence of a lesion in either the lumbar spine or hip which may make this position more desirable (see Fig. 9B). When an upper joint fixation is on one side and a lower joint fixation on the other, the upper joint fixation should be placed superior and a contact taken on the inferior angle of the sacrum. The thrust is delivered in an arching motion, rostrally and laterally as if to come over the buttock (Fig. 9C).

The manipulation of choice for a lower joint or extension fixation is accomplished by placing the fixated sacroiliac joint up and preparing the patient in a way similar to that described for an upper joint fixation. In this situation, however, the upper leg is flexed past 90° in order to take advantage of the force applied to the pelvis by the hamstring muscles (see Fig. 10A). The slack is taken up by moving the clinician's leg against the superior leg of the patient during exhalation. The contact hands are placed on the ischial tuberosity and the deltoid. The adjustive thrust is directed toward the midpoint between the patient's lower shoulder and chin. The extension fixation may also be adjusted by taking a direct contact on the posterior sacrum and using a thrust directed perpendicular to the sacroiliac joint toward the clinician (Fig. 10B). Alternately, a closed fist contact may be used in an attempt to draw the sacrum inferiorly. Following a successful manipulation of the pelvis, reexamination of the patient should reveal an immediate change in the movement palpation tests.

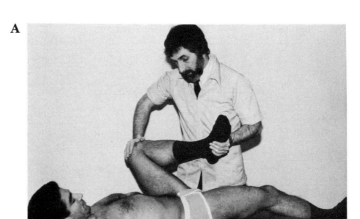

A

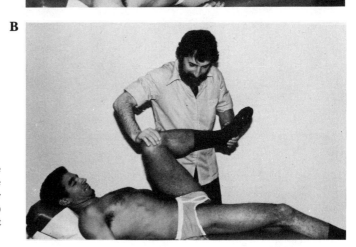

B

FIG. 5. Mobilizing techniques for the sacroiliac joint with the hip and knee flexed (see text). (A) Technique for upper sacroiliac joint mobilization. (B) Technique for lower sacroiliac joint mobilization.

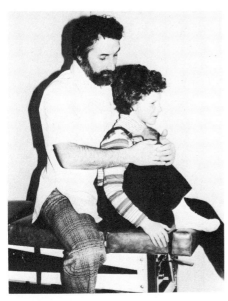

FIG. 6. A technique for mobilizing the sacroiliac joint in the sitting position.

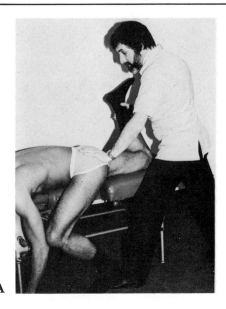

A

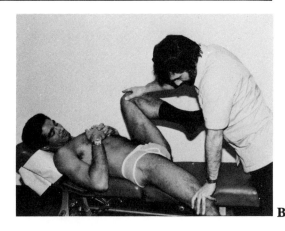

B

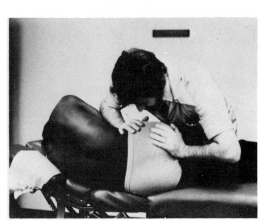

C

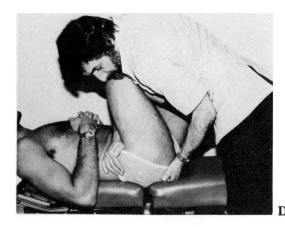

D

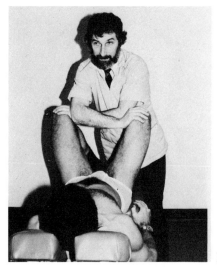

E

FIG. 7. Alternate techniques for sacroiliac joint mobilization. (A) Technique in prone position for right upper joint and left lower joint mobilization. (B) Technique in supine position for right upper joint and left lower joint mobilization. (C) Technique in side posture position for right lower joint mobilization. (D) Technique in supine position for right lower joint mobilization. (E) Technique in supine position using resisted bilateral adduction with repeated effort and increasing resistance.

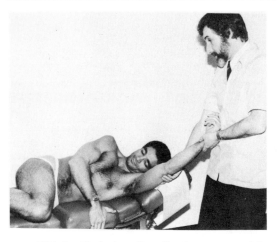
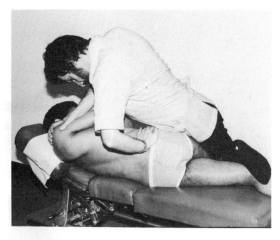

FIG. 8. Technique for adjusting an upper joint or flexion fixation of the sacroiliac joint. (Left) In preparation for this adjustment the inferior arm is tractioned beneath the patient who grips the side of the table with his superior hand. (Right) The adjustive thrust is given in the direction of the superior flexed femur of the patient.

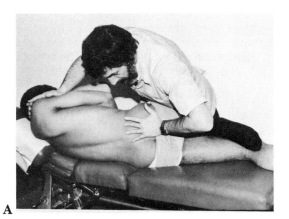
A

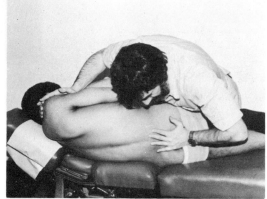
B

FIG. 9. Alternate contact points and direction of thrust for adjusting the various sacroiliac fixations. (A) Contact on the inferior aspect of the sacrum with thrust along the axis of the body for an upper joint fixation of the sacroiliac joint. (B) The same contact point and direction of thrust as in (A), but with the fixed sacroiliac joint (left) placed inferior. (C) Technique for adjusting a combination right upper sacroiliac fixation and left lower sacroiliac fixation. An arching motion is used during the thrust.

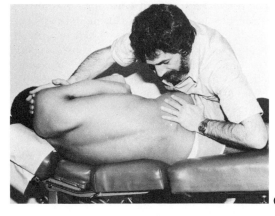
C

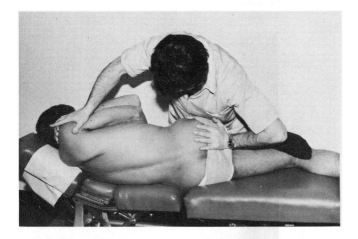

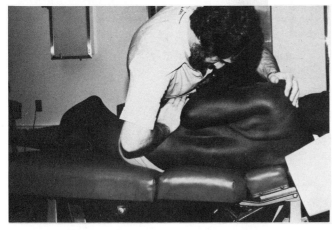

FIG. 10. **Techniques for adjusting a lower joint or extension fixation of the sacroiliac joint. (Top) The contact point is taken on the ischium and the thrust directed at a point between the patient's lower shoulder and chin. (Bottom) The contact point is taken on the posterior aspect of the sacrum and the thrust directed perpendicular to the sacroiliac joint.**

Facet Syndrome

The original term "facet syndrome" was introduced into the literature by Gormley (1933) one year before Mixter and Barr (1934) described the pathology of nucleus pulposis protrusion. These two lesions, however, do not represent separate chapters in the degenerative process of the lumbar spine. Farfan (1973) introduced the concept of the three joint complex and showed that torsional strains affect both the facet and the disc which are intimately related. One of the major causes of torsional strain is pelvic disrelationship. These strains are transferred to the lumbar spine by the muscles (sacrospinalis, multifidus, the abdominal muscles, and lumbodor-

sal facia) and by the lumbosacral disc and the iliolumbar ligaments which are placed under stress during movement of the ilia. Farfan (1978) has indicated that there are two major types of skeletal configurations important in disc degeneration. The first, thought to be important in L4-L5 disc degeneration, includes a high intercrestal line (the line drawn from the superior margin of one iliac crest to the superior margin of the opposite crest) which passes through the upper half of L4 and is commonly associated with a long transverse process on L5. In the second type, which may be of importance in L5-S1 degeneration, the intercrestal line passes through the body of L5 and is associated with short transverse processes on L5. This results in greater lumbosacral instability. It is therefore important that the static skeletal configuration be assessed in combination with dynamic factors such as sacroiliac fixation in order to more fully explain the dynamic stresses that may predispose to degenerative changes at the level of the L4-5 or L5-S1 joints (Vernon and Gitelman 1979). Biomechanical disturbances that result from sacroiliac fixation during locomotion could conceivably lead to hypertonicity or weakness of the lateral stabilizing muscles of the spine or even the oblique abdominal muscles and thereby leave the lumbar motion segments more vulnerable to torsional strain (Grice, 1976; Illi 1951).

The normal dynamic action of the spine during movement has been studied in some depth and the ranges, patterns, and axes of motion have been established (Allbrook 1957; Tanz 1953; Lysell 1971; Farfan 1973; Higley 1964; Sandoz 1965). Abnormal spinal movement has also been studied and a correlation between spinal lesions (including degenerative states) and disturbances of spinal movement has been postulated (Higley 1964; Gianturco 1944; Abel 1960; Knutsson 1944; Mensor et al. 1957, 1959; Sandoz 1965, 1971; Pennel 1972; Hasner 1957). Clinical observations have led to the suggestion that certain patterns of movement may be correlated with normal and abnormal muscle activity as well as ligamentous and discal change (Sandoz 1971; Hasner 1957; Gillet 1979; Grice 1976; Cassidy 1976; Hviid 1971; Stoddard 1959). The earliest and most reversible changes appear to take place in muscle (Illi 1951; Grice 1975; England 1972; Maigne 1972; Stoddard 1969; Denslow 1941).

Classification of Spinal Motion

Loss of motion in a vertebral segment has been classified according to a number of types of aberrant movement which can be observed on dynamic lateral flexion x-rays of the spine (Cassidy 1975; Grice 1979; Bonyon 1967; Watkins 1964). Cassidy (1976) and Grice (1979) have typed these aberrant motions and hypothetically correlated them to specific muscle and articular components. These aberrant move-

ments appear to be the earliest detectable x-ray change which can be seen in the process of lumbar spondylosis. These aberrant motions not only contribute to the production of the facet syndrome but also play a contributing role in the progressive degeneration of the lumbar spine.

X-ray studies on spinal motion are best carried out in the seated position (the same position in which movement palpation is conducted). The lumbar spine should be slightly flexed in order to flatten the lumbar lordosis. This diminishes the effect of the long postural muscles and accentuates the biomechanical effect of the smaller segmental muscles. Spinal movement is dependent upon normal coordination, tonicity, strength, and length relationships of the paraspinal muscles. During lateral bending the quadratus lumborum functions as the prime mover. Synergistic activity is provided by the sacrospinalis and iliopsoas as well as the small segmental muscles, multifidus, and intertransversarri. Since the axis of motion is near the posterior one-third of the lumbar disc (Farfan 1973) and the quadratus lumborum inserts posterior to that axis, the lumbar vertebral bodies rotate to the convexity of the curve formed during lateral bending. The spinous processes therefore appear to move toward the concavity and the wedging of the intervertebral disc has its apex on the side of the concavity. This is classified as type 1 movement and represents the normal mechanical action of the lumbar spine (Fig. 11A).

Type 2 movement occurs when the spinous process fails to rotate toward the concavity and may even rotate toward the convexity. Intervertebral disc wedging is, however, still toward the concavity (Fig. 11B). This type of movement is thought to result from hypertonicity of the multifidus, sacrospinalis, or psoas muscles or from weakness of the quadratus lumborum.

Type 3 motion shows normal spinous rotation toward the concavity but reversal or lack of normal disc wedging toward the concavity (Fig. 11C). Over activity of the quadratus lumborum, increased tension on the iliolumbar ligaments, hypertonicity of the intertransversarri, and internal derangement of the disc are a few of the postulated causes of this type of motion.

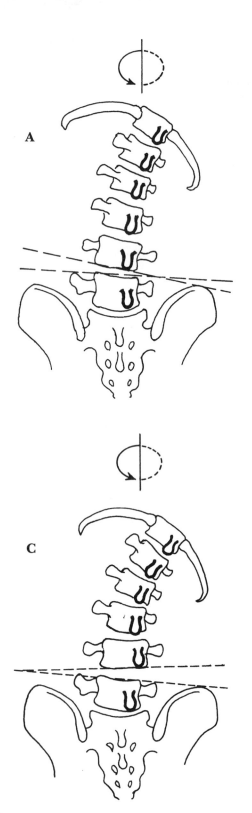

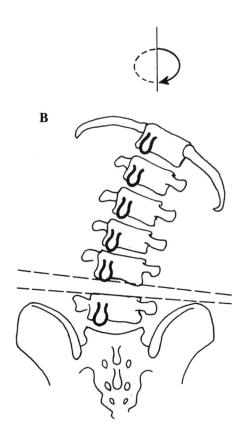

FIG. 11. The four types of lumbar spine motion as determined by lateral flexion x-rays in the sitting position. (A) Type 1 motion where the spinous processes move to the side of concavity and the intervertebral disc wedges to the side of concavity. (B) Type 2 motion where the spinous processes move to the side of convexity and the intervertebral disc wedges to the side of concavity. (C) Type 3 motion where the spinous processes move to the side of concavity and the intervertebral disc wedges to the side of convexity.

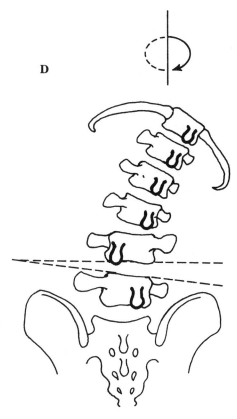

D

FIG. 11 (cont.). **(D) Type 4 motion where the spinous processes move to the side of convexity and the intervertebral disc wedges to the side of convexity.**

Type 4 motion occurs when the spinous process moves to the convexity in conjunction with intervertebral disc wedging toward the convexity (Fig. 11D). In this situation the multifidus or psoas muscles are thought to replace the quadratus as the prime mover of the lumbar spine. This type of motion is often seen in the presence of disc pathology.

Movement Palpation of the Lumbar Spine

Movement palpation techniques developed by Gillet and Liekens (1969) and advanced by Grice may be used to evaluate the spine in a manner similar to lateral bending x-rays.

With the patient seated in a relaxed posture

and the lumbar spine in slight kyphosis, the palpator places the flexed index finger supported by the thumb on the interspinous space. By rhythmically rocking the patient's upper body into flexion and extension over the forward moving interspinous contact (Fig. 12A,B) a smooth opening and closing of the interspinous spaces should normally be perceived. If movement cannot be felt, the same procedure can be performed laterally over the facets to determine if one or both sides are involved in the fixation complex. In order to test lateral bending of the lumbar spine, the patient is placed in the same position and the palpator hooks the lower spinous process with his middle finger and pushes the upper spinous process with his index finger or thumb. The patient then laterally flexes in the direction that the fingers are pointing (Fig. 12C). This movement should be passively assisted by the palpator with his/her free hand on the patient's shoulder. Normally, movement of the upper spinous over the lower spinous can be felt in the direction of the concavity. Absence of this movement is indicative of a lateral bending fixation of the superior segment. The test for rotation is done with the patient seated and his or her hands placed on the opposite shoulders. The palpator places his thumb alongside the spinous process of the motion segment to be palpated (Fig. 12D). With his other hand the palpator guides the patient's trunk into rotation by contacting the patient's elbow. Once again movement should be perceived with the superior spinous process rotating ahead of the inferior spinous process. Failure to perceive this steppage movement or the perception of a reversed movement at this segment would indicate a rotational fixation.

Mennell (1964) introduced the concept of joint play which he considers to be independent of voluntary muscle activity. Although Mennell's original tests were for peripheral joint movement, his method can be utilized when examining the spinal motion segments (Liekens 1969). Loss of joint play in the facets may compromise their function. In order to examine the joint play of facets the spinal segment is placed at the limit of the active range of movement and then slightly stressed. In flexion, extension, and

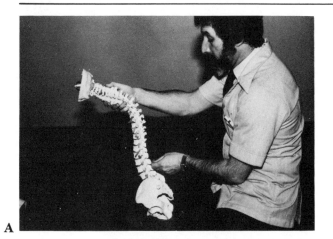

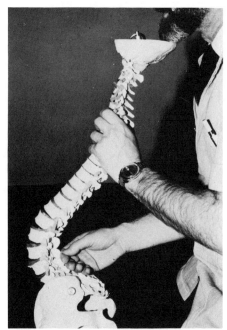

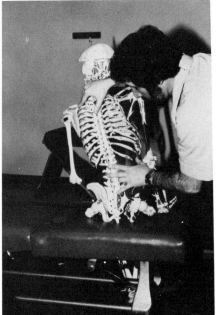

A

B

C

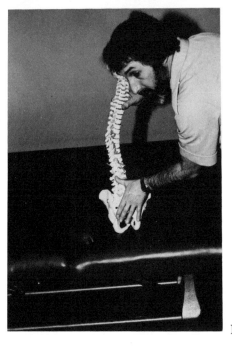

FIG. 12. **Palpation techniques for determining motion in the lumbar spine. Skeleton is used to illustrate the contact points: (A) flexion motion; (B) extension motion; (C) lateral bending motion; (D) rotation motion.**

D

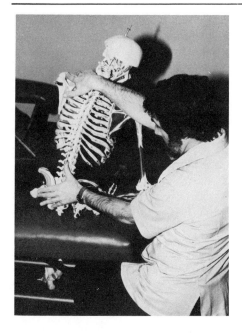
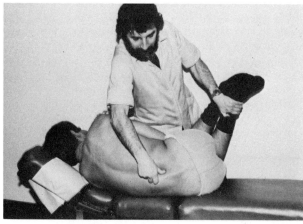

FIG. 13. **Palpatation techniques for determining lateral joint play in the lumbar spine in the sitting position (left) and in the side posture position (right).**

rotation it is convenient to simply exaggerate the movement palpation tests already described. However, in lateral bending, the patient should be laterally flexed toward the examining thumb which is placed on the lateral aspect of the spinous process to be tested (Fig. 13A). Lateral joint play may also be tested in the side posture position (Fig. 13B). In each case additional pressure is applied at the point of contact. A springy endfeel should be perceived by the palpator. If a hard endfeel is perceived, fixation of the ipsilateral facet in the presence of sacrospinalis hypertonicity should be suspected. A similar hard endfeel is present with fixation of the contralateral facet due to hypertonicity of the segmental muscles. This technique of motion palpation is especially useful in the presence of advanced spondylosis where chronic muscle contractures and structural change of the articulations have occurred.

The Clinical Picture of a Facet Syndrome

Asymmetric stresses to the posterior joints may produce synovial irritation and swelling and in this way be a cause of low-back pain. Degenera-

tive changes in the joint consist of loss of condroitin sulphate, fibrillation of the facet cartilage, and irregularity of the joint surfaces. As the degenerative process continues, further breakdown of the cartilage can result in loose body formation, synovial hypertrophy, and capsular laxity. This, in turn, may cause instability of the joint and osteophytosis. At this stage, recurrent low-back pain can be initiated by very minor stress to the lumbar spine and in this way produce the facet syndrome. The clinical picture commonly seen in the facet syndrome consists of low-back pain and/or leg pain. The pain follows a scleratogenous pattern rather than a dermatomal pattern (Kellgren 1938, 1939, 1972; Inman 1944; Feinstein 1977). In the early stages of the process the patient may show a direct straightline antalgic posture (laterally bending toward the side of pain). Movement of the trunk on lateral bending and rotation to the opposite side as well as extension are painful and limited. Extension tends to increase the lateral deviation of the pelvis. In forward flexion the patient usually deviates toward the side of pain but lateral deviation of the pelvis may decrease. The type 2 fixation, previously described as failure of the spinous process to deviate to the concavity on lateral bending, is often present in the initial stages of the facet syndrome. Therefore, movement palpation should indicate fixation of the involved segment on lateral bending and rotation as well as flexion. If the patient assumes an indirect antalgic position (the patient leaning away from the side of pain) then lateral bending and rotation to the painful side will be painful and limited. This is often seen in the presence of a type 3 fixation. Straight-leg raising may be limited to approximately 45 to 60° due to reflex spasm of the hamstring muscles. The deep tendon reflexes may even be diminished. The latter observation has been postulated to occur through inhibition of the anterior horn cells by noxious stimuli arising from the irritated facets (Mooney and Robertson 1976). The Bowstring test is negative and Bragard's sign is absent in the facet syndrome. Limited straight-leg raising and diminished tendon reflexes have been demonstrated clinically on a group of 100 patients by Mooney and Robertson (1976) using facet injections. They showed that one-third of these patients had a dramatic return of normal straight-leg raising and the reinstitution of tendon reflexes almost immediately after steroid injection into the offending facet.

It is common to find contraction of the psoas muscle on the side of the painful lesion in the acute initial episodes of facet pain. This is accompanied by a characteristic limitation of rotation of the hip and a positive Thomas test. Fixation of the thoracolumbar junction is also common in facet syndrome. Palpation of the psoas muscle through the abdomen should reveal fullness and tenderness when the thigh is flexed. The psoas contraction is often associated with contraction of the piriformis muscle and fixation of the lower sacroiliac joint. The presence of these muscle syndromes, which are commonly associated with the facet syndrome, should be suspected when the pain radiates to the anterior thigh and there is tenderness over the anterior acetabulum. This could be considered a pseudocoxalgia. Hyperesthesia and tenderness of the paraspinal musculature and the skin on the side of the lesion may be present (Glover 1960). Springing

of the individual facets is often painful at the level of involvement. In more chronic cases, skin rolling may cause exquisite pain and trophic changes of the skin have been noted (Gunn 1978). The selection of a manipulative procedure should be determined from the clinical picture and motion palpation findings. The major muscles involved in the limitation of motion at a particular spinal segment must be determined. Segmental problems revealed by lack of motion at one or two levels are commonly associated with contraction of the multifidus and/or intertransversarri muscles. It should be remembered that multifidus contraction on one side causes an approximation of the facets on that side. This can bring about a cantilever effect producing hypermotoricity of the opposite facet. If additional torsion strain is placed on this motion segment it is the hypermobile facet which will receive most of the insult and become painful. If a number of segments are involved, the major muscular components of the fixation usually include the quadratus lumborum, sacrospinalis, or psoas. The selection of the adjustment should be influenced by the muscle involved. The technique that places the involved muscle under passive stretch and at the same time gaps the offending facet and restores the compromised movements is the technique of choice. The selection of the technique of choice is also dependent on the direction of pain-free movement, bony anomalies, and facet facings.

Adjustment Techniques for the Lumbar Spine

All adjustive procedures require the proper positioning of the patient, a specific contact on the spine, and the removal of joint slack to the point where a controlled dynamic impulse can accomplish a specific movement of an articulation. The correction of a type 4 L4-L5 fixation determined by movement palpation will serve as an example of how this is accomplished. In this situation the vertebral body has rotated to the right and a multifidus muscle contraction exists on the left. There is failure of the disc to form a wedge on the right side on lateral bend-

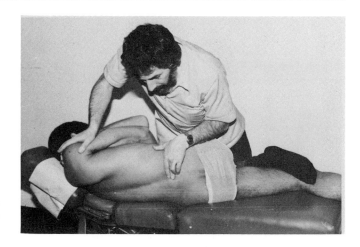

FIG. 14. **A technique for adjusting a type 4 L4-L5 fixation using a single spinous push (see text).**

ing to that side. The facet on the left is fixed in extension. In order to correct this problem the patient is placed in the side posture position with the left side up. The clinician places his or her fingers at the L3-4 interspace and rotates the lower shoulder girdle around the long axis of the body. The clinician should now be able to appreciate the progressive rotation and blocking that is occurring down through the spine. The patient's hands are placed comfortably on the anterior aspect of the opposite shoulder. The right leg is flexed slightly in order to reduce the lordosis of the lumbar spine. This is done in order to cause slight gaping of the facets which, in turn, assists in the restoration of intersegmental flexion. The upper leg is flexed to the point where the palpating finger can feel movement at the L5-S1 interspace. The upper leg is now rotated toward the floor until rotation of the pelvis and lower lumbar spine can be appreciated at the level of L4-5. The patient is now stabilized in his or her longitudinal axis around the contact point at L4-L5. Any increase in pressure through either of the long levers (the shoulder or the leg) will produce stress at the L4-L5 segment. Contact is now taken with the reinforced index finger on the lateral aspect of the spinous process of L4 (Fig. 14). Additional slack may be taken up at this time by having the patient take a deep breath. On expiration, a gentle stress on both the long levers will take the articulation to be manipulated into

the paraphysiological range. At the moment of maximal relaxation (end of expiration) a thrust is delivered in such a way as to dynamically separate the attachments of the involved multifidus contraction. This is done by thrusting toward the floor and slightly headward. This should cause a gaping of the upper facet and create a negative pressure within the disc. At the same time the multifidus muscle on the left is subjected to a dynamic stretching force. This adjustment, therefore, is aimed at reinstating the normal motoricity of the L4-5 motion segments by specifically applying a force in all the directions where motion was compromised, that is, rotation, lateral bending, and flexion.

There are a number of variations in the application of the thrust which can be made from this basic technique. A light thrust on the shoulder can give greater isolation of rotation in this distortion (Sandoz 1965). Additional kyphosis can be introduced by increasing thigh flexion in order to facilitate the restoration of intersegmental flexion. If more force is required, a pisiform contact can be used on the lateral aspect of the spinous process or a double index finger contact can be used by threading the clinician's arm through the flexed elbow of the patient (Fig. 15). In a situation where there is a specific discal component to the fixated motion segment, excess axial torsion should be avoided. This is done in order to minimize the stress on an already compromised annulus. The

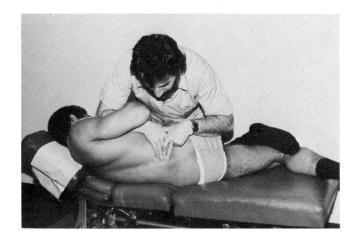

FIG. 15. **A technique for adjusting the lumbar spine using a reinforced double spinous push.**

correction of the same fixation can be accomplished from the opposite side using a hook contact on the spinous processes (Fig. 16A) or a mammillary contact (Fig. 16B). In this case the patient is placed on his/her opposite side with the fixation down. This procedure is less effective since one is forced to depend upon the passive introduction of one or more of the compromised coupled motions to achieve reduction of the fixation. Given these limitations, however, certain clinical situations make this technique the adjustment of choice. This is especially true when rotation to the left in the side posture position is not tolerated by the patient. The sacrospinalis stretch technique (Fig. 16C) is, in fact, a reverse lumbar roll where the specific contact made by the clinician is at the lateral aspect of the spinous process and an assisted thrust is given headward and anteriorly by the other hand. The application of a voluntary isometric contraction by the patient against resistance allows the clinician to take up additional slack when the patient relaxes. If this is repeated two or three times, the adjustment may be facilitated and hence make it more effective (Gaymans 1973). Each of the adjustments aimed at stretching the sacrospinalis, quadratus lumborum, or multifidus muscles may be accomplished in the seated position with the patient either straddling the treatment table or using a safety belt tightened across his/her thighs to provide stabilization.

Some of the earliest adjustments were given in the prone position with a thrust on either the spinous process or mammillary process with the direction of thrust usually given headward or straight through to the floor. The lower vertebra of the fixated segment is the one which is contacted and mobilized in this adjustment. This adjustment can be more effective when the pelvic section of a multisegmented adjusting table is elevated or when a roll or table with a drop abdominal section is used. This adjustment is of greater use for general mobilization, as a high force thrust in this position can be uncomfortable to the patient. The late Dr. Clarence Gonstead developed a sophisticated variation of this type of adjustment where the patient was positioned on a specifically designed lumbar knee posture bench (Fig. 16D). Research on the relative efficacy of all of these techniques has yet to be conducted.

Combined Facet and Sacroiliac Syndrome

There are subdivisions of the facet syndromes which have as yet to be clearly delineated on the basis of pathomechanics. In chronic patients better results from spinal adjustments can be expected if there is an active sacroiliac lesion in conjunction with the facet lesion. This might

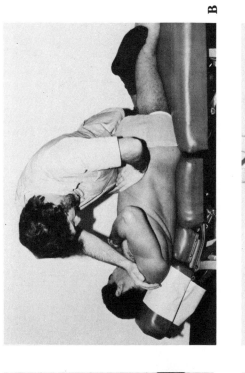

A

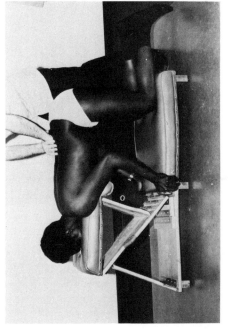

B

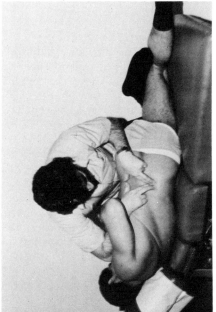

C

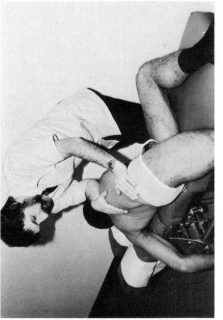

D

FIG. 16.   Alternate methods of adjusting the lumbar spine. (A) The double spinous hook technique. (B) The mammillary process rotary adjustment. (C) The sacrospinalis stretch adjustment. (D) The anterior to posterior adjustment in the kneeling position.

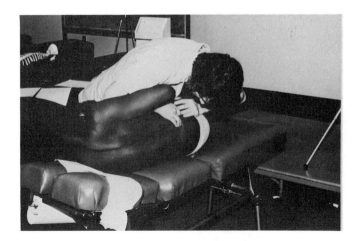

FIG. 17. **An adjusting technique for correcting a combined right multifidus contraction and right inferior sacrum fixation. A spinous push together with an inferior sacrum contact is used.**

suggest a causal relationship between these two problems or a constitution of different stages in a single pathomechanical process. The coupling of these two syndromes, as can be seen in many patients, makes it necessary to create combinations of adjustive procedures by applying the biomechanical principles that have already been discussed. At the same time, the syndromes must be considered individually. For example, a fourth lumbar multifidus contraction on the right with resultant spinous rotation to that side which is present in conjunction with an inferior sacrum on the same side may be adjusted in such a way as to correct both fixations at the same time. This technique is illustrated in Figure 17.

Intervertebral Disc Syndromes

The relationship of the pathomechanical effects of the posterior joint and sacroiliac dysfunction can be considered a critical factor with respect to the behavior of the anterior portion of the motion segment. Aberrant motion of these complexes can contribute to the displacement of the axis of motion of the entire motion segment as observed by Smith et al. (1906). This, in turn, could conceivably act as an initial factor in predisposing the posterior annulus to excess torsion strains. Farfan (1973) has observed that the end result of torsion strain is the development of circumferential tears. It is these circumferential tears and the effect on the attachments of the longitudinal ligaments which are responsible for the traction spurs that can be observed later on x-ray. The accumulation of additional torsion together with repeated minor trauma can further disturb the normal dynamic function of the disc. These stresses can produce radial tears in the area of the circumferential tears. These radial tears, when large enough, can lead to extrusion and even sequestration of the nucleus pulposis. This occurs either through the radial tear due to torsion or through end-plate fracture due to compression. If herniation does not occur, there may still be internal disruption of the disc with resultant bulging or protrusion and loss of disc height. This probably occurs more frequently than true herniation or sequestration of the nucleus pulposis. The disc will continue to degenerate internally until complete internal disruption of the architecture occurs. Kirkaldy-Willis (1978) has described the appearance of such a disc as looking like a deflated football.

Degenerated discal material will eventually become fibrotic due to resorption of the water content and hardening of the disc substance. The resultant loss of disc height produces a posterior inferior movement of the superior vertebra. This causes additional stress to be placed on the facet resulting in further compromise of its movements. Endstage disc degeneration can therefore be classified as a pathological fixation which, in turn, can compromise the mobility of the segments above and below, thus encouraging the same process to begin at other levels.

Clinical Picture

In the case of true disc herniation or sequestration, the patient usually reports a previous history of recurrent back pain. The acute incipient event is usually traumatic but often only minimal stress is involved. Backache progressing to leg pain is the inevitable early complaint. Later, the back pain may leave as the leg pain becomes more pronounced. The pain is aggravated by activity, straining, coughing, and sneezing as well as by sitting and rising from a chair. The pain is relieved by rest. Paraesthesias are common, but not necessarily associated with a demonstrable loss of sensation (at the periphery of the offending dermatone). The patient stands in either a direct or crossed antalgic position, the direct position being most common with the patient slightly flexed resulting in a loss of lumbar lordosis. The patient may stand with the hip and knee slightly flexed and even walk on the toes of the affected side in order to relieve tension on the sciatic nerve. The trunk movements are grossly limited in a pattern which is dependent on the nature of the spinal distortion, the site of the herniation, and its relationship to the irritated nerve root. Gross limitation of straight-leg raising is pronounced. Bowstring and Bragard's sign are positive and knee flexion usually relieves the pain. The contralateral sign where lifting of the healthy leg produces pain on the offending side is often positive. The healthy leg, however, can usually be taken higher than the other one. Neck flexion in the supine position may exaggerate the pain, especially if the herniation is on the

shoulder (the lateral aspect) of the nerve. All of these signs indicate that the nerve root is being compressed.

Springing of the lumbar spine commonly produces pain, and vertebral and sacroiliac fixation together with inequality of hip rotation is always present in this author's experience. Tenderness of the muscles related to the insulted nerve may be present. More severe or long standing nerve root compression can produce characteristic motor weakness, sensory impairment, and reflex changes depending on which nerve root has been insulted. Bladder and bowel paralysis indicates cauda equina pressure and should be considered a surgical emergency. If gross muscle weakness and progressive neural deficit occurs in spite of bed rest and conservative treatment, this too should be referred for surgical consultation.

Adjustment Techniques for Intervertebral Disc Syndrome

An adjustment directed to the specific level of herniation is one which involves a degree of risk. However, in conjunction with bed rest, adjustments may be given to other areas of the spine. Reflex and myofascial techniques may be applied as long as further torsional insult does not occur at the level of the lesion. Passive traction maneuvers may be helpful. Cox (1974, 1977), using a chiromanus table and gentle sucussion-like manipulations, reported 95.7 percent positive response in 89 cases which he classified as lateral disc protrusions and 87 percent positive response in 69 patients which he classified as medial disc protrusions. It should be pointed out, however, that in all likelihood, there was no sequestration or herniation of the disc in these cases. Further research is needed in this promising area.

In the intervertebral disc syndromes unaccompanied by herniation or sequestration, the following manipulative procedures represent a rational approach. Sandoz (1971) and Matthews and Yates (1969) have each described the effect of helicord traction which was previously demonstrated by Levernieux (1960). This adjustment is accomplished in the side posture position similar to the classical lumbar roll. A mammillary contact on the lower segment of the fixation complex is made which is used to resist a thrust to the shoulder which is directed headward and posteriorly. This adjustment is an attempt to produce negative intradiscal pressure by gapping the disc. Bonyon (1967) and Grice have described an adjustive maneuver designed to cause the closure of the disc on the superior side while opening the wedged disc on the inferior side. This adjustment avoids rotational strain. The patient is placed in the side posture position with both the pelvis and trunk elevated either by pillows or by adjusting the treatment table. A double mammillary or finger push contact is taken and the thrust is directed to the floor in order to open the lower facet and gap the disc on the lower side. The aim of this adjustment is to produce negative intradiscal pressure in the hope of reducing a radial protrusion on the superior side. Both of these adjustments are aimed at reducing the incarcerated nuclear material in radial annular tears. Reduction may conceivably also occur if nuclear material has fractured through the end plate. It is possible that an adjustment may result in the shifting of a sequestrated piece of discal material in such a way as to place it in a more innocent location.

Lateral Spinal Nerve Entrapment

The nerve root can be mechanically irritated in the lateral recess of the intervertebral foramen or subarticular gutter as a result of disc degeneration and protrusion. Degenerative changes of the facet joint and the guillotine-like lowering of the superior pedical can also cause lateral spinal nerve entrapment. These entrapment syndromes, as a rule, do not show the acute symptoms of disc herniation and therefore the straight-leg raising sign is not as limited. Bowstring's sign and Bragard's sign are both usually negative. There are a variety of clinical pictures

seen in nerve root entrapment syndromes. Their response to short-term manipulative treatment is poor. However, long-term management with proper spinal hygiene may be rewarding.

Central Spinal Stenosis

Hypertrophy and osteophytosis of facets and thickening of the adjacent lamina can encroach not only on the lateral recess but also on the posterior aspect of the spinal canal itself. This can be demonstrated radiographically. Kirkaldy-Willis and McIvor (1976), Kirkaldy-Willis (1978), and Arnoldi et al. (1976) have described and classified lumbar spinal stenosis and the nerve root entrapment syndromes. The typical patient with this problem is usually past 50, has a history of long-standing dull backache which commences some time before the leg pains begin. The leg pain may be claudic or sciatic in nature. The leg pain does not usually come on as acutely as that which accompanies a herniated disc. Morning pain and stiffness can be "worked out" in a few hours. However, fatigue and discomfort may return in the latter part of the day. This is unlike the herniated disc which is exaggerated by activity. The pain of stenosis is less localized than that which occurs in a disc lesion, and the patient may show signs resembling intermittent claudication. Walking can cause weakness of the legs, severe cramping, and numbness which can become severe enough to force the patient to rest. The symptoms then disappear on rest and reoccur once the patient resumes walking. The clinical picture usually suggests that more than one root is involved and the roots that are involved, unlike herniation of the disc, are often above the level of L5. Flexion of the spine usually relieves symptoms while extension may aggravate them. Pain on straight-leg raising is less remarkable and often closely symmetrical. Paraspinal muscle spasm is not as severe when compared to disc herniation. The circulation to the legs is normal. There may be sensory changes with muscle weakness and reflex changes consistent with the involved roots. Treatment should include isometric abdominal exercises. An elastic back support may be helpful. Adjustments can be attempted even in advanced cases.

The following typical case report has been presented by Professor Kirkaldy-Willis (1978):

A 63-year-old man had low back pain for 22 years. Two years before visiting our office he had a coronary bypass operation. He gave a seven year history of increasingly severe low back pain and pain in both legs to the feet. After walking three blocks he had to rest because of pain. On examination, straight leg raising was 30° on the right and 45° on the left. Sensation was decreased over the L5 dermatome and left extensor hallucis longus muscle was slightly weak. Plain radiographs suggested spinal stenosis. A myelogram done one year previously at another centre showed marked central spinal stenosis at the L5-S1 level, with an almost complete block. Because of the patient's cardiac condition, it was considered wise to avoid operative decompression. After two weeks of manipulations he reported that his back was 50% improved and that he had no leg pain at all. This was a most gratifying result although it is not common for manipulation to be so effective in such an advanced stage of spinal stenosis. Furthermore this relief may not be permanent.

Conclusion

The necessity of differentiating between the various pathological and biomechanical disorders of the lumbar spine prior to applying manipulative therapy cannot be overly stressed. A pilot project on the effectiveness of spinal manipulation on patients with chronic low-back pain has been undertaken by the interdisciplinary team of Kirkaldy-Willis, Gitelman, and Grice at the University of Saskatchewan. The results of this trial, as presented to the October 1978 meeting of the North American Academy of Manipulative Medicine, reviewed 208 patients who had previously tried most other forms of treatment. Eighty-eight percent of all patients with a diagnosis of sacroiliac syndrome became either symptom-free or were very much

improved following spinal manipulation. This contrasted markedly with the 55 percent of patients with a diagnosis of posterior facet syndrome, 22 percent with a diagnosis of herniated nucleus pulposis, 31 percent with lateral nerve entrapment, and 29 percent with central spinal stenosis who responded in a similar manner to spinal manipulative therapy. The apparent disappointing results in patients with facet syndrome may be related to the fact that all patients in the trial had suffered from low-back pain for an average of 5 years and received an average of only 6 manipulations. On the other hand, the results in patients with acute facet syndrome following spinal manipulation have indicated a better than 90 percent positive response rate (Fisk 1971; Potter 1978). This classification probably will need subgrouping to account for the hypermobility syndromes and other considerations such as architectural variations in the osseous structures. The proper examination of the patient is necessary to determine the nature of the spinal lesion and the biomechanical factors which influence the adjustive technique likely to be most effective. It is also the primary means of determining the degree of success one is likely to achieve with chiropractic care.

In our present state of ignorance the challenge is obvious. The future leaders of the field of manipulative therapy will be those who can combine intuitive philosophy with the scientific clinical method: that is, combine the principal of neurophysiological centrality in human health with an understanding of the static and dynamic behavior of the human locomotor system.

Acknowledgments

The assistance of Howard Vernon and David Brunarski in proofreading and the collection of material is greatfully acknowledged. The literature review on which this chapter was based was funded by the Foundation for Chiropractic Education and Research and the Canadian Memorial Chiropractic College.

REFERENCES

Abel MS: Oblique motion studies and other non-myelographic rentgenographic criteria for diagnosis of traumatized or degenerated lumbar intervertebral discs. Am J Surg 99:717, 1960

Allbrook D: Movements of the lumbar spinal column. J Bone Joint Surg 39B:339, 1957.

Arnoldi A, et al: (1976) Lumbar spinal stenosis and nerve root entrapment syndromes—definition and classification. Clin Ortho Rel Res 115:4, 1976

Bergquist-Ulmann M, Larsson U: Acute low-back pain in industry. Acta Orthop Scand [Suppl] 170, 1977

Bonyon J: Lumbar instability. Toronto, Postgraduate Seminar Canadian Memorial Chiropractic College, 1967

Breen AC: Chiropractors and the treatment of back pain. Rheum Rehabil 16:46, 1977

Cassidy JD: Reotgenological examination of the functional mechanics of the lumbar spine in lateral flexion. J Can Chiropr Assoc 20, 2:13, 1976

Chrisman OD, Mittnacht A, Snook G: A study of the results following rotatory manipulation in the lumbar intervertebral disc syndrome. J Bone Joint Surg 46A:517, 1964

Colachis SC, Warden RE, Bechtol CO, Strohm BR: Arch Phys Med Rehabil 44:490, 1963

Cox JM: The lumbar disc syndrome: A chiropractic evaluation. Presented at Spinal Research Symposium (notes). Troy, Michigan, 1977

Coyer B, Curwen HM: Low back pain treated by manipulation. Br Med J 1:705, 1955

Denslow HS, Clough GN: Reflex activity in the spinal extensors. J Neurophysiol 4:430, 1941

DeJarnette MB: Sacro-occipital technic. Unpublished notes, 1967

Doran DML, Newel DJ: Manipulation in treatment of low back pain. A multicentre study. Br Med J 2:161, 1975

Edwards BC: Low back pain and pain resulting from lumbar spine conditions. A comparison of treatment results. Aust J Physiother 14:104, 1969

Edwards FO: Piriformis syndrome. In Year Book. Academy of Applied Osteopathy, 1962

Egund N, Olsson TH, Schmid H, Selvick G: Movements in the sacroiliac joint demonstrated with roentgen stereophogrammetry. Acta Radiol 19:883, 1978

England RW, Deibert PW: Electromyographic studies. Part I: Consideration of the evaluation of steopathic therapy. J Am Osteop Assoc 72:162, 1972

Evans DP, Burke MS, Lloyd KN, Roberts EE, Roberts GM: Lumbar spinal manipulation on trial. Parts I and II. Rheum Rehabil 17:46, 1978

Farfan HF: Mechanical Disorders of the Low Back. Philadelphia, Lea & Febiger, 1973

Farfan HF, MacGibbon B: Are all lumbar spines the same. In preparation

Feinstein B: Referred pain for paravertebral structures. In Buerger AA, Tobis JS (eds): Approaches to the Validation of Manipulative Therapy. Springfield IL, Thomas, 1977

Fick R: Handbuch der anatomi und mechanik der gelenke und bercksightigung der benegenden musken. Jena, Bardeleben 1911

Fisk JW: Manipulation in general practice. NZ Med J 74:172, 1971

Frigerio NA, Stowe RW, Howe JW: Movement of the sacroiliac joint. Clin Orthop Rel Res 100:370, 1974

Gaymans F: Neue mobilisations prinzipien und techniken an der wirbelsaule. Man Med 11:35, 1973

Gillet H, Liekens M: A further study of spinal fixations. Ann Swiss Chiropr Assoc 4:41, 1969

Gillet H, Liekens M: Belgian Chiropractic Research Notes. Brussels, 1979

Gitelman R: The treatment of pain by spinal manipulation. In Goldstein M (ed): The Research Status of Spinal Manipulative Therapy. NINCDS Monograph #15. Bethesda MD, DHEW, 1975

Gianturco C: A roentgenographic analysis of the lower lumbar vertebrae in normal individuals and in patients with low back pain. Am J Roent 52:261, 1944

Glover JR: Back pain and hyperaesthesia. Lancet 1:1165, 1960

Glover JR: Back pain: A randomized clinical trial of rotational manipulation of the trunk. Br J Ind Med 31:59, 1974

Gravel P, Gravel AL: Integrated Chiropractic Methods. Montreal, 1966

Grice A: Muscle tone change following manipulation. J Can Chiropr Assoc 18, 4:29, 1975

Grice A: Harmony of joint and muscle function in the prevention of lower back syndromes J Can Chiropr Assoc 20, 2:7, 1976

Grice A: Radiographic, biomechanical and clinical factors in lumbar lateral flexion. Part 1. J Manip Phys Ther 2, 1:26, 1979

Gunn CC, Milbrant WE: Early subtle signs in low back sprain. Spine 3, 3:267, 1978

Hackett GS: Ligament and Tendon Relaxation Treatment Procotherapy. Thomas, Springfield IL, 1956

Hagen R: Pelvic girdle relaxation from an orthopaedic point of view. Acta Orthop Scand 45:545, 1974

Hasner E, Schalintzer M, Snorrason E: Roetenological examination of the function of the lumbar spine. Presented at the Congress of Northern Association for Medical Radiology. Copenhagen, June 1957

Henderson RS: The treatment of lumbar intervertebral disc protrusion: an assessment of conservative measure. Br Med J 2:597, 1952

Heyse-Moore GG: A rational approach to the use of epidural medication in the treatment of sciatic pain. Acta Orthop Scand 49:366, 1978

Hviid H: The influence of Chiropractic treatment on the rotatory mobility of the cervical spine. Ann Swiss Chiropr Assoc 5:31, 1971

Higley NG, Goodick T: Report of study of spinal mechanics L3, L4, L5. Des Moines, Foundation for Chiropractic Education and Research, 1964

Illi F: Highlights of 45 Years of Experience and 35 Years of Research. Geneva, 1971

Illi F: Sacroiliac mechanism keystone of spinal balance of body locomotion. Chicago, National College of Chiropractic, 1940

Illi F: The Vertebral Column, Lifeline of the Body. Chicago, National College of Chiropractic, 1951

Inman VT, Saunders JB: Referred pain from skeletal structures. J Neurol Med Dis 99:660, 1944

Janse J, Houser TH, Wells BF: Chiropractic Principles and Technic. Chicago, National College of Chiropractic, 1947

Janse J: The clinical biomechanics of the sacroiliac mechanism. J Am Chiropr Assoc 15, 1:27, 1978

Kane RL, Fischer FD, Leymaster C et al: Manipulating the patient, a comparison of the effectiveness of physician and chiropractor care. Lancet 1:1333, 1974

Kellgren JH: Observation in referred pain arising from muscle. Clin Sci 3:175, 1938

Kellgren JH: On the distribution of pain arising from keep somatic structures. Clin Sci 4:35, 1939

Kellgren JH: Anatomical source of back pain. Rheum Rehabil 16:3, 1977

Kirkaldy-Willis WH: Common back disorders, how to diagnose and treat them. Geriatrics December 1978, p 32

Kirkaldy-Willis W, Yong-Hing K, Reilly J: Pathology and pathogenesis of lumbar spondylosis and stenosis. Spine 3:319, 1978

Kirkaldy-Willis WH, McIvor GWD: Lumbar spinal stenosis. Clin Orthop Rel Res 115:2, 1976

Knutsson F: The instability associated with disc degeneration of the lumbar spine. Acta Radiol 25:593, 1944

LeVernieux J: Les traction vertebrales l'expansion. Paris, 1960

Logan VF: Logan Basic Methods. St. Louis, Logan College, 1956

Lysell E: The pattern of motion in the cervical spine. In Hirsch C, Zotterman Y (eds): Cervical Pain. Oxford, Pergamon Press, 1971

Maigne R: Orthopedic Medicine—A New Approach to Vertebral Manipulation. Springfield IL, Thomas, 1972

Matthews JA, Yates EAH: Reduction of lumbar disc prolapse by manipulation. Br Med J 3:692, 1969

Maxwell TD: The piriformis muscle and its relation to the long legged sciatic syndrome J Can Chiropr Assoc 22, 2:51, 1978

Mennell J: Back Pain. Boston, Little, Brown, 1960

Mennell J: Joint Pain. Boston, Little, Brown, 1964

Mensor, MC: Non-operative treatment including manipulation for lumbar intervertebral disc syndrome. J Bone Jt Surg 37A:925, 1955

Mensor MC, Duval G: Absence of motion at the 4th and 5th lumbar interspaces in patients with and without low back pain. J Bone Jt Surg 41A: 1959

Mensor MC, Gross AJ, Duval G: Mobility studies of the lumbar spine in relation to low back pain. A preliminary report. J Bone Jt Surg 39A:448, 1957

Meyer GH: Des mechanisms der symphysis sacroiliaca. Arch Anat Physiol, 1878

Mitchell F: Structural pelvic function. In Yearbook. Academy of Applied Osteopathy, 1965

Mixter WJ, Barr JS: Rupture of the intervertebral disc with involvement of the spinal canal. N Engl J Med 210:211, 1934

Mooney V, Robertson J: The facet syndrome. Clin Orthop Rel Res 115:140, 1976

Parsons WB, Cumming JDA: Manipulation in back pain. Can Med Assoc J 79:103, 1958

Pennel GF, et al: Motion studies of the lumbar spine. J Bone Jt Surg 54B:442, 1972

Potter GE: A study of 744 cases of neck and back pain treated with spinal manpulation J Can Chiropr Assoc 21, 4:154, 1977

Potter GE: Summary of results in 1960 patients treated with spinal manipulation 1974-1975. J Can Chiropr Assoc, in press

Riches EW: End-results of manipulation of the back. Lancet May 1930, p 957

Robinson DR: Piriformis syndrome in relation to sciatic pain. Am J Surg 73:335, 1947

Sandoz R: Technique and interpretation of the functional radiography of the lumbar spine. Ann Swiss Chiropr Assoc 3:66, 1965

Sandoz R: Degenerative conditions of the lumbosacral spine. Ann Swiss Chiropr Assoc 1:77, 1960

Sandoz R: Newer trends in the pathogenesis of spinal disorders. Ann Swiss Chiropr Assoc 5:93, 1971

Sashin D: A critical analysis of the anatomy and pathological changes in the sacroiliac joints. J Bone Jt Surg 12:891, 1930

Siehl D, Bradford WG: Manipulation of the low back under general anesthesia. J Am Osteop Assoc, December 1952, p 239

Sims-Williams H, Jayson MIV, Young SMS, et al: Controlled trial of mobilization and manipulation for patients with low back pain in general practice. Br Med J 2:1338, 1978

Smith OG, Longworthy SM, Paxson NC: Modern Chiropractic. Cedar Rapids IA, Lawrence Press, 1906

Stoddard A: Manual of Osteopathic Technique. New York, Harper & Row, 1959

Tanz SS: Motion of the lumbar spine. Can J Roent 69:399, 1953

Vernon H, Gitelman R: A comparative study of the static and dynamic models of the mechanics of the lower lumbar spine, post graduate research in progress. Toronto, Canadian Memorial Chiropractic College, 1979

Warr A, Wilkinson JA, Burn JMB, Langdon L: Chronic lumbosciatic syndrome treated by epidural injection and manipulation. Practitioner 209:53, 1972

Weisl H: The movements of the sacroiliac joint. Acta Anat 23:80, 1955

Yeomen W: The relation of arthritis of the sacroiliac joint to sciatic with all analysis of 100 cases. Lancet 2:1119, 1928

CHAPTER FIFTEEN
A Biomechanical Approach to Cervical and Dorsal Adjusting
ADRIAN S. GRICE

Spinal manipulation has been utilized in some form throughout history prior to the emergence of chiropractic and osteopathy. Schafer (1976) has reviewed the ancient history of spinal manipulation, describing murals depicting crude manipulative maneuvers from as early as the Aurignacian period (17,500 B.C.) as well as from the ancient Chinese (2700 B.C.) and Greek (1500 B.C.) civilizations. He has provided references that manipulation was practiced by the Japanese Indians of Asia, the Egyptians, Babylonians, Syrians, Hindus, Tibetans, and Tahitians. Lomax (1975) and Hildebrandt (1978) have each presented a brief history of spinal manipulation up to more modern times. Although widely used throughout history, the development of more sophisticated techniques of spinal manipulation has occurred primarily in the last century with the interest of chiropractic, osteopathy, and medicine.

Osteopathic treatment as described by A.T. Still appears most often to have consisted of mobilization of the spine, ribs, and peripheral joints. The treatment was often pharmacologic in nature; i.e., each diagnosed condition had a complete series of maneuvers and remedies (Still 1910).

D.D. Palmer, the founder of chiropractic, on the other hand, appears to have been the first to use the spinous and transverse processes as levers (D.D. Palmer 1910). The adjustive thrust developed by D.D. Palmer was certainly a different method of spinal manipulative therapy (SMT) than that of Still and the early osteopaths. Osteopathy consisted of long-lever techniques of mobilization and manipulation, whereas chiropractic methods consisted of short-lever techniques utilizing specific contacts with a dynamic thrust of controlled depth and magnitude. Davis (1909) discussed this difference in therapy between the two professions and reviewed a number of early osteopathic techniques which demonstrated the emphasis on long-lever mobilization. Gregory (1912), on the other hand, reviewed a number of chiropractic techniques that demonstrated the short-lever adjustive techniques which were developed by early chiropractors. A close review of the early medical, osteopathic, and chiropractic literature shows that many of the practitioners held dual degrees which probably facilitated the exchange of concepts and techniques that has evolved.

One of the earliest texts, by Smith, Langworthy, and Paxson (1906), presented many concepts important in SMT that have stood the test of time. In this text, the chiropractic thrust was described as a specific contact on the spine utilizing a short, nonviolent, gauged, rapid pressure in a specific direction. A simple subluxation was defined as a condition in which the joint surfaces were slightly changed in position though the articular surfaces were still in contact (static subluxation). The authors felt that an intervertebral joint was capable of a certain field of motion and had a certain axis of motion. A subluxation was depicted as a wheel whose hub was off center. Diagnosis of this subluxation was accomplished by static and early forms of motion palpation, inspection, gait analysis, and nerve tracing. Correction of the vertebral subluxation took into consideration the muscular forces acting on the segments of the spine and the type of motion which was possible. The authors made a distinction between three forms of adjustive thrust: (1) fast delivery, rapid release as in the toggle recoil or dynamic thrust procedures; (2) fast delivery, slow release as in dorsal adjusting; and (3) slow delivery or pressure thrusts.

The development of modern chiropractic technique has taken several directions. W. Carver (1909), F. Carver (1938), and Beatty (1939) placed their emphasis on the development of a more general approach to spinal manipulative therapy (SMT). B.J. Palmer (1911), on the other hand, carried on his father's tradition and developed a specific full spine approach based on the meric system. In later years, B.J. Palmer (1934) went further by adopting the specific upper cervical technique sometimes referred to as "hole-in-one" (HIO). Since then a great many technique systems have developed. Only those technique systems which

have contributed to an overall biomechanical kinesiological understanding of SMT will be recognized in this chapter.

Classification of Spinal Manipulative Therapy

Adjustive Procedures

Spinal adjustive procedures remain the most important part of spinal manipulative therapy. The adjustive thrust is characterized by a transmission of force using a combination of muscular power and the body weight of the practitioner. The force is delivered with controlled speed, depth, and magnitude through a specific contact on a particular structure such as the transverse or spinous process of a vertebra. Control of the adjustive thrust requires practice and skill in order for the practitioner to deliver a thrust with exact amplitude, speed, and force. Common methods of developing the adjustive

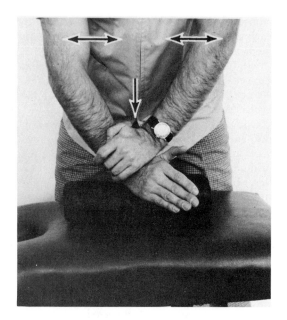 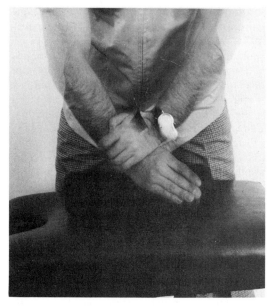

FIG. 1. **Recoil adjustment. (A) Arm-hand position. (B) Triceps motion.**

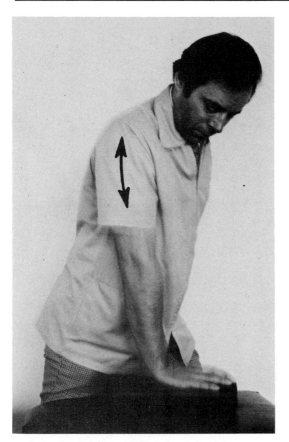

FIG. 2. **Straight-arm adjustment—shoulder thrust.**

thrust are: the recoil triceps motion (Fig. 1), shoulder–straight-arm thrust (Fig. 2), and body drop thrust (Fig. 3). All combinations of the above are possible and once skill is developed the thrust may be given in a variety of positions. For instance, rotary cervical adjustments may require the hands to move in opposite directions. In thoracic adjustments, however, both arms may move together in the same direction.

The mechanical goals of a spinal adjustment include: (1) correction of static misalignment; (2) correction of dysfunction of motion segment dynamics or general spinal curvature dynamics; and (3) correction of any combination of the above. These goals may be achieved through basic adjustment techniques.

Recoil Adjustment. The patient is in a neutral position, at rest and relaxed. The thrust is a dynamic adjustive thrust given in a specific direction with a specific depth, high velocity, and low amplitude. A free-fall head piece or table cushion may be used with a set spring reset release to take up part of the force and allow for counterresistance of the fixed vertebrae (Fig. 4).

Dynamic Thrust. This adjustment is given in two ways:

1. With the patient in the neutral position, specific contact or contacts are taken on a vertebral process and the thrust is given in a

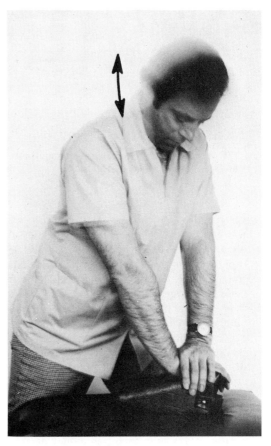

FIG. 3. **Body drop adjustment—body thrust.**

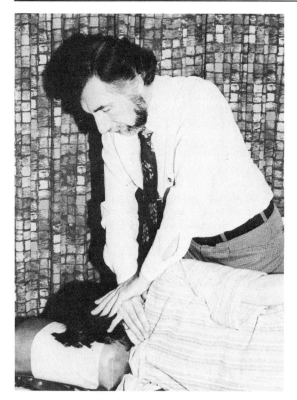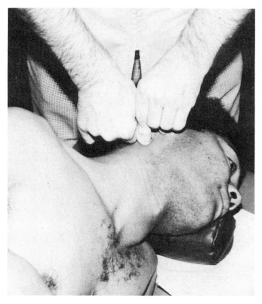

FIG. 4. **Side posture recoil adjustment. (Left) With drop headpiece and pisiform contact. (Right) Modified thumb contact on atlas.**

specific direction similar to the recoil adjustment; no recoil is involved nor is a drop mechanism utilized. The thrust may be rapid with either a slow or fast release. Neutral joint slack or tissue elasticity is taken out prior to delivering the thrust (see page 351).

2. The adjustment is given by moving the patient in a specific direction to take out the active and passive motion at that level. The thrust is then given beyond the passive range of motion. It is possible to vary the velocity and depth or amplitude depending on the area being adjusted (see page 346).

Specific Directional Adjustment to Holding Elements. This adjustment is aimed at correcting dysfunction of the static or dynamic forces that are causing static misalignment and/or functional impairment of the motion segment dynamics. That is, the adjustment is given to stretch muscles or ligaments that are causing static or dynamic motion-segment faults. The dynamic stretch, when applied to a muscle, may produce relaxation of that muscle (England 1972; Grice 1974).

Manipulation Procedures

Specific Motion Segment Procedures. Joint stressing or joint challenging procedures can be specific as far as direction and force are concerned (Fig. 5). A contact on the spinous or transverse process of the segment may be utilized and the joint forced in a specific direction.

Segmental directional mobilization involves

the forcing of the spinal segment in a specific direction. The motion segment is forced beyond the active range of motion to the end of the passive range of motion (Fig. 6). Mobilization procedures may be accomplished at a slower, more rhythmic speed than the adjustment. This may or may not include joint separation ("crack" or "pop").

General Motion Segment Procedure. A number of motion segments or a large area of the spinal column is mobilized as a block in a specific direction beyond the active to the end of the passive range of motion. This may include joint separation (Fig. 7).

General Mobilization. Mobilization through all ranges of motion may be directed at either (1) a single motion segment or (2) a block of motion segments, i.e., the entire cervical spine.

Exercise Procedures. Either active or passive exercise procedures can be used for mobilization or strengthening. Active exercise strengthens and tones muscle and thereby indirectly increases joint mobility, whereas passive

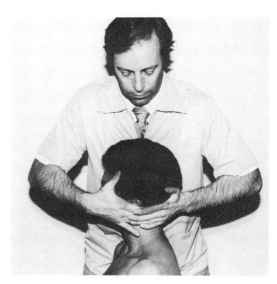

FIG. 6. **Segmental mobilization of the cervical spine in lateral flexion.**

exercise (e.g., yoga) stretches muscles and ligaments and specifically increases joint mobility.

Reflex Procedures

These procedures can be broken down into three groups: (1) pressure techniques including stimulation or stripping techniques for muscle relaxation or pain control, massage and trigger-point therapy; (2) acutherapy procedures, percussion and spondylotherapy; and (3) neural stimulation or inhibition procedures.

Mechanotherapy

A large number of appliances have been developed over the years which have been closely associated with SMT. These include:

1. Heel lifts, shoe lifts, foot appliances, correction braces, collars, etc.
2. Traction apparatus—harness, tables, reverse gravity units;
3. Locomotor apparatus, walkers, torso-locomotor apparatus, etc.

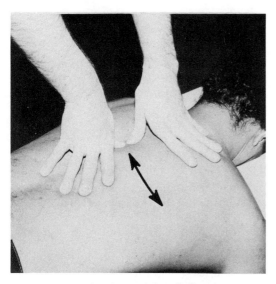

FIG. 5. **Joint stressing or joint challenging procedures for mobilization or palpation of the thoracic spine.**

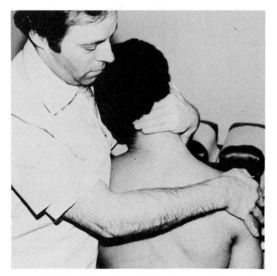 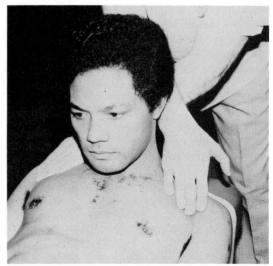

FIG 7. **General mobilization procedures aimed at producing muscular stretch and general joint separation of cervical spine (A) lateral flexion; (B) forward flexion.**

4. Adjustive or mobilization appliances such as percussors, vibrators, adjusting guns, stimulation devices, etc.

Determination of Where and How To Apply Spinal Manipulative Therapy

For primary contact practitioners applying SMT, a double diagnosis is necessary for proper and complete patient management. This double diagnosis concept is further developed by Gitelman in Chapter 14, this volume. The primary diagnosis is based on the subjective symptoms and objective signs which are elicited from the history and the physical examination as well as radiographic and laboratory examinations. This diagnosis describes the nature and extent of the pathological process causing the patient's symptoms and signs. The second diagnosis is a spinal structure evaluation. This latter diagnosis is primary to the application of SMT and has a direct bearing on where and

which manipulative procedure is to be given. This part of the double diagnosis establishes the environs of the lesion or syndrome and relates it to the total spinal or locomotor statics and dynamics.

Biomechanical Kinesiological Diagnostic Methods (Structural Diagnosis)

Inspection. This method consists of visualization of body posture and gross spinal movements. The nature and quality of joint motion is important, as well as the basic spinal curvatures and asymmetries. This examination procedure may help determine the chronicity of the structural deficit and the biomechanical interrelated nature of distortions or subluxations and the nature of gross body curvatures or segmental faults.

Palpation. The most important and most frequently utilized diagnostic evaluation procedure, palpation, determines not only surface bony architecture and position but also joint function. Static joint challenge techniques as well as dynamic motion palpation methods determine normal and abnormal motion segment dynamics.

Static Palpation. Static palpation is useful in evaluating skin, muscle, subcutaneous tissues, and osseous structures. Important factors include texture, tenderness, and pain as well as the position and shape of these structures. Static palpation can be enhanced by utilizing static joint challenge, joint springing, joint play, and gliding palpating techniques. Skin tenderness, texture changes, pigmentation, and changes in skin rolling perception have been considered important as indicators of a facilitated segment, subluxation, or area of somatic dysfunction. These abnormalities along with muscle tension and joint dysfunction are considered the primary sites for SMT. The latter information determines the direction and force of the adjustment.

Dynamic Palpation. Dynamic palpation is the evaluation of the dynamic range of motion, including active and passive motion followed by joint challenge, joint springing, or in some cases joint play. Dynamic palpation elicits information on the holding elements, particularly the muscles involved in movement. Information obtained from dynamic palpation may guide the direction of thrust and influence the choice of body position of the patient for SMT. Historically many chiropractors have attached importance to the fact that pain occurs in certain directions of joint motion and have emphasized the point that the adjustment should be given in the pain-free direction of motion (Overton 1958; Amodel 1958). Maigne (1972) more recently calls this the "no pain and free movement" rule. The range of motion in the nonpainful or nonacute direction may suggest the degree of chronicity of the case.

Plumbline Evaluation Methods. These methods include static postural evaluation for curvatures, body balance, spinal compensation, and decompensation which can be interpreted by static analysis. Dynamic evaluation of spinal movement as well as pre- and postadjustment evaluations may be accomplished with the plumbline.

Weight-Scale Analysis. Double weight scales (Chirotron, Inc.) can be used to evaluate body balance. Four-quadrant weight scales have been developed for accurate postural evaluation of body imbalance due to nonequilibrated torsions or nonbalanced torsions (Illi 1952). These nonbalanced torsions have been considered to be related to postural fatigue and may be helped by exercise or mechanotherapy in the form of shoe lifts or supports as well as by spinal manipulative therapy.

Radiographic Diagnosis
A Pathological and Morphological Evaluation. To determine whether spinal adjustments, mobilization, manipulation, or other corrective procedures are indicated or contraindicated a pathological and morphological evaluation may be used. The technique of spinal manipulative therapy may also be influenced by morphological changes seen on x-rays. For example, areas of hypermobility may require immobilization rather than mobilization. If mobilization procedures are indicated, the degree of force and the amplitude of this force may be altered by the x-ray findings. Mobilization procedures or nonforceful spinal adjustments may be indicated rather than dynamic adjustive thrusts in the presence of nondestructive pathological or morphological changes.

Static Postural Studies. Studies of this type include both segmental and gross evaluation of the position of the vertebrae relative to each other. A so-called "listing," i.e., a short-form description of vertebral malposition, has been developed to indicate the direction and contact point for the adjustive thrust. Careful static analysis may also give some indication of dynamic dysfunction. General static radiographic marking procedures have been presented by Logan (1950), Weinterstein (1971), and Hildebrandt (1977). On the other hand, clinicians such as Gonstead (1978), Pettibon (1968), Grostic (1966), Blair (1968), and B.J. Palmer (1934) have developed specific technique systems that utilize often unique spinal static marking procedures.

Dynamic or Stress Radiographs. These radiographs determine the functional aspects of vertebral motion, both segmental and general. Overlay marking systems in the cervical spine have been described by Grice (1977) and Conley (1974). Jirout (1973) and Lewit (1965) have discussed the clinical importance of dynamic analysis of the cervical joints in lateral flexion. Radiographic analysis produces an accurate evaluation of joint dysfunction and allows for the specific adjustment of the fixed or blocked motion segment and a selective approach to exercise and mobilization procedures.

Leg Length Analysis. This procedure is one of the most frequently utilized biomechanical evaluation methods and is often given too much importance. Most commonly, leg length is related to pelvic distortion (Chapter 14, this volume). However, certain techniques and methods of determining changes in leg length following head rotation and tipping are said to relate to cervical function. Changes in leg length with regard to cervical motion usually have been considered to indicate abnormalities in cervical biomechanics.

Reflex Analytical Methods. Surface reflex points have been utilized in chiropractic and osteopathy for analysis and treatment. Muscle-testing techniques, parietal and occipital trigger zones, challenge techniques, and leg length reflex points all use surface stimulation of the skin and subcutaneous tissue which are assumed to produce neurological phenomena in the body. Direct evaluation techniques are far more reliable than remote reflex tests which, at this point, require careful scientific evaluation before they can be considered for general use. Unfortunately many system techniques rely heavily on such evaluation methods.

Skin Temperature, Hyperemia, and Resistance Analysis. Over the years, many devices have been developed to measure skin temperature, hyperemia, or skin resistance. The physiological changes measured by these devices have been thought to reflect autonomic function or the activity of the so-called "facilitated segment" (Kuntz 1953; Muller 1954). These measurements were intended to aid the practitioner in locating areas of spinal "lesion" or "subluxation" and to monitor the response to spinal adjustive therapy. Unfortuantely, few of these instruments have been subjected to proper clinical evaluation.

Basic Principles of Cervical and Dorsal Manipulation Procedures

The mechanical basis for spinal manipulation involves:

1. Correcting aberrant motion segment statics; i.e., bony malposition or misalignment (the static subluxation);
2. Correcting aberrant motion segment dynamics; i.e., restoring joint range and axis of motion toward normal (the dynamic subluxation);
3. Correcting a combination of the above.

Techniques for spinal adjustment or manipulation have been developed over the years with reliance primarily on empirical results rather than controlled scientific studies. This has led to the evolution of numerous different systems and methods of approach. All techniques, however, can be evaluated on a biomechanical kinesiological basis. Figure 8 shows schematically the range of motion of a joint. A normal joint has a static accessory motion, an active range of motion, a passive range of motion, and a paraphysiological motion; i.e., a motion which is at the end of the passive motion is slight and has to do with ligamentous laxity and elasticity. Most exercises are aimed at restoring the passive range of motion. Articulating, mobilization,

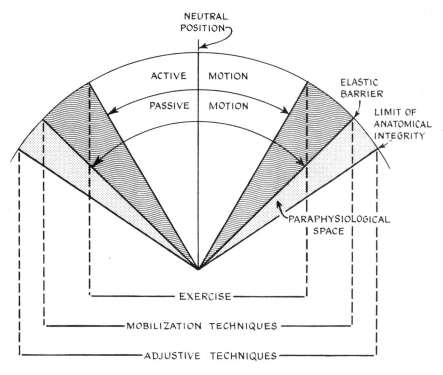

FIG. 8. The normal joint range of motion and the mechanical effect of exercise mobilization and adjustive procedures. (Modified from Sandoz 1976)

or manipulative procedures help to restore the active and passive ranges of motion while specific spinal adjustments help to restore the active, passive, and paraphysiological motion of joints. The spinal adjustment often produces joint separation (the "pop"). In this way neutral joint mobility (best determined by joint challenge or springing) and end fell mobility (best determined by dynamic palpation methods) is often restored. Some characteristics of the "joint crack" or "joint pop" elicited during an adjustment have been determined. Sandoz (1969) noted that there was an increased range of motion in all directions in the motion segment following an adjustment and the appearance of a radiolucent cavity in the joint space, thought to be intraarticular gas formation. The "crack phenomenon," which accompanies joint separation, is followed by a short refractory period of about 20 minutes before the "joint

crack" can be reproduced (Roston and Haines 1957).

General Biomechanical Concepts

The movements most often discussed in the application of spinal manipulative therapy are flexion and extension, lateral flexion, and rotation. Translatory or gliding motion also exists at certain joints. There are very few movements in the spinal column that take place in a single plane. White and Panjabi (1978) have discussed the coupled motions in the cervical, dorsal, and lumbar spine showing that during the individual motions of rotation and lateral flexion one motion cannot be produced without the other. Adjustments that are given for laterality correct rotation and rotation adjustments correct laterality. The overall shape of the motion segment and particularly the shape of the facets control the kinematics of the motion segment and therefore control the effect of manipulative or adjustive forces that are introduced into the spine. Coupled motions in vertebral motion segments, therefore, bring about a general increase in all ranges of motion following a vertebral adjustment. Thus, even poorly directed corrective procedures are able to have some positive effect. This is perhaps one reason why clinicians who are inexperienced or unskilled in the practice of spinal manipulative therapy often obtain satisfactory clinical results.

General Kinesiological Concepts

A motion segment is made up of two adjacent vertebrae with their ligamentous connecting tissues, including the intervertebral disc. In the thoracic spine the costovertebral joints are included, and in the cervical spine the joints of Lushka are included under this term. The typical motion segment consists of two posterior joints, the intervertebral disc, the ligaments (intrinsic factors), and the muscles (extrinsic factors). The latter two components combine to produce stability. Correction of motion segment dysfunction must consider both the intrinsic and extrinsic factors. Manipulative and adjustive procedures, in order to be most effective, must be given to: 1) the specific facet which is malpositioned (subluxated); 2) the facet which is blocked or restricted in its main motion (fixated); and/or 3) the holding elements by producing a dynamic stretch to the ligamentous or the more responsive muscular tissues. The adjustive thrust should therefore be directed toward the fixed facet with a line of thrust in the plane of the involved facet and in a direction which stretches the holding elements. An adjustment which includes these parameters should ensure a maximum corrective response.

The status of the various tissues in the motion segment allow for the selection of the proper manipulation technique as well as the amplitude and speed of the thrust. If joint degeneration or inflammation is present, slow mobilization or nonforce adjustive techniques may be employed. If ligaments are involved with contracture, articulating or mobilizing procedures and dynamic stretch techniques are indicated. If the dysfunction is largely due to muscular imbalance, dynamic adjustive thrusts are most effective. Hypermobile facets should not be manipulated or adjusted even in the presence of static misalignment. However, a hypermobile facet is frequently due to fixation of the opposite facet. For the same reason the interaction of various spinal levels must also be considered. For example, the relationship between the upper cervical spine and the pelvis may be clinically significant. Illi (1971) has stated that the atlas acts as a sort of hypermobile joint between the head and C2 and hence the rest of the cervical spine. He further observed that the C0, C1, and C2 segments, being the most mobile and situated on the end of a long lever arm (the spinal column), may produce static and dynamic changes throughout the whole column (Illi 1951). Adjustive procedures directed toward the upper cervical spine and the sacroiliac joint may therefore have a greater affect on general body posture than adjustments at other regions of the spine. Many techniques including the sacrooccipital (S.O.T., 1940) and Pierce-Stillwagon (1977) technique systems emphasize these relationships. In a study of 355 patients, Gregory (1978) reported a direct relationship between the correction of C1 laterality and the rotation and changes in pelvic distortion. These changes in pelvic distortion were measured with a so-called "anatometer" and were related directly to functional short-leg measurements. Similar clinical empirical observations on the effects of correcting one motion segment or area of the spine on other spinal areas are widespread. Experimental evidence for these changes, however, is not extensive. Stewart (1976) reported weight distribution changes following cervical and dorsal adjusting. My own supervised study of 53 subjects showed 56.4 percent improvement in balance on a four-quadrant weight scale measurement and plumbline postural analysis following a single adjustment. Similarly, Gillet (1975) reported that thoracic adjustive procedures caused improvement in the cervical lordosis. Controlled clinical studies are, however, necessary if we are to understand these effects.

The Upper Cervical Spine

Reports on the range of motion in the upper cervical region are quite varied. Part of the reason seems to be the variety of measurement methods utilized.

Flexion-Extension Motion. Cailliet (1964) states that there is a total flexion-extension range of motion of 35° between the occiput and atlas (10° flexion, 25° extension) (Fig. 9) while at the same time suggesting that no rotation takes place between C0 and C1. Werne (1957) using the palatine line on cadavers, showed a flexion-extension range of motion between C0 and C1 which averaged 13.4° with an additional 10° occurring between C1 and C2. Hahl (1964) and Kapandji (1974) further discuss this range of motion in flexion and extension, the former author suggests that there is 15° of flexion between C0 and C1 and 15° of extension between C1 and C2. Kapandji gives a figure of 15° total for flexion and extension between C0 and C1 using the axis of motion as a point and measur-

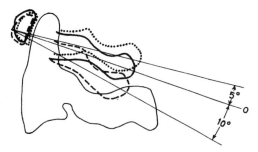

FIG. 10. **The flexion-extension range of motion between atlas (C1) and axis (C2).**

ing the angle formed by the excursion of the occipital condyle. Grice (1977) showed that flexion between C0 and C1 takes place early in the flexion motion of the cervical spine, particularly with chin retraction, and usually disappears or reverses with full forward flexion of the cervical spine. This rhythmic movement, showing first flexion of the occiput and then extension during full cervical flexion is important in radiographic functional analysis.

Flexion and extension between C1 and C2 is a complex motion taking place between the articular facets and the anterior arch of atlas and the odontoid. The motion involves rocking and gliding, and the center of motion is considered to be somewhere in the odontoid process. No single axis of motion exists. The range of motion between C1 and C2 may be up to 35° (Braakman and Penning 1971). However, the most commonly quoted range of motion is 15° (Fielding 1957) with 10° of extension and 5° of flexion (Fig. 10).

Another method of measuring flexion and extension of the upper cervical spine is to draw a line vertically through the tip and base of the odontoid process to form an angle of about 101° in the neutral position with a line drawn across the anterior and posterior lips of the foramen magnum. Braakman and Penning (1971) have demonstrated that during normal flexion and extension this angle changes a total of 11° whereas with chin retraction and chin extension (gliding movement) the angle changes a total of 31°.

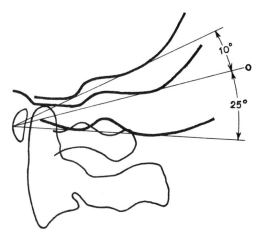

FIG. 9. **The flexion-extension range of motion between occiput (C0) and atlas (C1).**

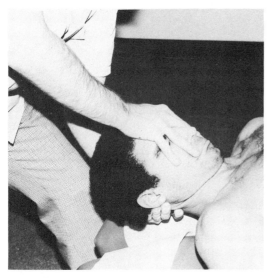

FIG. 11. **Occipital flexion traction adjustment. Thrust is given in the AP plane with traction on the occiput.**

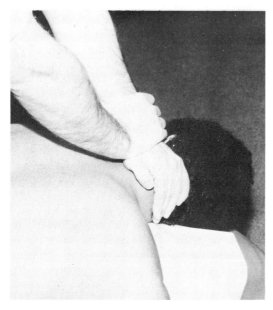

FIG. 12. **Suboccipital lift to produce flexion of the occiput.**

Flexion-Extension Adjustments of the Upper Cervical Spine. Mobilization and adjustive procedures aimed at producing a maximum range of motion in the flexion extension plane between C0 and C1 and between C1 and C2 must utilize chin retraction and chin jutting procedures. Figures 11 and 12 illustrate two suboccipital lift adjustments for the correction of flexion and extension fixations. Figure 13 demonstrates a technique which is more often utilized as an adjustment for lateral flexion and rotation of the upper cervical region. However, proper positioning can result in the centering of the adjustive force to produce flexion between C0, C1 and C2.

Lateral Motion Between C0 and C1 and C1 and C2. Lateral movement between C0 and C2 has been studied by Lewit (1965) who showed that an angulation of 5.5° takes place between the foramen magnum and C2. Braakman and Penning (1971) give a range of approximately 5° of lateral movement each between C0 and C1 and C1 and C2 (Figs. 14 and 15). Werne (1957) gives a figure of 8° between C1 and C2 while Bakke (1931) in an earlier study, gives a range of motion of 3 to 4°. Lewit (1965) states that although the main motion between C0 and C1 is flexion and extension, craniovertebral joints should be studied functionally in lateral flexion.

Laterality Adjustments of the Upper Cervical Spine. The most frequently utilized adjustment technique for occipital laterality has been presented by Janse (1947) and States (1967) and is a modification of the technique illustrated in Fig. 13. Grostic, Blair, Mears, Gregory and Pettibon are a few of the better known clinicians who have developed a specific approach to upper cervical analysis and correction. The Grostic (1966) technique which has been developed further by Gregory (NUCCA) uses a precise system of analysis and a meticulous adjusting approach. The adjustment is not given with a dynamic thrust but with a slower force of increasing magnitude. The adjustment attempts a specific correction of a subluxation through the application of a force with a con-

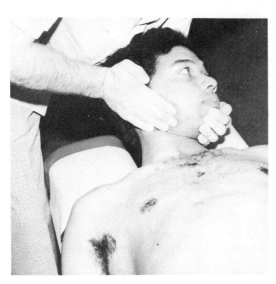

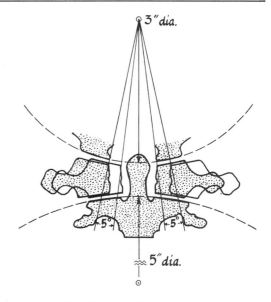

FIG. 13. **Occipital flexion adjustment given with minimal rotation, chin retraction, and a headward thrust. The inferior contact is on the occipital rim with the forearm and wrist. The fingers are lightly anchored on the mandible. This technique can be modified to give an occipital lateral flexion adjustment by applying slightly more rotation and a straight lateral flexion thrust.**

FIG. 14. **Five degrees of lateral flexion take place between C0 and C1 using the arc of the condyles to form a center of motion.**

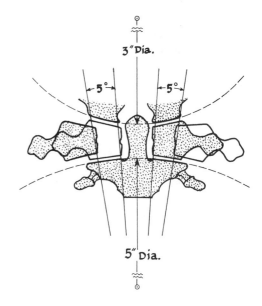

trolled direction and magnitude. The adjustment of the atlas by this tehnique has eight phases in the setup and delivery: "The Triceps Pull Phase is the final adjustive phase (Phase No. 8) in the series. The purpose of this phase is to activate the seven previous phases; to convert potential into kinetic energy" (Gregory 1978) (Fig. 16).

The technique developed by Blair (1968) is based on special radiographic analysis of the upper cervical region with emphasis on the relationship of the occipital condyle to the lateral mass of the atlas. Precise analysis of the condylar slope allows the adjustment to be given at the exact angle through the joint. The adjustment is given with torque for the simultaneous correction of anteriority or superiority (flexion and extension) as well as rotation and laterality. (Torque is a rotation component of the thrust that centers the force and attempts to impart

FIG. 15. **Five degrees of lateral flexion take place between C1 and C2 using the arc of the C2 facets to form a center of motion.**

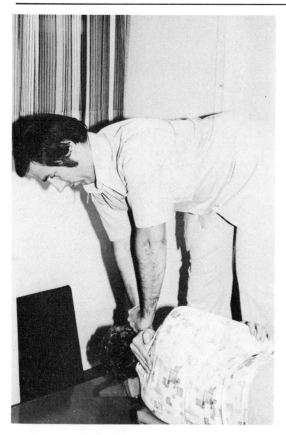

FIG. 16. **Grostic adjustment for laterality of the upper cervical spine.**

utilizes a special table with sectional drop units for the delivery of a high-velocity adjustive thrust. The table has a variable tension mechanism which can be set depending on the weight of the patient, thus allowing a lesser force to be utilized while ensuring maximum velocity.

Van Rumpt (1977) uses a light toggle thumb contact for his directional nonforce technique. The activator method, on the other hand, stresses speed and line of drive by using a small handheld adjusting gun which delivers a triggered, sharp percussion thrust.

The Palmer upper cervical toggle recoil technique utilizes a concussion of forces, applied by the hands, arms, and shoulders, to correct subluxations of the atlas and axis. The patient is placed in the side posture position with the side of C1 or C2 laterality up. The patient's head rests on a headpiece which can drop about one-half inch. The transverse process and the lamina of the axis are the usual contact points. The toggle adjustment is given with speed, di-

rotation to the motion segment.) Pettibon's method (1968) also utilizes radiographic analysis to establish a listing but the adjustment is given by means of an adjustive instrument. The technique recommended by Mears (1976) is also based on radiographic analysis. He uses a double pull-type opposing force to correct the lateral disrelationships between occiput and atlas, atlas and axis, or both. The fingers, hand, and thumb are used as directional contacts for the adjustment. The patient's position allows for a combined rotation-lateral flexion correction (Fig. 17). The Pierce-Stillwagon technique utilizes a drop headpiece for upper cervical adjustments which can be set for torque. The Thompson terminal-point technique (1977)

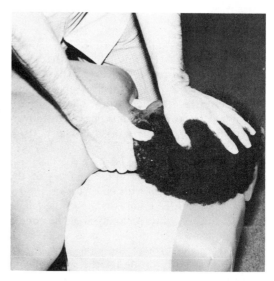

FIG. 17. **Mears technique for laterality adjustment of the upper cervical spine. Contact is on the axis with the fingers and on the atlas with the thumb, thereby producing a rotation lateral flexion correction.**

rection, torque, and recoil using the technique already demonstrated in Fig. 4A. The toggle recoil adjustment or side posture adjustments may also use the reinforced thumb for a contact (see Fig. 4B). Contacts on the articular pillars or spinous processes tend to convert this lateral thrust into a rotational adjustment. The utilization of the drop headpiece common to many of these specific techniques allows a high velocity thrust with minimal trauma to the patient.

Rotation Motion Between C1 and C2. Rotation between C1 and C2 is the major movement of the upper cervical spine and accounts for about 50 percent of the rotation of the entire cervical region. The total range of motion of the cervical region is considered to be 80 to 90° to each side (Kapandji 1974). Braakman and Penning (1971) give a total C1–C2 rotational range of motion of 100°. Werne (1975) on autopsy studies showed a rotational movement of 47° to each side while Fielding (1957) in cine radiographic studies gives a total rotational range of 90°. Selecki (1969) states that the first 30° of movement takes place between C1 and C2. Further rotation, up to approximately 45°, causes motion of the rest of the cervical spine. All of the above authors recognize the fact that lateral flexion takes place during rotation.

Rotational mobilization procedures are achieved by contacting the occiput bilaterally and performing left and right rotational movements of the cervical spine. DeJarnette's (1978) adjusting technique utilizes a figure-eight motion of the occiput with both hands on the blocked segment during the movement. Rotation adjustments of C1 and C2 are achieved in a similar manner to those of the lower cervical segments (Fig. 18). Recoil adjustments using the C2 spinous contact may also produce rotation corrections.

The Lower Cervical Spine

Pettibon (1972) suggests that the cervical lordosis from C1 to T1 usually has a radius of about 7 in. The normal cervical lordosis has an angulation of 30 to 45°, the curve being formed by the normal wedging of cervical discs. Flatten-

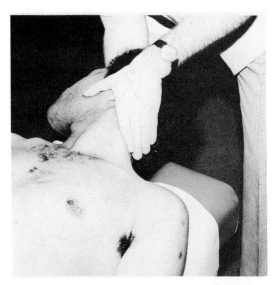

FIG. 18. **A pure rotation cervical adjustment (spine). Contact may be from C1 to T1 and a rotational thrust is used.**

ing of this curve in young women and the existence of a double lordotic curve appears to fall within the range of normal (Jochumsen 1970). The anterior-posterior visualization of the cervical spine is usually considered to be relatively straight. He found that the most common cervical curvature tended to be to the left. Similarly, Schmorl and Junghanns (1971) quote Farkas, who in 1932 suggested that 80 percent of spines show a physiological scoliosis with a left cervical, upper thoracic and lumbar curve and a right compensatory lower thoracic curve. Further studies are certainly necessary, but a mild left cervical curve would seem to be physiological.

The significance of the cervical curve in SMT is related primarily to the muscular holding elements. When the cervical curve flattens, increased activity of the splenius capitis muscle as well as the anterior cervical muscles produces flexion of the lower and midcervical vertebrae. Adjustments directed at the scalenii, longus coli, and capitis should, therefore, be from anterior to posterior (Grice 1977). A second group of muscles that may influence the cervical curve is the cervical-thoracic musculature, e.g., splenis

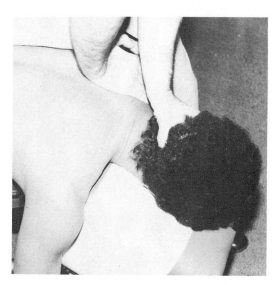

FIG. 19.   **Combination upper thoracic adjustment and cervical muscle release. Contact is on the transverse process of the thoracic segment or the angle of the ribs. A second contact is on the rim of the occiput, spinous, or transverse process of the cervical segment.**

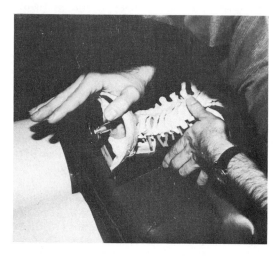

FIG. 20.   **Illustration using a bony spine of a combination cervical occipital adjustment. Contact on the transverse of the cervical segment (articular pillar). The patient's head is turned away from the contact. The second contact hand is on the occiput.**

cervicis and levator scapulae. Prone adjustments that affect thoracic and cervical correction simultaneously appear to be most effective (Figs. 19 and 20).

Increased cervical lordosis is not as common but when it exists the cervical vertebrae should not be adjusted with a rotatory "break" (rotation and lateral flexion) but with a pure rotation technique in order not to increase the extension motion of the cervical segments (see Fig. 18). Patients with an increased cervical lordosis often show an increase range of motion in lateral flexion and rotation as well as ligamentous laxity. Therefore, the adjustment should be given with minimal amplitude and force. Uniform scalenus involvement with an erect posture may also produce an increased cervical lordosis which can best be corrected by adjustments from anterior to posterior. (The scalenii muscles in the cervical region have a similar action to that of the psoas muscle in the lumbar region.)

Flexion and Extension.   In flexion and extension the superior vertebra moves forward and backward over an axis of motion located in the superior aspect of the inferior vertebral body (Fig. 21). This arc of motion is slightly flatter in the lower cervical region and the axis of motion has a longer radius than in the upper cervical region. When manipulating or adjusting a patient, the direction of thrust or motion as well as the patient's position must be such as to mobilize the cervical vertebrae along this arc of motion. During flexion, the superior vertebra tilts and glides forward over the vertebra below. The intervertebral disc is compressed on the anterior and opens on the posterior while the whole disc is stretched in a ventral direction. The superior facet slides upwards and separates slightly in its inferior aspect and, at the limit of the range of motion, the capsule is tightened. The rhythm of the motion is such that tilting and gliding occur simultaneously. Extension of the cervical spine biomechanically is similar to flexion except that it is in the reverse direction. The flexion:extension ratio is usually 2:1.

When adjusting to produce flexion the thrust

should come from inferior to superior. Slight cervical flexion prior to the thrust is advisable. Since there is a 2:1 ratio of flexion to extension, most fixations develop in the plane of the greatest range of motion, i.e., flexion. Therefore, an adjustive force should be directed from posterior to anterior. An adjustment directed from anterior to posterior is possible with the patient sitting, the cervical spine slightly ex-

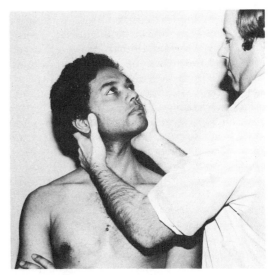

FIG. 22. **The sitting anterior to posterior adjustment. Contact is made on the anterior transverse process. The patient's head is cradled in both hands which produces extension and traction. The thrust is given from inferior to superior. The muscles are stretched and the motion segment is released along the arc of motion of the joints of Luschka. Contact may be made as high as the mastoid or as low as C6.**

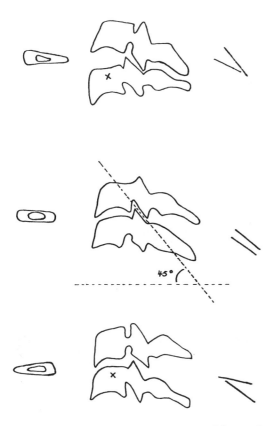

FIG. 21. **Flexion-extension movement of the cervical spine. In the neutral position there is a 45° angle facing. Flexion causes anterior compression of disc with tightening of posterior fibers due to forward gliding. The facets move by gliding and tilting. The axis of motion illustrated with an X is located in the superior aspect of the lower motion segment. Extension causes disc compression posteriorly. The facets move by posterior gliding and tilting. The axis of motion shown by X in inferior motion segment.**

tended, and the adjustive force directed from inferior to superior along the first half of the arc of motion of the segment (Fig. 22).

Lateral Flexion and Rotation. Lateral flexion motion is always combined or coupled with rotation. During lateral flexion, rotation occurs in such a way that the spinous process moves toward the side opposite that of lateral flexion. Braagman and Penning (1971) have observed that the deviation is minimal at C7 and maximal at C2. Jirout (1971) suggested that there are three types of coupled motion in the sagittal plane. Lateral flexion Type I motion is characterized by ventral tilting of the vertebra, Type II by caudal tilting, and Type III by no tilting or by maintenance of a neutral position. They noted that Type I motion was the most common. The nature of tilting relates to the forces acting on the cervical vertebrae through the cervical ligaments (ligamentum nuchae) and muscles. If the cervicocranial forces are more active (via the craniocervical muscles) ventral tilting (Type I) would occur. However, if cervicodorsal forces (via the cervicothoracic muscles) were more active dorsal tilting (Type II) would occur. Equalization of these forces would result in no tilting (Type III) motion.

A muscle in contraction could, therefore, produce fixation or aberrant action at its origin and at its insertion. Therefore adjustive procedures should locate areas of possible subluxation as well as related or paired fixations. Ventral tilting Type I biomechanical changes may lead to loss of the cervical curve, whereas Type II caudal tilting may lead to an increase in the cervical curve. This phenomenon may explain the clinical observation that thoracic adjustments tend to reduce cervical lordosis (Gillet and Liekins 1968; Watkins 1969).

The range of motion in rotation varies from about 5 to 10° at each segment of the lower cervical spine while the amount of lateral flexion varies from about 6° to 10°. Lateral flexion and rotation show a direct and reciprocal relationship (Lysell 1971). During full flexion the cervical facets are in a state of almost complete separation and therefore cervical adjustments should never be given during full flexion of any segment. Bard and Jones (1964) showed that during traction slight separation of the facets takes place. During cervical manipulation or adjustment, slight traction should therefore make correction easier.

A few manipulative procedures for rotation and lateral flexion have already been described: Figure 7B shows mobilization in flexion, Figure 7A shows a muscle technique for the lateral cervical musculature, and Figure 6 shows a lateral flexion mobilization procedure. Additional techniques for adjusting the spine in various positions have been developed since certain problems such as acute torticollis, severe pain, vertigo, chronic illness, or disability make it difficult for a patient to assume certain positions of the cervical spine. Cervical spine adjustments can therefore be applied in the seated, supine, or prone positions. In recent years techniques have been developed which have fairly minor

biomechanical, kinesiologic, and/or neurologic differences. A selective approach to their application is becoming increasingly important. The plane of the vertebral articulations has been considered the most important factor in determining the direction of the adjustive force by many early chiropractors such as Smith et al. (1906) and Palmer (1911). Although this factor is still considered to be of major importance, increased emphasis is now being placed on the arc of motion of the motion segment and on the muscular holding elements. Cervical adjustive techniques may be carried out with the active and passive motion being eliminated and the thrust directed through to the elastic range of the motion segment. Janse (1947) and States (1967) demonstrate lateral flexion adjustments referred to as cervical "break" techniques. These maneuvers are performed to create lateral movement in the cervical spine. The patient's position is such that the head is held straight and the contact made in such a way as to produce straight lateral movement of the

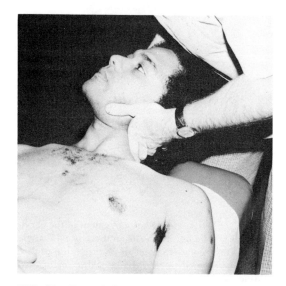

FIG. 23. **Lateral flexion cervical adjustment. Patient's chin is kept in neutral upright position. Lateral flexion slack is taken out and the thrust is given from superior to inferior with slight headward traction.**

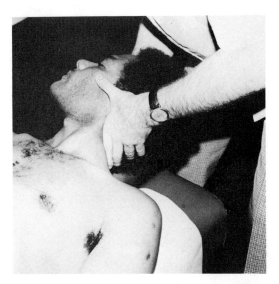

FIG. 24. **Combined lateral flexion· and rotation cervical adjustment. Patient's head is rotated about 45°; the adjustment is given similarly to that shown in Figure 23.**

selected segment (Fig. 23). A combined rotation and lateral flexion maneuver can be achieved by rotating the head 45° with simultaneous lateral flexion of the cervical vertebra being adjusted. This maneuver is called a "rotary break." These adjustments are usually given with a dynamic adjustive thrust of small amplitude and the minimal effective force (Fig. 24).

Adjustments in lateral flexion should consider the arc of motion of the joints of Luschka as illustrated in Figure 25. It is especially important that patients with degenerative changes, angulated, or deep joints of Luschka be adjusted with this arc of motion in mind in order to produce a pain-free adjustment. In supine adjustments where the thrust comes from superior to inferior, consideration of this plane of motion can be achieved by utilizing finger push spinous or articular pillar contacts. Sitting adjustments from the anterior utilizing thrusts coming from inferior to superior also relate to this arc of motion. Since degenerative cervical spines are more easily and painlessly adjusted in

the supine or sitting positions, selectivity and expertise in a variety of techniques is important.

Restricted gliding or flexion movement of the cervical motion segments can best be corrected by partial flexion and rotation of the cervical spine. Certain patients with long supple cervical spines are more easily adjusted in rotation. Adjustments in lateral flexion or half lateral flexion may stress the ligaments which are often slack in these patients. At the same time the joints of Luschka are often deep and angulated due to increased mobility.

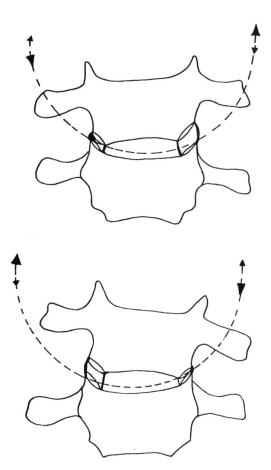

FIG. 25. **Cross section of the bodies of a cervical motion segment showing the arc of motion produced by the joints of Luschka.**

The Thoracic Spine

The thoracic curvature is formed at birth. This is in contrast to the cervical curve which forms by extension as the baby learns to lift its head and develop head control. The normal thoracic kyphosis may be influenced by muscle and gravitational forces acting on the thoracic curve as well as muscular responses to viscerosomatic and psychosomatic reflexes. The depth of the thoracic curve is often considered to be associated with the depth of the lumbar curve. However, the posture or position of the occiput in relation to the gravity line and the influence of the postural muscles (e.g., the semispinalis capitis, which extends from the occiput down as far as T7) may also have a significant effect on the dorsal kyphosis.

Study of the mechanics of motion in the thoracic spine has been largely neglected. White (1969) probably has the best study available in this area. In the thoracic spine, the kyphotic curve is formed by wedging of the vertebral

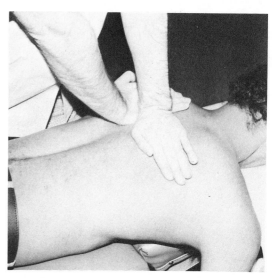

FIG. 27. **Cross bilateral thoracic adjustment. Contact on transverse process of motion segment on opposite sides produces counterrotation correction.**

bodies. The thoracic disc margins are parallel to each other in the lateral plane while the vertebral bodies are 1 to 2 mm narrower on anterior than on posterior measurement. The height of the disc in relation to the body of the vertebra is about 25 percent, suggesting that there is less mobility than in the cervical or lumbar region. This is due primarily to the rib attachments which limit flexibility in the thoracic spine. These factors make it important to limit the depth or amplitude of dorsal and rib adjustments. The thoracic facets are coronal in orientation, those of the lower dorsal spine being slightly more oblique than in the upper dorsal region. Lines drawn perpendicular to each facet intersect anterior to the thoracic body indicating an axis of rotation anterior to the vertebral body (Fig. 26).

The thoracic spine has well-developed rotatory and multifidus muscles both of which aid to produce sharp segmental rotation. Adjustments such as the crossed bilateral technique with its multiple modifications which attempt to correct rotation fixations are therefore important (Fig. 27).

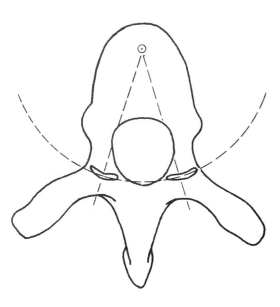

FIG. 26. **Superior view of a typical thoracic segment showing the facets which form an arc of rotation whose center is the anterior body.**

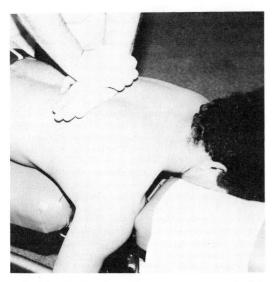

FIG. 28. **Knife-edge spinous contact producing flexion of the superior segment. Angulation of the contact may introduce simultaneous rotational correction.**

Flexion-Extension Motion. Little or no interest has been shown in the range or motion of the thoracic spine. White (1978) presents a median of 4° of motion for the upper thoracic segments and 12° of motion each for the T11, T12, and L1 segments. The instantaneous axis of motion for flexion is located in the anterior lower aspect of the body of the vertebra below and for extension in the anterior superior aspect of the body of the vertebra below .

Since the axis for extension is located in the superior aspect of the body below a knife edge contact on the spinous process becomes an important adjustment (Fig. 28). During this adjustment the contact is taken with pressure below the spinous process. A soft contact is used since the patient's spinous tip is often exquisitely tender. The thrust is given from inferior to superior. Single, double, or bridge contacts on the transverse process may be used for flexion fixations in the dorsal spine.

Lateral Flexion Motion. As in other areas of the spine, lateral flexion is accompanied by ro-

tation and movement in the sagittal plane. Lateral motion totals about 52° to each side with intersequential movement of about 5 to 6° in the upper segments and 8 to 9° in the lower segments. During lateral flexion the instantaneous axis of motion is located in the body of the vertebra below. This author's studies suggest that, in general, the upper thoracic vertebrae behave similar to a cervical motion segment while the lower thoracic vertebrae behave similar to a lumbar segment.

Mobilization procedures may be performed in the side posture position (Fig. 29) (Grecco 1953; Maigne 1972). These techniques can be modified by incorporating a dynamic thrust for the adjustive correction of a specific motion segment. Lateral flexion adjustments that

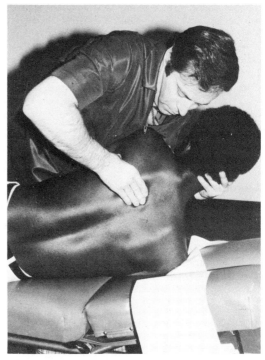

FIG. 29. **The side posture lateral flexion spinous contact may be utilized for mobilization of the thoracic spine employing slow rhythmic traction or as an adjustment by introducing traction, lateral flexion, and a dynamic thrust.**

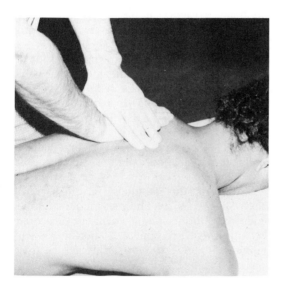

FIG. 30. **Single pisiform lateral flexion transverse process contact. The dynamic adjustive thrust is given from inferior to superior. The procedure may be modified to correct costovertebral fixations by taking a contact on the angle of the rib and thrusting from either inferior to superior or superior to inferior.**

utilize the transverse process as a lever may be performed with either a single pisiform (Fig. 30) or double pisiform (Fig. 27) contact.

Rotation Motion. Rotation in the thoracic spine is coupled with lateral flexion and occurs primarily during lateral flexion in the lower thoracic spine. The normal rotation movement in this region is similar to that of the lumbar spine, i.e., spinous rotation is toward the concavity (Type I motion) (Grice 1979). In the upper thoracic spine, rotation during lateral flexion is similar to that in the cervical spine; i.e., the rotation of the spinous process is toward the convexity (Type II motion) (Grice 1979). Clinically, there is an additional coupled motion in the sagittal plane during rotation. In the lower thoracic region this motion appears to be extension, whereas in the lower thoracic region it is flexion. The transition point for these movements in the transverse and sagittal plane

is approximately T6. This transition point is a key area for spinous tenderness and subluxation. A flattening or saucer effect may also occur in the area.

The rotation range of motion for the whole thoracic spine is 41°. Each vertebral segment in the upper area moves about 8° with the lower three thoracic segments moving only about 2° (White 1978).

Many adjustments for the correction of rotational subluxations may also be effective for the coupled lateral flexion or flexion-extension subluxations. Sitting and prone rotational mobilization techniques are also effective for costovertebral fixations (Fig. 31; see also Fig. 18). There are many variations of this procedure described in the literature (States 1967; Grecco 1953; Janse 1947). In the upper thoracic region where rotational fixations are very common a TM (thumb move) adjustment may be very effective (Fig. 32).

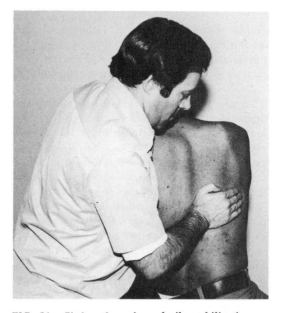

FIG. 31. **Sitting thoracic and rib mobilization or adjustive procedure. Contact is taken on the transverse or angle of the ribs. The patient's arms are crossed in front. A second contact is taken on the elbow of the superior arm.**

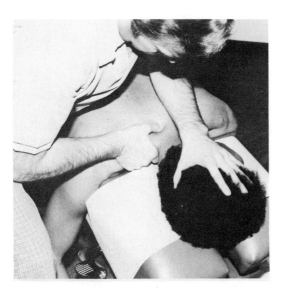

FIG. 32. **Upper thoracic thumb move (TM) rotation adjustment. The direction of the thrust is straight lateral through the spinous of the upper thoracic vertebrae. The second contact is on the occiput and/or the spinous of the cervical motion segment.**

Manipulative and adjustive procedures in the thoracic spine have tended to be more general in their application than is the case for other areas of the spine and, thus, fewer specific adjustive techniques have been developed.

Costovertebral and Costocostal Articulations. There are two basic movements of the rib cage: a bucket-handle-type motion and a caliperlike motion. These are the basic movements during respiration. During quiet breathing, minimal activity of the ribs is present. Forced breathing causes greater movement with elevation and expansion of the chest cage. The upper ribs move anterior and superior while the lower ribs widen the chest cage with a caliper effect. Subluxations of ribs appear as posterior movement abnormalities (opening of the caliper) (Fig. 33) or as superior or inferior coupled motions (the bucket handle effect) (Fig. 34). It is important to ascertain which muscles are producing the abnormality. This will allow for a more correct line of drive during the adjustment. Spinal curvatures may also deform the rib cage and vice versa. Therefore, costothoracic adjustments must take into consideration both the rib cage and thoracic spine.

Figures 35 and 36 demonstrate general thoracic manipulative procedures in the supine and standing positions. The latter procedure utilizes the more general contact. Both of these procedures are referred to as anterior thoracic adjustments and have been demonstrated in texts by B.J. Palmer (1911), Gregory (1912), Janse (1947), States (1967), Stoddard (1969), Fryette (1959), Mennel (1960), Maigne (1972), and Fisk (1977). The standing adjusting tech-

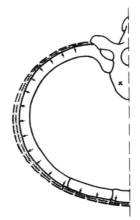

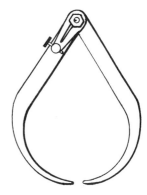

FIG. 33. **Caliper-like motion of the lower ribs. Costovertebral fixations may appear as a posterior displacement.**

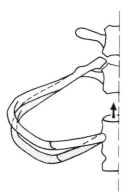

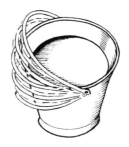

FIG. 34. **Bucket-handle effect on the upper ribs may result in costovertebral or costo-costal fixations (superior or inferior ribs).**

nique produces flexion of the vertebra as well as costovertebral mobilization. It can be applied in the sitting position, using the clinician's chest or knee as a contact. The contact may be reinforced by a roll or pillow (Fig. 37). This procedure is corrective for flattening (common saucer) in the mid-upper-dorsal region. It separates the ribs at the same time flexing the thoracic segments.

Cervical thoracic adjustive procedures such as the prone combination contact shown in Figure 19 are indicated when the cervicothoracic musculature is producing a postural or fixation fault. The fact that active postural muscles from the occiput and cervical spine attach as far down as T6 or T7 must be kept in mind. Semispinalis capitus contraction may produce direct effects in the thoracic as well as the upper cervical region. Semispinalis cervicis, splenius capitis, and cervicis, as well as the sacrospinalis muscles, may also be involved in combined cervical and thoracic subluxations.

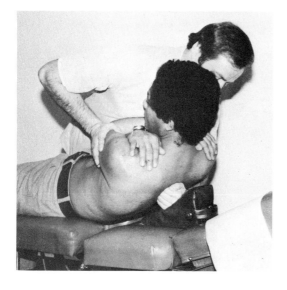

FIG. 35. **Supine costovertebral adjustment. This adjustment may be utilized during pregnancy.**

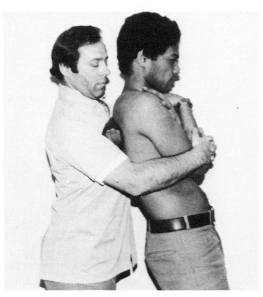

FIG. 36. **Standing costovertebral adjustment.**

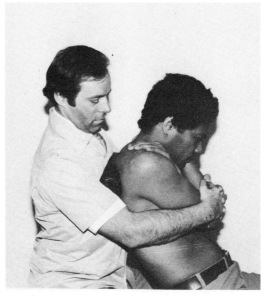

FIG. 37. **Sitting costovertebral adjustment.**

The pelvic and lumbar thoracic musculature (sacrospinalis longissimus) may be involved in fixations of the lower thoracic spine and rib cage in addition to lumbar or sacroiliac fixations. The latter fixations may be adjusted by combined pelvic-thoracic moves (Fig. 38) and/or sitting thoracic or rib adjustments (see Fig. 31).

Thoracic vertebra and rib techniques are, in many cases, similar in that the only variation is the point of contact. There are, in addition, mobilization procedures which correct rib static or dynamic subluxations from the lateral or anterior aspect of the rib cage. These procedures are carried out in the sitting or supine positions. Deep breathing is utilized during rib adjustments in order to facilitate the motion. Lower rib subluxations may be related to diaphragm activity and techniques to release diaphragm spasm and elevate the rib cage may be beneficial (Figs. 39 and 40). A side posture adjustment (Fig. 41) allows unrestricted correction of rib subluxations. The direction of thrust and traction may be varied during this adjustment.

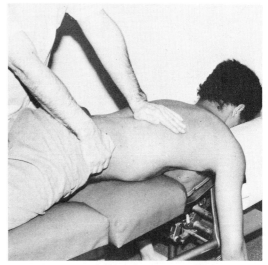

FIG. 38. **Prone vertebral or rib adjustment for correcting rotational subluxations and stretching sacrospinalis musculature.**

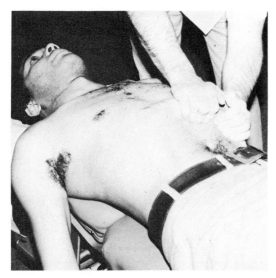

FIG. 39. **Anterior rib technique for mobilization of the lower ribs in the presence of intercostal and diaphragm muscular involvement.**

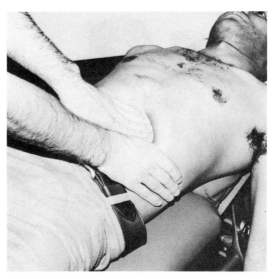

FIG. 40. **Diaphragm and abdominal muscular technique for mobilization of lower ribs.**

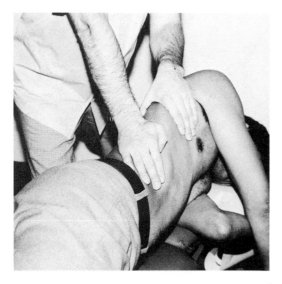

FIG. 41. **Side posture rib technique for intercostal musculature and bucket-handle mobilization.**

Acknowledgments

I would like to express my gratitude to Dr. R. Johnston for his advice and Cornelius Klamer for the art work. My thanks to Beryl Davidson for her many corrections, Johanna Klamer for assembly of the materials, my wife for many hours of help, and the students at C.M.C.C. for their assistance.

REFERENCES

Amodel JE: A technique for the painless correction of torticollis. J Nat Chiropr Assoc, December 1958, p 17

Bard G, Jones M: Cineradiographic recording of traction of the cervical spine. Arch Phys Med Rehabil, August 1964, p 403

Bakke SN: Rontgenologische beobachtungen uber die bewegungen der wirbelsaule. Acta Radiol [Suppl] 13, 1931

Beatty HG: Anatomical Adjustive Technique. Denver, 1939

Blair WC: Research for Evaluation for Progress. Int Rev Chiropr Part I, February 1968; Part II, April 1968

Braakman R, Penning L: Injuries of the cervical spine. Excerpta Med 1971

Cailliet R: Neck and Arm Pain. Philadelphia, F. A. Davis, 1964

Carver F: The Postural Method of Chiropractic Diagnosis and Adjusting. Wichita, 1938.

Carver W: Carver's Chiropractic Analysis of Chiropractic Principles as Applied to Pathology, Relatology, Symptomatology and Diagnosis. Oklahoma City, Self-published, 1909

Conley RN: Stress evaluation of cervical spinal mechanics. J Clin Chiropr 1(3) Special Edition, 1974

Davis AP: Neuropathy. Baker City OR, F. L. Rowe, 1909

DeJarnette MB: Sacro-Occipital Technique of Spinal Therapy. Nebraska City, NB, Self-published, 1940

DeJarnette MB: Sacro-OccipitalTechnic. Nebraska City, NB, 1978

England RW, Deibert PW: Electromyographic studies: Part I. Consideration in the evaluation of osteopathic therapy. J Am Osteop Assoc, October 1972, p 162

Fielding JW: Cineroentgenography of the normal cervical spine. J Bone Joint Surg 39A:1280, 1957

Fisk JW: The Painful Neck and Back. Springfield, IL, Thomas, 1978

Gillet H, Liekens ME: Belgian Chiropractic Research Notes. 10th ed. Brussels, Belgium 1973

Gillet XM: Investigation into the effect of upper thoracic manipulation on the cervical lordosis in the elderly. Bournemonth, Anglo European Chiropractic College, 1975

Glover JR: Characterization of localized back pain. In Buerger AA, Tobis JS (eds): Approaches to the Validation of Manipulative Therapy. Springfield, IL, Thomas, 1977

Gonstead CS: Gonstead Chiropractic In Herbst TW (ed): Science and Healing Art. Mt. Horeb, WI, Sci-Chi Publications, 1968

Gravel P, Gravel A: Gravel Integrated Chiropractic Methods. Montreal, 1966

Grecco MA: Chiropractic Technique Illustrated. New York, Jarl, 1953

Gregory AA: Spinal Treatment. 2nd ed. Oklahoma City, Palmer-Gregory College, 1912

Gregory R: The A.S.C. and Leg Imbalance. The National Upper Cervical Chiropractic Association News. Vol 1, No. 7, 1969

Gregory R: The Upper Cervical Monograph. Vol 2, No 4, 1978

Gregory R: The Upper Cervical Monograph. Vol 2, No 5, 1978

Grice AS: Muscle tonus change following manipulation. J Can Chiropr Assoc, December 1974, p 29

Grice AS: Preliminary evaluation of 50 sagittal cervical motion radiographic evaluations. J Can Chiropr Assoc, March 1977, p 33

Grice AS: Scalenus anticus syndrome: diagnosis and chiropractic adjustive procedure. J Can Chiropr Assoc, March 1977, p 5

Grice AS: Radiographic biomechanical and clinical factors in lumbar lateral flexion. J Manip Physiol Therapeut 2, 1:26, 1979

Grostic J: Unpublished notes, 1966

Hahl M: Normal motions in the upper portion of the cervical spine. J Bone Joint Surg 46:1777, 1964

Haldeman S: The importance of research in principles and practice of chiropractic. J Can Chiropr Assoc 20, 3:7, 1976

Hildebrandt RW: Chiropractic Spinography. A Manual of Technology and Interpretation. Des Plaines, IL, Hilmark Publications, 1977

Hildebrandt RW: The scope of chiropractic as a clinical science and art: an introductory review of concepts. J Manip Physiol Therapeut 1, 1:7, 1978

Homewood AE: The Neurodynamics of the Vertebral Subluxation. Toronto, 1962

Illi FWH: The Vertebral Column: Life-Line of the Body. Lombard, National Chiropractic College, 1951

Illi FWH: Chiropractic, Locomotion Static Vertebrale. Geneva, 1952

Illi FWH: Highlights of 45 Years of Experience and 35 Years of Research,Presented at European Chiropractic Union Convention. May, 1971

Janse J, Houser R, Wells B: Chiropractic Principles and Technique. Lombard, IL, National College of Chiropractic, 1947

Jirout J: Patterns of changes in the cervical spine on lateroflexion. Neuroradiology 2:164, 1971

Jirout J: Changes in the atlas-axis relations on lateral flexion of the head and neck. Neuroradiology 6: 215, 1973

Jochumsen OH: The curve of the cervical spine. ACA J Chiropr, August 1970, p 49

Kapandji IA: The physiology of the joints. Vol. III. The Trunk and Vertebral Column. Churchill Livingstone, London. 1974.

Kotheimer WJ: Applied Chiropractic in Distortion Analysis. Philadelphia, Dorrance, 1976

Kuntz A: Autonomic Nervous System. Philadelphia, Lea & Febiger, 1953

Lewitt K. Krausova: The mechanism and the measuring of the mobility in the craniocervical joints during lateral inclinations. Acta Univ Carol, Med, [Suppl] 21:123, 1965

Logan HB: Textbook of Logan Basic Methods. St. Louis, Logan Chiropractic College. 1950

Lomax E: Manipulative therapy: A historical perspective from ancient times to the modern era. In Goldstein M (ed): The Research Status of Spinal Manipulative Therapy. NINCDS Monograph No. 15. Washington, DHEW, 1973

Lysell E: The patterns of motion in the cervical spine. In Hirsch C, Zotterman Y (eds): Cervical Spine. Vol 19. New York, Pergamon Press, 1971

Maigne R: Orthopedic Medicine. Springfield, IL, Thomas, 1972

Mears DB: The Mears Technic. St. Albans, VT, 1976

Mennell JM: Back Pain. Boston, Little, Brown, 1960

Müller RO: Autonomics in Chiropractic. Toronto, Chiro, 1954

Overton RM: Explanation of a technique for eliminating torticollis. J Nat Chiropr Assoc, September 1958, p 19

Palmer BJ: The Science of Chiropractic. Vol III. Davenport, IA, Palmer School of Chiropractic. 1911

Palmer BJ: The Subluxation Specific The Adjustment Specific. Davenport, IA, Palmer School of Chiropractic, 1934

Palmer DD: The Science Art and Philosophy of Chiropractic. Portland Printing House, 1910

Petersen AP: Segmental Neuropathy. Toronto, Candian Chiropractic College, 1970

Pierce W, Stillwagon G: Pierce-Stillwagon Technique. In Kfoury PW (ed): Catalog of Chiropractic Techniques. St. Louis, Logan Coll Chiropr 1977

Pettibon BR: Pettibon Method Cervical X-ray Analysis and Instrument Adjusting. Tacoma, B. R. Pettibon and Associates Inc. 1968

Pettibon BR: The concept of cervical unit subluxations. Dig Chiropr Econ March/April 1972, p 48

Roston JB, Haines WR: Cracking in the metacarpophalangeal joint. J Anat 81: 1947

Sandoz R: The significance of the manipulative crack and of other articular noises. Ann Swiss Chiropr Assoc 4:47, 1969

Sandoz R: Some physical measurements and effects of spiral adjustments. Ann Swiss Chiropr Assoc 6:92, 1976

Schafer RC: Chiropractic Health Care. 2nd ed. Des Moines, IA, Foundation for Chiropractic Education and Research. 1976

Schmorl G, Junghanns H: The Human Spine in Health and Disease. New York, Grune & Stratton, 1971

Selecki BR: The effect of rotation of the atlas on the axis: experimental work. Med J Austr, May 1969, p 1012

Smith OG, Langworthy SM, Paxson MC: Modernized Chiropractic. Cedar Rapids, IA, Laurence Press, 1906

States A: Spinal and Pelvic Technics. Lombard, IL, National Chiropractic College. 1967

Stewart GD: A Statistical Analysis of Variations in Weight Distribution due to Chiropractic Adjustment. Bournemouth, Anglo European Chiropractic College. 1976

Still AT: Osteopathy Research and Practice. Kirksville, MO, 1910

Stoddard A: Manual of Osteopathic Practice. New York, Harper & Row, 1969

Thompson C: Thompson Terminal Point Technique. In Kfoury W (ed): Catalog of Chiropractic Techniques. St. Louis, Logan Chiropractic College, 1977

VanRumpt R: Directional Non-force Technic (D.N.F.T.). In Kfoury W (ed): Catalog of Chiropractic Techniques. St. Louis, Logan Chiropractic College, 1977

Verner JR: The Science and Logic of Chiropractic. Self-published. Englewood, NJ, 1941

Watkins RJ: Upper Cervical Mechanics. J Clin Chiropr 2, 2:18, 1969

Werne S, Munksgaard E: Studies in Spontaneous Atlas Dislocation Acta Orthop Scand [Suppl] 13, 1957

White AA: Analysis of the mechanics of the thoracic spine in man. Acta Orthop Scand [Suppl] 127, 1969

White AA, Panjabi MM: The Clinical Biomechanics of the Spine. Philadelphia, Lippincott, 1978

Winterstein JF: Chiropractic Spinographology. Lombard, IL. National College, 1971

CHAPTER SIXTEEN
Complications of and Contraindications to Spinal Manipulative Therapy
ANDRIES M. KLEYNHANS

One of the great advantages of manipulations is that they are harmless. Why do we often repeat this statement, which we know to be false?—Because the severe dangers, sometimes fatal ones, that weigh heavily upon treatment by manipulations, are really extremely rare, and all factors taken into consideration, can nearly always be avoided.

Lescure 1954

An old adage in chiropractic claims, "It is more important to know when not to adjust than when to adjust" (Palmer BJ 1934). It has also been suggested that poorly executed adjustments may generate all the symptoms usually corrected by these maneuvers. (Lescure 1954; Maigne 1972; Sandoz and Lorenz 1960).

In accordance with these observations, the complications of spinal adjustments, the mechanisms by which they occur, and the cautions and contraindications which should be observed in applying spinal manipulative therapy will be discussed.

For present purposes, the terms *adjustment, chiropractic. adjustment, chiropractic manipulation,* and *manipulation* will be used interchangeably and refer to dynamic thrusts applied to the spinal column. These procedures are included under the abbreviation SMT (spinal manipulative therapy) and are differentiated from "mobilization" as described by Maitland (1973).

Complications from SMT may be classified as follows (Livingstone 1971):

Accidents—serious impairments, permanent or fatal, resulting from SMT
Incidents—consequences of SMT which are noticeable by their seriousness or their long duration

Reactions—consequences of SMT which are slight and short lived
Indirect complications—consequences of SMT resulting from delayed diagnosis and rational treatment

Incidents and accidents are similar and represent mainly a difference in severity—accidents being the more serious (Lescure 1954).

Frequency of Accidents and Incidents From Spinal Adjustments

Brewerton (1964) stated that "even though deaths have occurred following manipulations, it has to be pointed out that the mortality rate, when compared with the number of manipulations carried out daily, is indeed negligible." Members of the French League Against Rheumatism were questioned on chiropractic and 46 out of 375 responded. Twenty-five had observed no accidents caused by chiropractors in their own practice. Twenty-one had personally observed severe accidents or serious and long-standing incidents following chiropractic treatment. These complications of SMT included three cases of quadriplegia, four cases of paraplegia, six cases of worsened vertebral pain with persistent neurological disturbances, five cases of fracture, and a number of cases in which lumbago and sciatica were aggravated. The symptoms in 5 out of 1000 patients are reported to be exacerbated permanently or temporarily through SMT applied by physiotherapists (Paris 1965; Nwuga 1976). Referring to a fatal vertebrobasilar accident resulting from slight head rotation induced by a patient's wife "to relieve cervical tension," Maigne commented that such accidents are exceptional in view of the great number of manipulations that are carried out, correctly or incorrectly, every day. "There is probably less than one death of this nature out of several tens of millions of manipulations." He also reported that an examination of the records of 10,000 patients treated over a 15-year period in the institution with which he is associated, showed that there was not one single undesirable result (Maigne 1972). It may therefore be concluded that "manipulation is a good therapeutic procedure with few complications, provided high standards of manipulative therapy are applied." (Lewit 1972).

A statistical breakdown of the total number of accidents from SMT reported in literature is given in Table 1. Analysis of these statistics reveals that the prime age range for SMT accidents is 35 to 49 years, and that disability occurs considerably more often than death.

Accidents and Incidents Caused by Cervical SMT

Accidents Resulting in Vertebrobasilar Insult

It has been stated that vertebrobasilar accidents comprise the most severe complications of spinal manipulative therapy (Maigne 1969). A literature review of accidents resulting in vertebrobasilar insult is presented in Table 2. These figures suggest that the use of combined rotation and hyperextension during the adjustment is a common etiological factor. The incidence of complications appears to be highest in the 35 to 42-year-old age group.

Thrombosis appears to be the major cause of vertebrobasilar insult. Its manifestations de-

TABLE 1. **Analysis of Cited Accidents From SMT**

	Nature of Injury			
	Vertebrobasilar Insult	Unclassified Vascular and Neurological Complications	Spontaneous or Self-Inflicted Verbetral Artery Accidents	Total
No. of cases	25	25	8	58
Male	8	11	6	25
Female	17	14	2	33
Mean age	33–42	33–45	40–60	35–49
Adjustment performed by				
Chiropractor	7	19	0	26
Medical chiropractor (Germany)	10	4	0	14
Medical manipulator	8	2	0	10
Nonmanipulative trauma	0	0	8	8
Deaths (%)	39	4	25	22
Permanent disability (%)	59	96	75	76
Full recovery (%)	2	0	0	2

TABLE 2. **Accidents Due to Vertebrobasilar Insult from Cervical Adjustments***

Author/Year	Case Age/Sex	Adjusted/ Manipulated by*	Etiology/Mechanism of Injury	Sequelae
Boudin et al. 1958	32 F	C	Hyperextension of cervicals probably responsible for partial thrombosis of collaterals of basilar trunk	Uneasiness with headache; disturbance of sleep (first 24 hr); sudden quadraplegia, nuclear paralysis (III & IV right) and central left facial paralysis; after 4 wk, right hemiplegia remained
Davidson et al. 1975	42 F	C	Adjustment causing persistent pseudoaneurysm of right vertebral artery at C2	Neurological deficit
Green and Joynt 1959	31 F	C	Adjustment of patient with disseminated sclerosis caused vascular accident of cerebral trunk	Vertigo, nausea, vomiting, speech impediment, diplopia, motor, and sensory disturbances of left upper and lower extremities and horizontal nystagmus
Hardin and Cole (Cited by Masson and Cambier)	50 M	C (?)	Stenosis of right vertebral artery, level C5/C6, caused by osteophyte, with complete obstruction on rotation of head to right	Neurological symptoms typical of vertebrobasilar insufficiency
Heyden 1971	29 F	MC	Hyperextension, hyper-flexion and side rotation assumed to have caused vertebral artery injury	Neurological deficit
Kanshepolsky et al. 1972	39 F	C	Adjustment of the cervical spine resulting in spasm of vertebral artery (left at C2/C3)	Neurological deficit
Kunkle et al. 1952	35 M	M	Series of adjustments with unusually forceful extension and rotation of neck and head resulted in right vertebral artery insult; blockage not confirmed	Wallenberg's syndrome
Lorenz et al. 1972	39 F	MC	Attempted chiropractic adjustment resulted in basilar artery injury	Death (after 58 days)

(continued)

TABLE 2 *(continued)*

Author/Year	Case Age/Sex	Adjusted/ Manipulated by*	Etiology/Mechanism of Injury	Sequelae
Lyness et al. 1974	20 F	C (?)	Head rotation to both sides led to neurological deficit; angiography showed narrowing of basilar and vertebral arteries, possible closure left vertebral artery; aneurysm right internal carotid at C1 level	Neurological deficit
Mehalic et al. 1974	40 M	MC	Forceful rotation of head to both sides along with extension caused segmental narrowing of the right vertebral artery at C1/C2	Neurological deficit
Miller et al. 1974	52 F	MC	Repeated adjustments with painful head rotation caused posteroinferior cerebellar arterial thrombosis	Permanent neurological impairment (Wallenberg's syndrome)
	35 M	MC	Forced rotational manipulation caused left posterior cerebral arterial insult	Unconsciousness; full recovery
Mueller et al. 1976	38 M	MC	Several mechanical spinal treatments produced a deficit of posteroinferior cerebellar artery—right vertebral arterial irregularly filled in end portion	Neurological deficit
Nick et al. 1967	48 F	M	Probable cervical adjustment for suboccipital headaches and depression; arteriography showed obliteration of left vertebral artery at occipital foramen	Diplopia; violent suboccipital pain; instability standing; trigeminal anesthesia
	—M	M	Cervicobrachial nerve pain after violent lifting effort. Subsequent traction and manipulation caused incident; left vertebral artery smaller and deviated at C5/C6 disc due to osteophyte—worse on right head rotation	Feet and hands paresthesia; "electric shocks" in spine and extremities on neck flexion and coughing; left spastic gait; pyramidal hypertonus of left leg; consequent Brown-Sequard syndrome on left below T_4 and left cerebellar disturbances

TABLE 2 *(continued)*

Author/Year	Case Age/Sex	Adjusted/ Manipulated by*	Etiology/Mechanism of Injury	Sequelae
Pratt-Thomas et al.1947	32 M	M	Manipulation for persistent headaches injured basilar artery, left anteriorinferior cerebellar, right postero-inferior cerebellar artery	Death after 24 hr preceded by spasmodic quadraplegia, respiratory difficulties
	35 F	C	Adjustment injured right vertebral artery, lower quadrant basilar artery, left cerebral artery, postero-inferior cerebellar artery	Death after approximately 10 hr preceded by unconsciousness
Schmitt et al. 1973	35 F	MC	Forceful pull of head followed by rotation injured left vertebral artery and part of basilar artery	Death after approx. 3 hr
Schmitt 1976	51 M	MC	Extension of the cervical spine caused intermittent thromboses with ultimate collapse of left vertebral artery	Death after 4 wk preceded by neurological deficits
Unpublished cases	3 cases	MC	Adjustment caused vertebral arterial damage	Death in all 3 cases
Schmitt 1978	35 F	MC	Adjustment for neck pain produced rupture of left vertebral artery	Death
Smith and Estridge 1962	33 F	M	Cervical manipulation produced softening of cerebral trunk and cerebellum	Vertigo, vomiting, lack of coordination of extremities; coma—death after 3 days
	48 F	M	Cervical manipulation causing posteroinferior cerebellar arterial thrombosis	Vertigo, nausea, headache; Wallenberg's syndrome

*C, chiropractor; M, medical manipulator; MC, medical practitioner using chiropractic adjustment (largely in Germany).

pend on the vessel which is affected, the usual area of involvement being the brainstem and cerebellum (Fig. 1). Once the injury has occurred, permanent neurological deficit is the rule. However, progression to death is not uncommon. Common symptoms of vertebrobasilar insult include vertigo, nausea, vomiting, dysarthria, nystagmus, and partial facial paralysis. The Wallenburg syndrome is a common sequel and involves thrombosis of the posterior inferior cerebellar artery giving rise to symptoms of vertigo, nausea, and contralateral hemiparesis and hemianesthesia.

Spontaneous or Self-Inflicted Vertebrobasilar Accidents. A search of the literature reveals that nonmanipulative, often minor cervical movements, postures, and maneuvers may also

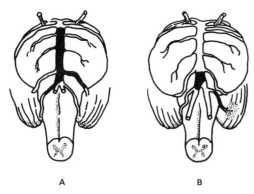

FIG. 1. **Diagrammatic representation of vertebrobasilar system. (A) Thrombus (black) in basilar, left anterior inferior, and right posterior inferior cerebellar arteries. (B) Thrombus (black) in basilar, right vertebral, and left posterior inferior cerebellar arteries with softening of left cerebellar tonsil. (From Pratt-Thomas HR et al. 1947)**

produce vertebrobasilar ischemia (Table 3). This suggests that preexisting conditions are present in a number of patients which may result in severe damage even if SMT is not given. It also emphasizes the need to adequately evaluate each patient for such preexisting conditions prior to administering a spinal adjustment in order to exclude those patients where referral may prevent serious disability or death (Miller and Burton 1974; Maigne 1972; Sandoz 1965).

Mechanisms of Vertebrobasilar Insult

Structural Factors. A review of the anatomy of the cervical spine reveals that the relationship of the vertebral arteries to neighboring structures makes these arteries susceptible to mechanical compression and trauma (Fig. 2).

Variations in the caliber of the vertebral arteries are common and thought to contribute to obstruction and thrombosis following SMT (Gowers 1899; Thane 1899; Hutchinson and Yates 1956; Virtama and Kivalo 1957; Green and Joynt 1959). In addition, attention has been drawn to the fragility of the vertebral arteries at the occipitocervical junction (Nick et al. 1967). There are four areas where the vertebral arteries are susceptible to compression:

1. At the posterior atlantooccipital membrane which is dense and inelastic. In this region the vertebral artery is surrounded by a fibrous tissue ring which is very firmly attached to the artery. This ring can be distorted to cause arterial obstruction during hyperextension with rotation (De Kleyn et al. 1927; Tissington Tatlow et al. 1957; Toole et al. 1960; Schneider and Schemm 1961; Jones 1966).

2. Between the occiput and posterior arch of atlas where the interval may become reduced to a mere slit during extension of the occipitoatlantal articulation and be further compromised by osteophytosis (Pratt-Thomas et al. 1957; Schneider and Schemm 1961; Jones 1966).

3. Between the lateral mass of the atlas and the transverse process of the axis where occlusion can occur at the limits of rotation, especially when accompanied by extension (Ford and Clar 1956; Jones 1966).

4. The posterior musculoskeletal venous plexus may become markedly engorged. In some instances, this engorgement resembles the gross varicose veins of the lower limbs and may fill the depths of the suboccipital triangle, the interlaminal spaces, and the posterior condylar fossae and extend along the canal for the hypoglossal nerve. This may cause intermittent or partial vertebral artery occlusion (Jones 1966). Venous congestion provides a fluid mass through which pulsations are transmitted. These pulsations may affect osseous structures leading to changes such as osteoporosis, osteophytosis, osteoarthrosis and bony erosion, which can further compromise the region (Jones 1966; Kleynhans 1970).

The Influence of Head Movements on Vertebral Artery Flow. Circulation through one vertebral artery is reduced when the head is hyperextended and rotated to the opposite side (De Kleyn et al. 1927; Pratt-Thomas et al. 1947; Tissington-Tatlow et al. 1957; Toole et al. 1960). In normal individuals there is adequate collateral circulation from the other vertebral artery. In the presence of vascular anomaly,

TABLE 3. **Spontaneous or Self-Inflicted Vertebral Artery Accidents**

Author/Year	Case Age/Sex	Incident or Etiology	Site/Mechanism of Injury	Sequelae
Alajouanine et al. 1957	34 M	Sustained extension and lateral flexion of the neck.	Suspected thrombosis of the terminal part of the vertebral artery	Vertigo, instability immediately followed by neck pain, nausea, intense vertigo, and hemiplegia
	60 M	Sustained extension and lateral flexion of the neck	Thrombosis either of vertebral artery or of the artery of the lateral bulbar fossa	Immediately—vertigo, instability, vomiting, swallowing difficulties; 48 hr later—Wallenberg's syndrome
	45 M	Sustained lateral flexion and extension of neck	As above	Vertigo and dull neck pain followed by complete Horners and Wallenberg's syndromes
Easton and Sherman 1977	38 F	Turning of the head	Infarction of pons and rostral medulla	Vertigo, ataxia, dysarthria, dysphagia, blurred vision
Ford and Clark 1956	37 M	Cervical torsions (by wife) "to release tension"	Thrombosis of basilar, left posterior cerebral, and left posteroinferior cerebellar arteries	Retinal hemorrhage, cervical sympathetic paralysis; cerebellar ataxia; facial analgesia; dysarthria; partial nerve deafness; death 60 hr after accident
Grinker et al. 1927	15 M	Yawn with arms stretched vigorously up and outward	Thrombosis of anterior spinal artery	Total tetraplegia followed by death
Tissington-Tatlow, et al. 1957	63 M	Turned head to left	Vertebral artery incompetence	Decreased vision, left-eye pain, dizziness
	67 F	Arose from seated position	Vertebral artery incompetence	Unsteadiness, unconscious periods

arteriosclerosis, or unilateral vertebral artery occlusion, however, the vertebrobasilar system may suffer relative embarrassment during head movements (Tissington-Tatlow et al. 1957; Green and Joynt 1959; Masson and Cambier 1962; Maigne 1972).

On rotation, the atlas pivots on the atlanto-axial joint on the side to which the head is turned. This results in anterior movement of the lateral mass on the opposite side, thus caus-ing traction on the vertebral artery (Tissington-Tatlow et al. 1957; Ford and Clark 1956; Schneider and Schemm 1961). This may pre-dispose to kinking or tearing of the vessel, particularly when there is a superimposed vascular injury or osseous abnormality (Fig. 3). Cervical osteophytes may be a further complicating factor (Tissington-Tatlow et al. 1957; Green and Joynt 1959; Masson and Cambier 1962; Maigne 1972). Considerable increase in retinal arterial

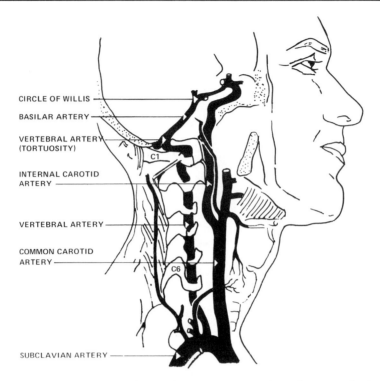

CIRCLE OF WILLIS

BASILAR ARTERY

VERTEBRAL ARTERY
(TORTUOSITY)

INTERNAL CAROTID
ARTERY

VERTEBRAL ARTERY

COMMON CAROTID
ARTERY

SUBCLAVIAN ARTERY

FIG. 2.   **Diagram illustrating the relationship between the cervical vertebrae, vertebral artery, and internal carotid artery. Note the tortuosity of the vertebral artery at the occipit-C1 level.**

pressure may occur on the side of bending during hyperextension, lateral flexion, and rotation. A concomitant reduction of flow may then occur on the side opposite lateral flexion.

The Influence of Degenerative Joint Changes on Vertebral Artery Flow. Loss of disc height can cause the cervical spine to become shorter, forcing the vertebral artery to become more tortuous and sinuous in its course. This may produce a reduction in the effective lumen of the vessel. Degenerative changes which occur predominantly in the lower cervical spine can, therefore, conceivably result in vascular changes in the atlantooccipital region.

Osteophytic outgrowths, especially from the zygapophyses, can displace the vertebral artery along its course. Obstruction in this case is induced by extension and rotation to the side where the osteophyte is present. This is in contradistinction to obstruction due to atlantoaxial

rotation where obstruction takes place on the side opposite extension and rotation (Bowden et al. 1967; Hutchinson and Yates 1956; Sheehan et al. 1960; Gortvai 1964).

Vertebral Artery Aneurysm. While rare, vertebral artery aneurysms may cause plain x-ray film findings of erosion with expansion of the transverse foramina (Fig. 4).

Atlas Compression of the Internal Carotid Artery Due to SMT

The internal carotid artery (Fig. 5), as it ascends to the cranium, lies in very close approximation to the anterolateral aspect of the atlas (Fig. 5A). When the head is rotated or held in a turned position, the atlas transverse process may press against the artery or cause an irritative reflex vasospasm, thus simulating a temporary vascular obstruction (Fig. 5B). Cervical manipulation

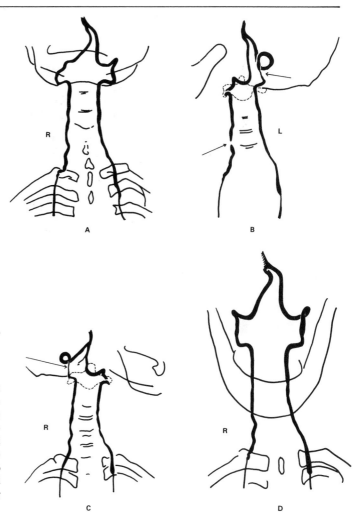

FIG. 3. **Diagrammatic representation of vertebral arteries. (A) In anteroposterior plane before head rotation; (B) effect of right head rotation on the vertebral arteries; (C) effect of left head rotation on the vertebral arteries; (D) the vertebral arteries have returned to their normal configuration. (Adapted from Tissington-Tatlow and Bammer 1957)**

may also force the carotid artery onto the transverse process of axis (Beatty 1977). Relative stasis may precipitate thrombus formation giving rise to obstruction or emboli (Boldrey et al. 1956) or result in intramural hematoma formation (Schneider et al. 1952).

Obstruction of the internal carotid system, even as transitory as from head rotation, or sleeping prone with the head rotated, can lead to thrombosis in the middle cerebral artery and therefore be a major etiological factor in the so-called "hypotensive stroke" (Boldrey et al. 1956). Adhesions, such as may occur from

chronic pharyngitis in adults can bind the carotid sheath to the carotid artery and adjacent tissues and interfere with the mobility between the carotid and adjacent tissues, "particularly the atlas transverse process." This may predispose to intimal damage and in this way induce thrombosis (Boldrey 1956).

Hematomyelia Due to Cervical Hyperextension

Hematomyelia is defined as bleeding into the spinal cord. During cervical hyperextension,

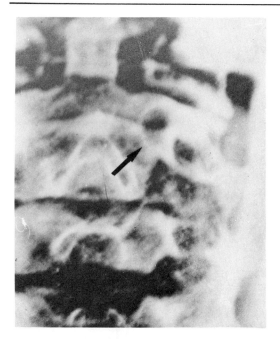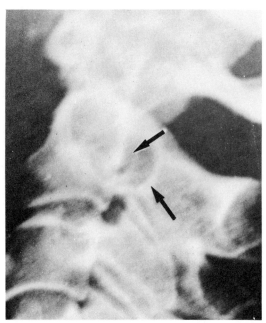

FIG. 4. **Vertebral artery aneurysm. Anteroposterior and lateral x-rays of the cervical spine to show well-demarcated expansion of the transverse foramen and erosion of a transverse process and pedicle from a vertebral artery aneurysm.**

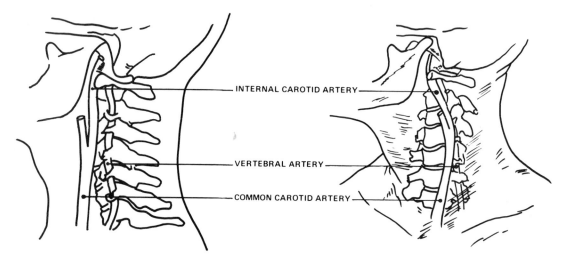

FIG. 5. **Diagrammatic representation illustrating displacement and compression of the internal carotid artery by the lateral process of the atlas when the head is turned sharply. Normal anatomical position (left); Head turned to side (right). (From Boldrey et al. 1956)**

the ligamentum flavum has been shown to bulge anteriorly, compressing the posterior cord by as much as 30 percent of its width. In the presence of osteophyte formation from the posterior aspect of the vertebral bodies, the amount of compression has been shown to increase. It is by this mechanism that hemorrhage into the cord is thought to occur. The syndrome is characterized by disproportionately more weakness of the upper extremity, bladder incontinence, and sensory disturbances (Schneider et al. 1954; Reid 1960).

Spinal Meningeal Hematoma Due to SMT Administered to Patients on Anticoagulant Therapy. Of 34 recorded accidents following SMT prior to 1963, spinal hematoma (most commonly extradural) occurred in six patients who had been receiving anticoagulant therapy. In such cases physical strain appeared to be the precipitating factor, with SMT producing the

actual bleeding. Intraspinal bleeding results in localized pain and is followed by "patchy" sensory and motor deficit which can progress to paraplegia, quadriplegia, or death (Dabbert et al. 1970).

Dislocation Due to SMT

Anterior Dislocation or Subluxation of Atlas on Axis. Dislocation of atlas on axis, caused by SMT, has been reported in the literature (Blain 1925). The following mechanisms for anterior dislocation of atlas on axis have been proposed (Yochum 1978).

Agenesis of the Transverse Ligament. A significant number of cases of mongoloidism (as high as 50 percent) may present agenesis of the transverse ligament of atlas creating tremendous instability and allowing for anterior dislocation of C1 on C2 (Fig. 6).

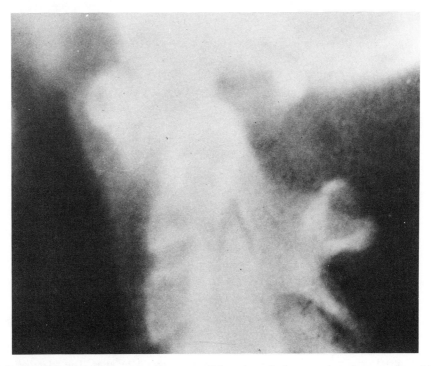

FIG. 6. **Lateral cervical x-ray showing gross dislocation of atlas on axis and an os odontoideum in a case of mongoloidism.**

Arthritides Leading to Rupture of Transverse Ligaments of C1. Ankylosing spondylitis, rheumatoid arthritis, psoriatic arthritis, and Reiter's syndrome are the four most common arthritides to cause inflammatory rupture of the transverse ligament with dislocation of the atlas.

It is therefore extremely important that flexion x-rays of the cervical spine be taken of such patients prior to SMT so as to accentuate any increase in the atlantoodontoid interspace (AOI) that may be present (Figs. 7–10). Similarly, any patient with ankylosing spondylitis

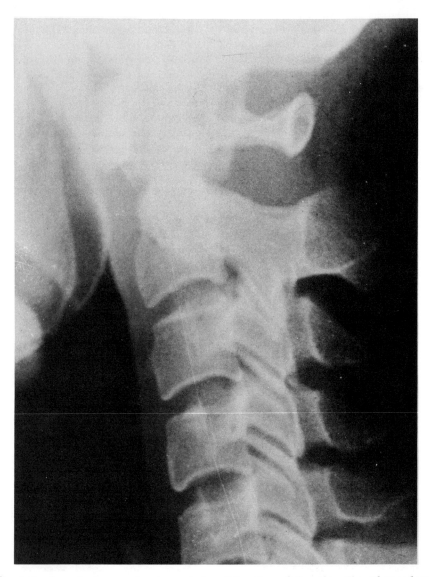

FIG. 7. **Lateral cervical x-ray showing anterior dislocation of the atlas. The atlantoodontoid interspace measures 6 to 7 mm. Rupture of the transverse ligament of C1 due to ankylosing spondylitis has occurred.**

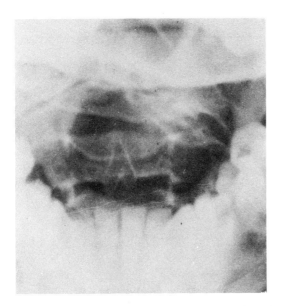
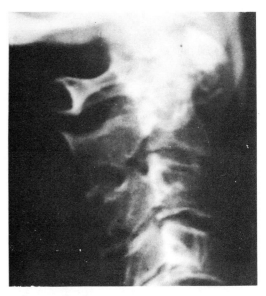

FIG. 8.   Anteroposterior-open-mouth (left) and neutral-lateral (right) x-rays of the upper cervical spine showing increased atlantoodontoid interspace and anterior slippage of atlas due to rheumatoid arthritis.

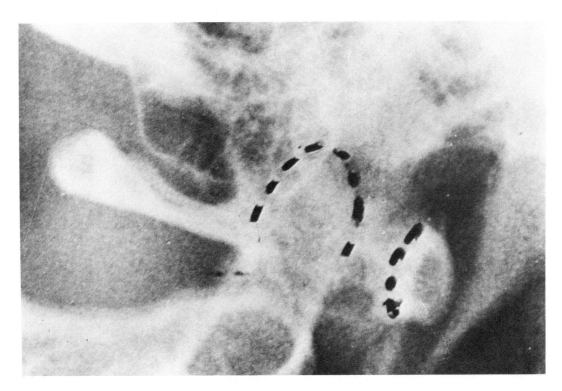

FIG. 9.   Lateral x-ray of the upper cervical spine showing rupture of the transverse ligament with increased atlantoodontoid interspace resulting from rheumatoid arthritis.

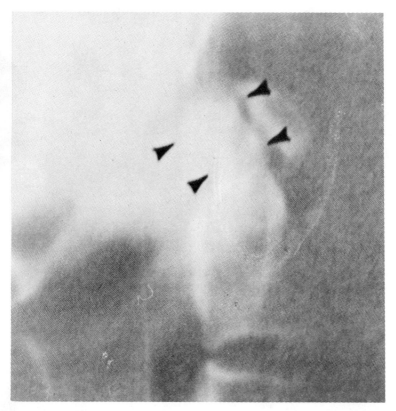

FIG. 10. **Lateral x-ray of the upper cervical spine showing dislocation of atlas on flexion with increased atlantoodontoid interspace. Note erosion of the odontoid process due to psoriatic arthritis.**

primarily involving the low back, any patient who complains of cervical symptoms, or any patient displaying symptoms that will require cervical SMT, should have a neutral lateral and flexion view of the cervical spine included in the radiographic examination (Yochum 1978).

The normal AOI in adults measures up to 3 mm, and in children up to 5 mm at a focal film distance of 72 in. Measurements in excess of these figures is indicative of anterior slippage of atlas on axis (Yochum 1978).

Agenesis of the Odontoid. Extensive excursion of the atlas on axis occurs in agenesis of the odontoid (Figs. 11 and 12). Evaluation of such patients is not complete without cervical flexion views which must be taken with great care to avoid cord compression.

Posterior Dislocation of Atlas on Axis. The most common causes of this serious derangement are agenesis of the odontoid and the condition known as os odontoideum. Rheumatoid arthritis with odontoid erosion may result in posterior subluxation.

The following instances demonstrate the importance of a proper case history and x-ray examination prior to the application of an adjustive thrust to the upper cervical spine.

Case 1—Ankylosing Spondylitis with Dislocation of the Atlas. There are no radiographic changes of ankylosing spondylitis in the cervical spine except for anterior dislocation of the atlas (Fig. 7). The AOI measures 6 to 7 mm.

The patient had been complaining of low-back pain and headaches. The low-back radio-

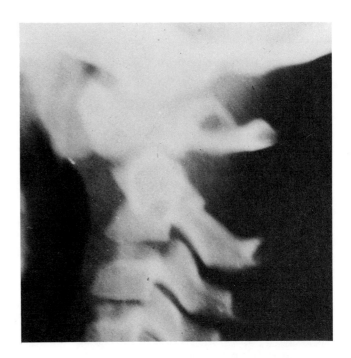

FIG. 11. Lateral x-ray of the cervical spine showing agenesis of the odontoid. Atlas is in an accentuated flexion position causing a highly unstable condition.

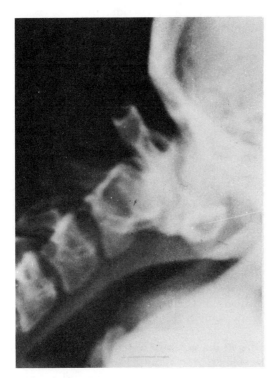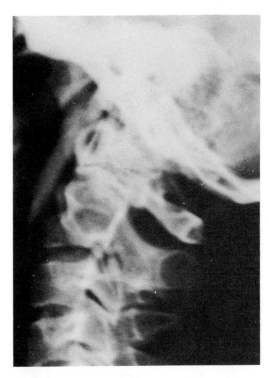

FIG. 12. Flexion and extension lateral x-ray views of the cervical spine. Absence of an odontoid process allows considerable excursion of atlas—anterior in flexion and posterior in extension. This is a highly unstable condition.

graphs revealed sacroiliac joint ankylosis and minimal vertebral body and facet joint ankylosis at the lower lumbar motor units.

Case 2—Rheumatoid Arthritis. The adult patient had a longstanding rheumatoid arthritis (Fig. 8). The joint articulations between the atlas and axis in the lateral cervical radiograph show loss of integrity with marginal erosion. There is an increase in the atlanto-odontal interspace (AOI) indicating that the atlas has slipped anterior on axis. The cortical white line at the spinal laminar junction of the posterior tubercle of the atlas is anterior to the cortical white lines of the remainder of the cervical spine at the spinal laminar junctions.

Case 3—Rheumatoid Arthritis. Increase in AOI and anterior dislocation of C1 is seen in the lateral radiograph of the cervical spine (Fig. 9). This patient had extensive rheumatoid arthritis in the extremities.

Case 4—Psoriatic Arthritis. There is erosion of the odontoid process noted on the extension cervical radiograph (Fig. 10). This patient had an increase in the AOI on flexion, consistent with dislocation of the atlas.

Case 5—Agenesis of the Odontoid. An adolescent male complaining of cervical headaches and suboccipital tension requested chiropractic care (Fig. 11). The lateral cervical radiograph reveals a posterior ponticle at the atlas with a large gap between the posterior tubercle of atlas and the spinous process of C2. A sharp peg is present at the base of the odontoid area and no odontoid process can be visualized. The cortical white lines at the spinal laminar junction are in alignment throughout the cervical spine except at the atlas, which has slipped anterior, creating a highly unstable area.

Case 6—Agenesis of the Odontoid. A 35-year-old male requesting chiropractic care complained of cervical spine pain with headaches (Fig. 12). Flexion and extension lateral x-ray views of the cervical spine from a Davis series reveal a posterior ponticle at the atlas. Considerable excursion of the atlas, anterior in flexion and pos-

terior in extension, is possible and can result in a highly unstable area.

SMT of the Thoracic Area: Costovertebral Sprain

The most common complaint of SMT in the thoracic region is straining of the costovertebral joints. These painful incidents may be due to excessive or severe SMT with poorly taken contacts, poor stabilization, or an incorrect line of thrust and are often difficult to correct (Maigne 1972).

Accidents and Incidents From SMT of the Low Back

The lumbar spine is considerably more capable of withstanding the thrusts and twists of SMT than is the cervical spine. This is probably the reason why reports of low-back injury following SMT have been few (Richard 1967).

Disc Herniation and Prolapse

Stoddard (1969) has divided disc disease into two categories, based on the degree of disc protrusion.

Disc Herniation. Small sections of the disc can bulge beneath the posterior longitudinal ligament. This degree of disc herniation is probably reducible by SMT. On the other hand, a disc herniation is likely to progress to a complete prolapse of the disc. It is a relative contraindication to SMT and has been considered an absolute contraindication to rotational adjustments in the side-lying position (Janse 1976; Winterstein 1971).

Disc Prolapse. Disc prolapse suggests a larger degree of protrusion than herniation and displays disruption of the annulus and posterior longitudinal ligament with nuclear material entering the spinal canal. This should be considered a contraindication to high velocity or

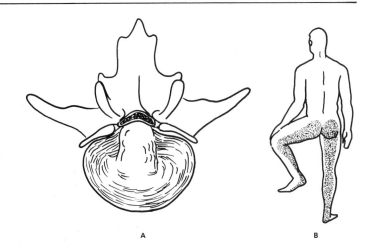

FIG. 13. **(A) Diagram illustrating that massive herniation at the level of the third, fourth, or fifth disc may cause severe compression of the cauda equina. Pain is confined chiefly to the buttocks and the back of the thighs and legs. (B) Numbness is widespread from the buttocks to the soles of the feet. Motor weakness or loss is present in the legs and feet with loss of muscle mass in the calves. The bladder and bowels are paralysed. (From DePalma and Rothman 1970.)**

long-lever manipulation techniques especially in the side-lying position. The manipulation of patients with disc prolapse may have disastrous consequences in the form of cauda equina compression (Jennett 1956; Richard 1967; Stoddard 1969; Winterstein 1971).

The most frequently described severe accident from SMT in the lumbar spine is compression of the cauda equina by a massive midline nuclear herniation at the level of the third, fourth, or fifth intervertebral disc. Pain from these lesions is confined chiefly to the buttocks and the back of the thighs and legs. Widespread numbness may be present over the buttocks, the posterior aspect of the legs, and the soles of the feet (Figure 13B). It may also result in weakness of the muscles in the legs and feet with atrophy of the calves. The bladder and bowels may become paralyzed (De Palma and Rothman 1970; Hooper 1973) (Fig. 13).

The risk of precipitating a cauda equina compression syndrome through SMT in uncomplicated cases of sciatica secondary to prolapsed intervertebral disc is always present. In fact, most cases of sciatic radiculopathy due to intervertebral disc herniation could be considered to be partial cauda equina lesions. These lesions are, however, usually unilateral with muscular weakness, wasting, reflex abnormalities, and sensory impairment referable to compression of one or more roots (Jennet 1956). Bilateral radiculopathies with distal paralysis of the lower limbs, sensory loss in the

sacral distribution, and sphincter paralysis represents the caudal equina syndrome. It does not respond to spinal manipulative therapy and should be considered a surgical emergency (Jennet 1956).

Miscellaneous Incidents Resulting From SMT

It has been stated that the poorly executed adjustment may generate all the symptoms usually corrected by these techniques (Lescure 1954; Maigne 1972). Therefore, the list of incidents from spinal adjustments could conceivably be quite extensive. There have been a number of extremely unusual and difficult to explain complications of SMT reported in the literature which are included for completion. It is possible that these symptoms are unrelated to SMT, simply occurring concomitantly with the manipulation by coincidence.

Skin Conditions

Petechial Rash of the Leg. A 42-year-old male received SMT for acute back pain two days after minor trauma. One day later, a petechial rash involving both lower extremities developed which extended from the thighs to the ankles. There was also a large effusion of the right knee joint and both ankles. Under observation, the rash and joint symptoms subsided within two days (Tomlinson 1955).

Purpura Over the Shoulder. Osteopathic SMT for a cervical lesion resulted in two patches of purpura over the shoulder in the area supplied by nerves arising from the vertebral levels manipulated. Blood fragility and clotting tests were normal and the rash faded within 2 days (Tomlinson 1955).

Endocrine Conditions

Thyrotoxicosis (Acute Basedow's Syndrome). A case that was successfully adjusted for severe low-back pain and headache developed acute thyrotoxicosis (an apparent exacerbation of a latent condition) after the third chiropractic adjustment. It subsided when SMT was discontinued and was attributed to a sympathetic reflex reaction (Rettig 1955).

Cardiorespiratory Arrest

One case of possible cardiorespiratory arrest following a cervical adjustment without anesthesia has been reported. The patient survived following cardiopulmonary resuscitation. No possible mechanism was given (Gorman 1978).

Reactions to SMT

Reactions to spinal adjustments may be either "normal" reactions that are expected to occur after successful SMT or "adverse" reactions, resulting from factors such as poor technique or the substitution of force for finesse. They can be classified (following Maigne 1972) into "functional" and "painful" reactions (Table 4).

Practitioner-Related Causes of Accidents, Incidents, and Adverse Reactions

A review of practitioner-related causes of accidents, incidents, and adverse reactions suggests three major factors:

Lack of Knowledge

Application of SMT where contraindicated or nonindicated has been responsible for many past accidents and incidents. These could, in many cases, have been avoided and were often due to lack of a proper diagnosis, which, when coupled with lack of skill or rational technique, caused considerable harm (Bollier 1960; Cyriax 1964, 1971, 1975; DeSeze 1955; Livingston 1971; Rubens 1958). It is recognized, however, that accidents can occur even when proper precautions are taken (Oger et al. 1966).

The importance of an exact diagnosis and the determination of the proper indications for spinal manipulation has been repeatedly stressed (Kaiser 1973; Kuhlendahl and Hansell 1958; Levernieux 1962). The diagnostic skills necessary for the practice of SMT extend beyond procedures normally used by clinicians who do not use spinal manipulation. It is necessary to be familiar with the clinical manifestations of the various spinal disorders and to become skilled in diagnosis of the locomotor system, particularly of the axial skeletal (Wolff 1972). It is unacceptable to apply SMT indiscriminately without knowledge and understanding of the underlying conditions for which it is indicated (Smart 1946). The mere fact that a patient is referred for SMT by a medically trained physician does not mean, a priori, that this constitutes a good indication. The final decision about the indication of SMT must always be taken by the practitioner himself (Sandoz 1960).

Lack of Skill

Excellent diagnostic acumen accompanied by a lack of skill in the application of SMT poses just as great a threat to the patient as does the application of SMT by persons untrained in the diagnostic sciences (Bollier 1960; Kewit 1972). In fact, the international medical literature lists many cases of damage and death which have resulted from poorly applied SMT by manipulators who replaced lack of experience and skill with brutal force (Bollier 1960). Livingston appropriately stated that, "Medical and

TABLE 4. **Reactions to Spinal Adjustments and Manipulations**

	Incidence	Latent Period	Duration	Mechanism or Cause/Sequelae
*Functional Reactions**				
Perspiration over trunk and axilla	Very common	0	Brief	Action on sympathetic nervous system; need not modify treatment
Episodes of generalized tremor (not due to fear or nervousness) with trembling and chills at times	Rare	0	Several minutes	Cervicodorsal manipulation
Meteorism with or without diarrhea	?	Brief period	Hours	Following lumbar or lower dorsal manipulation
Early or heavy menstruation	Often	1 day	4 days	Manipulation of cervical and cervico-brachial area
Epigastric pain (abdominal or pelvic pain)	Not rare	Within 24 hr	Several hours	Patients usually complained of such symptoms during their illness
"Sympathetic storm" (fainting, palpitation, cold perspiration and nausea)	1–2 cases out of 1000	Brief	24–48 hr	Unstable autonomic nervous system; subsequent manipulations 10 days or so later may not elicit reaction and results will generally be excellent with relief of other mild functional disturbances
Painful Reactions				
Post-manipulative diffuse pain lasting less than 2 days*	40% of cases	Brief	6–48 hr	After first session; usually does not recur after subsequent session;* release of strong adhesions†
Postmanipulative muscular aches and pains‡	Frequent in patients with good results	Brief or some delay	Half a day to 1 week; average 2–3 days	Ligamentous and muscular stretching, mild articular and disc strain; sympathetic irritation after first 1 or 2 treatments only (usually a good prognostic sign)‡

(continued)

TABLE 4. *(continued)*

	Incidence	Latent Period	Duration	Mechanism or Cause/Sequeale
Postmanipulative diffuse pain lasting more than 2 days†	?	Brief	Days	Manipulation was too forcible Manipulation was incorrectly applied (mechanical diagnosis was misconstrued and wrong technique was chosen) Joint was inflamed or the soft tissues were too irritable Patient resisted and the adhesions were merely stretched painfully Manipulation provoked a late reaction in a degenerated disc The joint was already hypermobile†
Transitory exaggerations of original pain*; temporary exaggeration of pain§	?	Few hours after treatment with relief of pain	6–24 hr	Normal recovery response (?)
Recurrence of pain in "attenuated form"	?	Days	Until subsequent treatment	Attenuated pain returns since additional treatment is required

*Maigne 1972; †Stoddard 1969; ‡Sandoz and Lorenz; subsequent manipulation should not be attempted until reactions generated by previous treatment are extinguished.

paramedical personnel would do well to either study spinal manipulation thoroughly or avoid it. Anesthesia may increase the hazard" (Livingston 1971).

Lack of Rational Attitude and Technique

Inadequate Diagnostic Habits. Doctrinal antipathy toward diagnosis (Sandoz 1965), or toward the use of x-ray (Livingston 1972), and failure to make a proper mechanical evaluation of the spine and to adjust accordingly (Maigne 1972) have been considered potential causes of injury.

Inadequate X-ray Evaluation. Failure to obtain x-rays of adequate quality (especially of the upper cervical complex), failure to obtain an adequate number of views in the area of primary complaint, or failure to obtain x-rays at all could result in misdiagnosis and injury from SMT (Maigne 1972; Schmorl and Junghanns 1971).

Delay in Referral. Early in this century, Timbrell Fisher pointed out that not only may there be danger in SMT itself, but also when it was not indicated, this form of therapy may prevent a patient from seeking proper medical advice until the favorable time for treatment has irretrievably passed (Fisher 1925; Livingston 1972).

Delay in Reevaluation. If a patient does not improve from SMT, treatment should be discontinued and the patient carefully reevaluated (Maitland 1973).

Lack of Interprofessional Cooperation. Failure to determine whether the patient is on anticoagulant or other types of concurrent therapy and lack of interprofessional cooperation (Dabbert et al. 1970) may have disastrous consequences when SMT is used.

Ignoring Patient Intolerances. Practitioners must be selective in their choice of treatment in view of patient intolerances and body type (Lescure 1954; Stoddard 1969; Maigne 1972). This is especially true when applying SMT in patients with unstable autonomic nervous systems without first warning the patient of the possibility of a "sympathetic storm" (Maigne 1972).

Poor Technique Selection. The use of untested "innovative" techniques instead of classical "proven" techniques (Maigne 1972) or the selection of a faulty or poor technique increases the risk of inducing injury.

Poor Technique Implementation. Forced or powerful SMT in the wrong direction (Maigne 1972) with failure to grade the manipulation according to the situation can be dangerous. Failure to apply proper leverage and traction further increases the risk.

Excessive Use of SMT. Applying SMT too frequently, or giving a subsequent treatment before reactions of the previous one are extinguished, can be detrimental (Gonstead 1972; Maigne 1972; Palmer BJ 1934).

Contraindications to SMT

Contraindications to SMT have been defined as "the presence of frank bone or joint disease or the absence of joint dysfunction" (Mennell 1960). Absolute contraindications are conditions that preclude the use of the dynamic adjustive thrust. These contraindications do not, however, in all cases preclude the use of soft tissues and mobilizing techniques such as Nimmo's triggerpoint therapy and Maitland's mobilization (Maitland 1973). The major contraindications to SMT are listed in Table 5.

Articular Derangements

The Arthritides. Potential or actual rupture of the transverse ligaments of atlas preclude forceful cervical SMT in patients with ankylosing spondylitis, rheumatoid and psoriatic arthritis, and Reiter's syndrome (Yochum 1978). In the acute inflammatory phase of ankylosing spondylitis, SMT and exercise is contraindicated and bed rest may be necessary (Stoddard 1969; Mathews 1972). Gentle, specialized techniques may be used once the condition has stabilized. Forceful adjustment is, however, strictly contraindicated because of possible luxation with cord injury (Rinsky et al. 1976).

It is important to remember the general rule that if pain improves with movement and heat the patient will usually benefit from SMT. On the other hand, if the pain is aggravated by the least movement, inflammation or acute injury may be present and the area should be placed in a state of physiological rest (Janse 1961).

Patients with severe cervical spondylosis or symptoms of vertebrobasilar insufficiency (particularly vertigo, nausea, dysphagia, dysarthria, syncope, or visual disturbances) should not undergo forceful SMT. Should these symptoms appear during SMT the procedure should be immediately discontinued (Miller and Burton 1974; Robertson 1968).

Articular Trauma. Dislocation, ruptured ligaments, and recent trauma, such as whiplash, preclude SMT since these merely add insult to injury. In whiplash, forceful SMT is usually not indicated during the first 6 weeks. This does not preclude the use of soft-tissue techniques (Stoddard 1969).

Joint Hypermobility. Often the result of long-term microtrauma, joint hypermobility is a contraindication to high-velocity adjustments but not to gently mobilizing or soft-tissue techniques (Maitland 1973).

Bone-Weakening Disease

Diseases which weaken bone include fracture, primary or secondary malignancy, osteomalacia, osteoporosis, and osteomyelitis. Any bone-weakening process, whatever its etiology, constitutes an absolute contraindication to forceful SMT but does not in all cases preclude mobilizing, light adjustments and soft-tissue techniques. There are no warning signs to indicate that an osteoporotic bone or a weakened ligament will respond adversely to the strain from an adjustment until the bone actually collapses.

Patients on long-term steroid therapy should be carefully assessed for iatrogenic osteoporosis which would preclude adjustment. This is especially true in the thoracic area because of the great susceptibility of osteoporotic ribs to fractures.

Circulatory Disturbances

Most of these disturbances have been discussed previously. Aneurysms involving any blood vessel, especially the abdominal aorta, represent an absolute contraindication to spinal adjustments in that region. An adequate physical examination, including palpation and auscultation, are essential to the diagnosis of such underlying conditions. Radiographic evaluation does not necessarily reveal the presence of such abnormalities.

Neurological Dysfunction

Sacral Nerve Root Involvement. Involvement of the sacral nerve roots from disc protrusion implies a medical and/or massive protrusion of the intervertebral disc into the spinal canal. SMT applied in this instance may result in disastrous consequences.

Excessive Pain. Response to pain varies among patients and ethnic groups. Any significant pain associated with manipulation should

TABLE 5. Contraindications to Spinal Adjustments

Condition	Authors
Articular Derangements	
Arthritides	
Acute arthritis of any type	Hauberg (1967), Janse (1976), Maigne (1972), Maitland (1973), Stoddard (1969), Yochum (1978)
Rheumatoid arthritis	Bourdillon (1973), Janse (1976), Maigne (1972), Stoddard (1969), Yochum (1978)
Acute ankylosing spondylitis	Bollier (1960), Droz (1971), Hauberg (1967), Janse (1967), Nwuga (1976), Stoddard (1969)
Cervical spondylosis with vertebrobasilar ischemia	Miller and Burton (1974)
Dislocation	Heilig (1965), Timbrell Fisher (1948)
Hypermobility	Gutmann (1978), Kaltenborn (1976), Maitland (1973), Stoddard (1969)
Ruptured ligaments	Gutmann (1978), Stoddard (1969)
Trauma of recent occurrence—whiplash	Gutmann (1978), Stoddard (1969)
Bone Weakness and Destructive Disease	
Calve's disease	Lindner (1960)
Fracture	Gutmann (1978), Heilig (1965), Maigne (1972), Nwuga (1976), Rinsky (1976), Siehl (1967), Stoddard (1969)
Malignancy (primary or secondary)	Bourdillon (1973), Gutmann (1978), Maigne (1972), Maitland (1973), Nwuga (1976), Timbrell Fisher (1948), Stoddard (1969)
Osteomalacia	Lindner (1960)

TABLE 5 (continued)

Condition	Authors
Osteoporosis	Bollier (1960), Bourdillon (1973), Maigne (1972), Nwuga (1976), Siehl (1967), Stoddard (1969)
Osteomyelitis	Hauberg (1967), Nwuga (1976), Sandoz (1960), Stoddard (1969)
Tuberculosis (Pott's disease)	Bourdillon (1973), Hauberg (1967), Maigne (1972), Siehl (1967), Stoddard (1969), Timbrell Fisher (1948)
Circulatory Disturbances	
Aneurysm	Dabbert (1970)
Anticoagulant therapy	
Atherosclerosis	Boshes (1959)
Vascular insufficiency of vertebrobasilar area or vertebral artery disease	Bourdillon (1973), Davidson (1975), Heilig (1965), Maigne (1972), Maitland (1973), Mehalic (1974), Miller and Burton (1974), Nwuga (1976), Sandoz (1965)
Disc Lesions	
Prolapse with serious neurological changes (including cauda equina syndrome)	Bourdillon (1973), Cyriax (1971), Jaquet (1978), Jennet (1956), Nwuga (1976), Odom (1970), Stoddard (1969)
Neurological Dysfunction	
Micturition with sacral root involvement	Cyriax (1971), Stoddard (1969)
Painful movement in all directions	Maigne (1972)
Vertigo	Maitland (1973)
Unclassified	
Infectious disease	Maigne (1972), Nwuga (1976)
Psychological intolerances	Lescue (1954)

be avoided. Pain intolerances and pain in all directions of spinal movement have been considered contraindications to forceful adjustments (Janse 1961; Lescure 1954; Maigne 1972). Anesthesia removes this barrier but represents a greater risk in causing more serious accidents (Morey 1973; Maigne 1972; Rumney 1968; Siehl 1967). The use of other forms of conservative procedures such as ice and gentle mobilization have been recommended for use with these patients (Maigne 1972).

Vertigo. Exploratory movements or postural tests (Maigne 1972; Maitland 1973; Bradford and Spurling as cited by Sandoz 1965) should be made prior to cervical SMT in the presence of vertigo. Any position of the head which is held for 40 to 50 seconds or less and which causes vertigo and/or nystagmus can be considered a contraindication to SMT in that direction until fully evaluated. It is usually only when vertigo is secondary to headache that mobilization techniques will be of benefit (Ryand and Cope 1955 as quoted by Maitland 1973). Functional intolerances (Lescure 1954) such as dizziness during certain movements and positions of the neck may occur. Patients who cannot lie down or get up from the table and who cannot tolerate the postural positions of the neck should not receive SMT. However, very careful mobilizing techniques within the range of tolerance may be of some value (Lescure 1954; Maigne 1972; Maitland 1973).

Psychological Intolerance

Psychological intolerance (Lescure 1954) relates to the patient's fear of pain or discomfort. This is often overcome by a partial or gentle demonstration of the painlessness of a maneuver. Explanation of the aim and effects of SMT using radiographs or spinal models of the problem in language understandable to the patient may help to allay this fear. SMT applied in the absence of such counseling and without complete cooperation of the patient increases the chances of causing injury (Lescure 1954; Maigne 1972; Stoddard 1969).

Factors That Reduce the Number of Complications From SMT

Many contraindications to SMT may be regarded as restricted indications for SMT (Gutmann 1978) and the extent to which they preclude the use of SMT may be influenced by the following factors:

1. *Finesse.* As the finesse and skill in the application of the various techniques of SMT increases, so the list of relative contraindications decreases.
2. *Knowledge.* As knowledge of the mechanisms of action of the various forms of SMT increases and the exact nature of the spinal lesion which responds to SMT becomes better understood, the number of relative contraindications decreases.
3. *Area of the spine adjusted.* An absolute contraindication for SMT in one area of the spine may not apply to another area of the spine unaffected by the condition, e.g., fracture.
4. *Technique.* Specific techniques may be contraindicated in a particular patient but not SMT per se (Stoddard 1969; Maigne 1972; Kleynhans 1976).
5. *Positioning of the patient.* Contraindications to SMT in certain patient positions do not apply in other positions (e.g., sitting instead of side-lying position for lumbosacral facet asymmetry and acute lumbar disc protrusion) (Janse 1950; Kleynhans 1976; Winterstein 1971).

REFERENCES

Alajouanine MMTh, et al.: The role of abnormal and sustained positions of the head and neck in the determination and assessment of certain vascular accidents of the cerebral trunk. Bull Mem Soc Med Hopit Paris 1957

Attali P: Severe accidents after an untimely manipulation by a chiropractor. Rev Rheum 24:n.p., 1957

Beatty RA: Dissecting hematoma of internal carotid artery following chiropractic cervical manipulation. J Trauma 17:3, 1977

Beyeler W: Scheuermann's disease and its chiropractic management. Ann Swiss Chiropr Assoc 1:170, 1960

Blaine ES: Manipulative (chiropractic) dislocation of the axis. JAMA 85:1356, 1925

Boldrey E et al.: The role of atlantoid compression in the etiology of internal carotid thrombosis. J Neurosurg 13(2):127, 1956

Bollier W: Editorial: Chiropractic and medicine. Ann Swiss Chiropr Assoc 1:11, 1960

Bollier W: Inflammatory, infectious and neoplastic disease of the lumbar spine. Ann Swiss Chiropr Assoc 1:112, 1960

Boshes LD: Vascular accidents associated with neck manipulation. JAMA 171:1652, 1959

Boudin G et al.: Severe syndrome of the cerebral trunk following cervical manipulations (Translated from French). Bull Mem Soc Med Hopit Paris 73:562, 1958

Bowden REM, et al.: Anatomy of the cervical spine membranes, spinal cord, nerve roots and brachial plexus. In Brain WR, Wilkinson M (eds): Cervical Spondylosis. London, Heinemann, 1967

Bourdillon JF: Spinal Manipulation. London, Heinmann, 1973

Brewerton DA: Conservative treatment of painful neck. Proc R Soc Med 57, 16, 1964

Cyriax J: Cervical Spondylosis. London, Butterworths, 1971

Cyriax J: Textbook of Orthopaedic Medicine. Vol. 1. London, Cassell, 1962

Cyriax J: Treatment by manipulation, massage, and injection. Textbook of Orthopaedic Medicine. vol. 2. London, Balliere Tindal, 1971

Cyriax J: The Slipped Disc, 2d ed. Epping, Essex, Gower Press, 1975

Dabbert O et al: Spinal meningeal hematoma, warfarin therapy and chiropractic adjustment. JAMA 214:11, 1970

Davidson KC et al.: Traumatic vertebral artery pseudoaneurysm following chiropractic manipulation. Neuroradiology 115:651, 1975

De Kleyn A, Niewenhuyse P: Schwindelanfalle und nystagmus bei einer bestimmten stellung des koppes. Acta Oto-Laryngol 11:155, 1927

De Palma AF, Rothman RH: The Intervertebral Disc. Saunders, Philadelphia, 1970

De Seze S et al.: Vertebral manipulations. Rev Rhum Mal Osteo-Articulaires 22:633, 1955

Deshayes P et al.: A case of superior plexus paralysis, accident resulting from a cervical manipulation. Rev Rhum 29:137, 1962

Droz JM: Indications and contraindications of vertebral manipulations. Ann Swiss Chiropr Assoc 5:81, 1971

Easton JD et al.: Cervical manipulation and stroke. Stroke 8:5, 1977

Fisher AGT: Treatment by Manipulation. H.K. Lewis, 1948

Ford FR et al.: Thrombosis of the basilar artery with softening of the cerebellum and brain stem due to manipulation of the neck. Bull Johns Hopkins Hosp 98:37, 1956

Gonstead C: Unpublished notes, 1972

Gorman RF: Cardiac arrest after cervical mobilization. Med J Aust 2:169, 1978

Gortvai P: Insufficiency of vertebral artery treated by decompression. Br Med J 2:233, 1964

Gowers WR: A Manual of Disease of the Nervous System, 3d ed. Vol I, London, Churchill, 1899

Green D et al.: Vascular accidents to the brain stem associated with neck manipulation. JAMA 170:522, 1959

Grillo F: Anomalies of the lumbar spine. Ann Swiss Chiropr Assoc 1:56, 1960.

Grinker RR, Guy CC: Sprain of cervical spine causing thrombosis of anterior spinal artery. JAMA 88:1140, 1927

Gutmann G: Chirotherapie, Grundlagen, Indikationen, Gegenindikationen and Objektivier barkeit. Med Welt 29:653, 1978

Hauberg GV: Contraindications of the manual therapy of the spine. Hippokrates, 231, 1967

Heilig D: Whiplash—mechanics of injury, management of cervical and dorsal involvement. 1965 Year Book, Academy of Applied Osteopathy.

Heyden S: Mater Med Nordmark 23:24 1971

Hooper J: Low back pain and manipulation. Paraparesis after treatment of low back pain by physical methods. Med J Aust 1:549, 1973

Hutchinson EC, Yates PO: The cervical portion of the vertebral artery. A clinicopathological study. Brain 79:319, 1956

Janse J: Principles and Practice of Chiropractic: An anthology (R. Hildebrandt, ed). Lombard, IL, National College of Chiropractic, 1976

Janse J: Unpublished notes, 1961, 1974

Jaquet P: Clinical Chiropractic—A Study of Cases. Geneva, Grounauer, 1978

Jennet WB: A study of 25 cases of compression of the cauda equina by prolapsed IVD. J Neurol Neurosurg Psychiatry 19:109 1956

Jones RT: Vascular changes occurring in the cervical musculoskeletal system. S Afr Med J 40:388, 1966

Kaiser, G: Orthopedics and traumatology. Beitr Orthop 20:581, 1973

Kaiser VG: The manual therapy of the spine and its indications. Orthop Traumatol 11, 1973

Kaltenborn FM: Manual Therapy of the Extremity Joints, Oslo, Norlis, 1976

Kanshelpolsky, J et al.: Vertebral artery insufficiency and cerebellar infarct due to manipulation of the neck. Bull Los Angeles Neurol Soc 37:2, 1972

Kleynhans AM: Vascular changes occurring in the cervical musculo skeletal system. J Can Chiropr Assoc 14:19, 1970

Kleynhans AM: Unpublished notes, 1976

Kuhlendahl H et al.: Nil Nocere. Shaden bei Wirbelsaulenreposition 1? Munch Med Wochenschr 100:1738, 1958

Kunkle E et al.: Traumatic brain thrombosis. Ann Int Med 36:1329, 1952

Lescure R: Incidents, accidents, contreindications des manipulations de la colonne vertebrale. Med Hyg [Geneva] 12:456, 1954

Levernieux J: Risks involved in the manipulation and traction of the vertebral column. Rev Prat 12:2725, 1962

Lewit K: Complications following chiropractic manipulations (Translated from German). Dtsch Med Wochenschr 97:784, 1972

Lindner H: A synopsis of the dystrophies of the lumbar spine. Ann Swiss Chiropr Assoc 1:143, 1960

Livingston M: Spinal manipulation causing injury. Br Columb Med J 14:78, 1971

Lorenz R et al.: Basilar artery thrombosis after chiropractic manipulation of the cervical spine. Dtsch Med Wochenschr 97:36, 1972

Lyness SS et al.: Neurological deficit following cervical manipulation. Surg Neurol 2:121, 1972

Maigne R: Les Manipulations vertebrales et les thromboses vertebro basilaires. Angeiologie 21:287, 1969

Maigne R: Orthopaedic Medicine: A New Approach to Vertebral Manipulation. Springfield, IL, Thomas, 1972

Maitland GD: Vertebral Manipulation. London, Butterworths, 1973

Masson M, Cambier J: Vertebro-basilar circulatory insufficency. Presse Med 70:1990, 1962

Mathews JA: The scope of manipulation in the management of rheumatic disease. Practitioner 208:107, 1972

Mehalic T et al.: Vertebral artery injury from chiropractic manipulation. Surg Neurol 2:125, 1974

Mennell JM: Back Pain. Diagnosis and Treatment Using Manipulative Techniques. Boston, Little, Brown, 1960

Miller RG et al.: Stroke following chiropractic manipulation of the spine. JAMA 229:189, 1974

Morey LW: Osteopathic manipulation under general anesthesia 1973 Year Book. Academy of Osteopathy

Mueller SS: Brain stem dysfunction related to cervical

manipulation. Neurology (Minneap) 26:547, 1976

Nagler W: Vertebral artery obstruction by hyperextension of the neck. Arch Phys Med Rehab 54:237, 1973

Nick J et al.: Neurological incidents and accidents caused by cervical manipulations (in reference to three observations). Soc Med Hopit Paris 5:435, 1967

Nwuga VC: Manipulation of the Spine. Baltimore, Williams & Wilkins 1976

Odom GL: Neck ache and back ache. In Gurdjian ES (ed): Proceedings of NINCDS Conference on Neck Ache and Back Ache. Springfield, IL, Thomas, 1970, p 150

Oger J et al.: The dangers and accidents of vertebral manipulations. Rev Rhum 33:493, 1966

Palmer BJ: The subluxation specific—the adjustment specific. Davenport, IA, Palmer School of Chiropractic 1934

Paris SV: Spinal Lesion. Christchurch, New Zealand, Pegasus Press, 1965

Pratt-Thomas HR et al.: Cerebellar and spinal injuries after chiropractic manipulation JAMA 133:600, 1947

Pribek RA: Brain stem vascular accident following neck manipulation. Wis Med J 62:141, 1963

Reid JB: Effects of flexion-extension movements of the head and spine upon the spinal cord and nerve roots. J Neurol Neurosurg Psychiatry 23:214, 1960

Rettig H: Observation of an acute Basedow's syndrome after chiropractic treatment of the cervical spine. Med Klin 36:1528, 1955

Richard J: Disc rupture with cauda equina syndrome after chiropractic adjustment. NY State J Med 67:2496, 1967

Rinsky LA et al.: Cervical spinal cord injury after chiropractic adjustment. Paraplegia 13:223, 1976

Robertson AHM: Manipulation in cervical syndromes. Practitioner 200:396, 1968

Rubens-Duval A: Chiropractors activities and misdeeds (Translated from French). Rev Rhum Mal Osteo-Articulaires 25:438, 1958

Rumney IC: Manipulation of the spine and appendages under anesthesia: an evaluation. J Am Osteop Assoc 68:235, 1968

Sandoz RW: About some problems pertaining to the choice of indications for chiropractic therapy. Ann Swiss Chiropr Assoc 3:201, 1965

Sandoz R et al.: Presentation of an original lumbar technic. Ann Swiss Chiropr Assoc 1:43, 1960

Schmitt HP et al.: Disseziierende rupture der ateria vertebralis mit todlichem vertebralis und basilaris verschluss. Rechtsmed Z 73:301, 1973

Schmitt HP: Rupturen und thrombosen der arteria vertebralis nach gedetchen mechaniseh insulten. Schweiz Arch Neurol Psychiatry 119:363, 1976

Schmitt HP: Manuale therapie der halswirvelsaüle. Z FA [Stuttgart] 54:467, 1978

Schmorl G, Junghanns H: The Human Spine in Health and Disease. Besemann EF (trans). 2d ed. New York, Grune & Stratton, 1971

Schneider RC, Schemm LJ: Traumatic internal carotid artery thrombosis secondary to non penetrating wounds of the neck. A problem in the differential diagnosis of craniocerebral trauma. J Neurosurg 9:495, 1952

Schneider RC et al.: The syndrome of acute central cervical spinal cord injury. J Neurosurg 6:546, 1954

Schwarz GA et al.: Posterior inferior cerebellar artery syndrome of Wallenberg after chiropractic manipulation. Arch Int Med 97:352, 1956

Sheehan S, Bauer RB, Meyer JS: Vertebral artery compression in cervical spondylosis. Neurology (Minneap) 10:968, 1960

Siehl D: Manipulation of the spine under anesthesia. 1967 Yearbook. Academy of Osteopathy

Siehl D: Manipulation of the spine under general anesthesia. J Am Osteop Assoc 62:881, 1963

Smart M: Manipulation. Arch Phys Med 27:730, 1946

Smith RA et al.: Neurological complications of head and neck manipulations. Report of two cases. JAMA 182:528, 1962

Stoddard A: Manual of Osteopathic Practice. London, Hutchinson, 1969

Thane GD: Quain's Elements of Anatomy, 10th ed. London 1899

Tissington-Tatlow WF et al.: Syndrome of vertebral artery compression. Neurology (Minneap) 7, 5, 331, 1957

Tomlinson KM: Purpura following manipulation of the spine. Br Med J 1:1260, 1955

Toole JF, Tacker SH: Influence of head position upon cerebral circulation. Arch Neurol 2:616, 1960

Valentini E: The occipito-cervical region. Ann Swiss Chiropr Assoc 4:225, 1969

Virtama R, Kivalo E: Impression of the vertebral artery by a deformation of the uncovertebral joints. Acta Radiol 48:410, 1957

Winterstein JF: Acute lumbar disc syndrome (lecture notes) National College of Chiropractic, Lombard, Illinois, 1971

Wolff HD: Remarks on the present situation and further development of manual medicine with special regard to chirotherapy. Presented to the Deutscher Gesellschaft fur Manuelle Medizin, February 1972

Yochum TR: Radiology of the arthritides (lecture notes) International College of Chiropractic, Melbourne, Australia, 1978

Index